Prescription
DRUGS

Prescription
DRUGS

Reader's Digest

Reader's Digest Association, Inc.
Pleasantville, New York / Montreal

Reader's Digest Project Staff

Senior Editor
Marianne Wait

Senior Designer
Judith Carmel

Production Technology Manager
Douglas A. Croll

Reader's Digest Health Publishing

Editorial Director
Christopher Cavanaugh

Art Director
Joan Mazzeo

Marketing Director
James H. Malloy

Vice President and General Manager
Shirrel Rhoades

The Reader's Digest Association, Inc.

Editor-in-Chief
Eric W. Schrier

President, North American Books and Home Entertainment
Thomas D. Gardner

Reader's Digest Book Produced by Rebus, Inc.

Publisher
Rodney Friedman

Editorial Director
Evan Hansen

Senior Editor
Sandra Wilmot

Contributing Editor
Marya Dalrymple

Consulting Editors
Jeremy D. Birch, Andrea Peirce, Carol Weeg

Chief of Information Resources
Tom Damrauer

Production Database Manager
John Vasiliadis

Art Director
Timothy Jeffs

Art Associate
Bree Rock

Address any comments about Guide to Drugs and Supplements: Prescription Drugs to
Reader's Digest, Editorial Director, Reader's Digest Health Publishing
Reader's Digest Road
Pleasantville, NY 10570

To order additional copies of Guide to Drugs and Supplements: Prescription Drugs,
call 1-800-846-2100

Visit our website at www.rd.com

1 3 5 7 9 10 8 6 4 2

Library of Congress Cataloging-in-Publication Data

Guide to drugs and supplements : prescription drugs.
    p. cm.
    Includes index.
    ISBN 0-7621-0365-5
    1. Drugs–Popular works. 2. Drugs–Encyclopedias. I. Reader's Digest
Association.

RM301.15 .G85 2002
615'.1–dc21
                                                    2001048893

CONTENTS

▼

HOW TO USE THIS BOOK

▼

This book presents the essential facts on hundreds of the most common generic and brand name drugs in use today. With all the prescription and nonprescription drugs that are now available, it's more important than ever to be well informed on the safe and proper use of medications—whether for yourself, an aging parent, or a sick child. This book will help you to do that. It presents the facts in clear, easy-to-understand language, and in a context that will help you to make the best decisions and to use your medicines in the safest and most effective way possible.

THE BOOK CONSISTS OF THREE MAIN SECTIONS:

A General Medication Overview. The introductory portion of the book contains essential information to help you use medicines wisely. It has practical advice on *Understanding Your Medications*, including valuable tips on drug safety, traveling with medications, proper storage, as well as dozens of other relevant topics. It also features a comprehensive listing of *Common Disorders and the Drugs Prescribed for Them.*

A-to-Z Individual Drug Profiles. The core of this book is an A-to-Z resource of more than 170 individual drug profiles, encompassing hundreds of generic and brand name medications. Here you'll find all the information you need about a particular drug and its proper use—including why it's prescribed, how it works, dosage guidelines, precautions, side effects, what to do in the case of an overdose, and food and drug interactions. Each drug profile is clearly organized for you in a one- to two-page format for quick, easy lookup.

A Glossary, Directories, and Index. The back pages of the book contain a comprehensive *Glossary of Drug Terms*, a state-by-state directory of *Certified Poison Control Centers*, a directory of *Health Information Organizations*, and an *Index* to help you quickly and easily find the appropriate drug profile.

Remember, you are part of a health-care team. This book will help you to become better informed about your drugs and medications. Use it to work closely with your doctor, pharmacist, and other trusted health-care professionals, to help answer any questions you may have about getting the most out of your medications and to obtain the best possible medical care and advice.

▼ THE DRUG PROFILE

Each of the medications covered in this book is given a drug profile, which contains the essential facts about it in an easy-to-follow, standardized, one- to two-page format. The profile will give you the various names and formulations for a drug, information on its proper use or uses, guidelines for taking the drug, side effects and precautions associated with the drug, any potentially dangerous interactions with food or other medicines, and additional facts that you need to know to manage your medications.

The individual components of each drug profile are discussed below, with a brief description of the topics covered under each heading. General tips and suggestions for using your medicines safely and effectively are provided here as well. You can use this overview to get acquainted with how the profiles are organized and to obtain important general advice about your medications. Refer to it again to answer any questions you may have about general drug safety after consulting a specific drug profile, or whenever you begin a new course of medication.

◆ *Generic and Brand Names*

The drug profile identifies each drug in large, bold type at the top of the page by its generic name—a unique and standardized scientific designation that is recognized worldwide. In addition, many drugs are commonly known by one or more brand names—the name that the drug manufacturer selects to market its product. For example, ibuprofen is the generic designation for a commonly used pain reliever; Motrin, Nuprin, Medipren, and Advil are four of the brand names for ibuprofen. The drug profile includes brand names that are commonly available in the United States. Unlike generic designations, brand names (also referred to as trade names) may vary from country to country. Generic drug names are listed alphabetically in the main portion of the book. If you know the generic name of a drug, you can use this A-to-Z resource to quickly locate the relevant information. Note that some profiles include combinations of two or more generic drugs, formulated as a single preparation. Also, terms such as "hydrochloride" or "sodium" are sometimes included in a generic

GENERIC VERSUS BRAND NAME: WHICH IS BETTER?

Generic drugs have become increasingly popular since the 1980s, when the generic drug approval process was expanded and safety guidelines were issued by the Food and Drug Administration (FDA). About 250 new generic drugs are approved by the FDA each year. Generics are less expensive than brand name drugs. But are they as effective?

Ongoing supervision by the FDA helps to assure that generics sold in this country *are* as safe and effective as their brand name counterparts. The FDA requires that all generic drugs be bioequivalent to their brand name counterparts—that is, they must deliver the same amount of active ingredient to the body in a similar time frame. Furthermore, they must have similar chemical stability, so that they maintain their potency under normal circumstances for an equivalent period of time.

In addition, all drugs, including generics, must meet specifications set by the U.S. Pharmacopeial Convention, a private scientific organization that sets standards for drugs and drug products in the United States. Although there are stories in the media from time to time about the sale of substandard generic drugs, such occurrences are rare. The FDA maintains strict standards and inspection practices as well as extensive testing and monitoring of all drug manufacturing processes. About 80 percent of generic drugs sold in this country are manufactured by brand name firms in state-of-the-art plants.

You and your doctor can discuss whether generic or brand name drugs are right for you. Once you have started on a new drug therapy, it's best to stick with what you've been using—be it generic or name brand—unless your doctor says it's okay to change. There are subtle variations between some generic and brand name drugs that may make one type preferable for your situation. Switching from one form to the other could, for example, slightly alter the dose that your doctor has determined to be most suitable for your needs.

drug's name. In many instances the modified formulation (sometimes called a "salt") is not important, because the drug will break down into a single active ingredient in the body.

The pain reliever naproxen, for example, is sold by prescription simply as naproxen, whereas the version of the drug that has been approved for nonprescription use is formulated as naproxen sodium; both versions act identically once the common active ingredient (naproxen) is released in the body, and hence both are combined in a single drug profile. In other cases, though, a chemical modification is significant. Acetaminophen with codeine phosphate, acetaminophen and oxycodone, and acetaminophen and propoxyphene all act differently enough in the body to qualify as separate drugs, so each has its own profile.

If you know a drug by its brand name, you can find its profile quickly by consulting the index at the back of the book, which lists both generic and brand names for drugs and the appropriate page number for their profiles. Of course, due to space constraints, not every single medicine sold around the world is included in this book. We have selected the generic and brand name drugs most commonly used in the United States today.

◆ Available Forms

The drug profile lists the available forms of a drug, such as tablet, capsule, liquid, or inhalant. Each form has certain properties that may make it preferable for your condition or that can make taking your medications easier, safer, or more effective. If you have a skin infection, for example, you may need an antibiotic skin cream; an eye or ear infection, on the other hand, may call for ophthalmic or otic drops or ointment.

TIPS FOR TAKING YOUR MEDICATIONS

TABLETS AND CAPSULES

Tablets come in many forms besides the standard round pill. Capsules and caplets (oblong-shaped tablets) are preferred by some people because they are easier to swallow than most round tablets. Chewable tablets are good for those who have trouble swallowing any type of pill; they should be chewed thoroughly to avoid stomach upset and should not be given to children younger than age 2 (who can't chew them properly).

Some people prefer crushing tablets and mixing them with juice, water, or soft foods like applesauce to make them easier to swallow. This may be okay for some drugs, but certain medications are not designed for this. Enteric-coated tablets, for example, have a protective layer that allows the pill to dissolve in the intestine rather than the stomach. Crushing the tablet could cause stomach irritation.

Similarly, pills that have a sustained-release, timed-release, or extended-release formulation are designed to disintegrate slowly within the body and should be swallowed whole. Capsules, too, are not supposed to be broken up or cut into pieces. Check with your doctor or pharmacist before crushing any pills or tablets.

Additional Tips

- To make a pill easier to swallow, it may be helpful to drink some water before taking it and a glass of water after. It's also a good idea to stand up while swallowing.

- If a pill gets stuck in your throat, try eating a soft food such as a banana. Swallowing the food may help to carry the pill down.

EYE AND EAR MEDICATIONS

Always wash your hands before and after administering eye (ophthalmic) or ear (otic) medications. In addition, be careful not to touch the tip of the dropper or applicator to any surface, including the ear canal or eye lids, to avoid contamination. Following are additional tips for applying these medications.

Using an Eyedropper
- Tilt the head back.

- Pull the lower eyelid downward using a finger or by pinching and pulling with the thumb and index finger, creating a pocket between the eye and lower lid.

- Drop the medication into this eyelid pocket. Blink to disperse.

Applying Eye Ointments
- Pull the lower eyelid downward using a finger or by pinching and pulling with the thumb and index finger to create a pocket.

- Squeeze the tube and apply a thin strip (about a third of an inch) of ointment into this eyelid pocket. Blink to disperse.

Administering Ear Drops
- Lie down or tilt the head so that the affected ear faces up.

- For adults, pull the ear lobe up and back to straighten the ear canal. In young children, pull the ear lobe down and back.

- Drop the medication into the ear canal, but don't insert the tip of the dropper any deeper than the outer ear.

- Keep the ear facing up for a few minutes so the medication can reach the bottom of the ear canal.

RECTAL SUPPOSITORIES

A rectal suppository is a relatively large, bullet-shaped drug preparation that is designed to be inserted into the rectum. Once inside, it melts with body heat and the drug is released. Suppositories may be useful for very ill patients, young children, or for others who cannot take oral medications. Lubricant suppositories may also be helpful for the treatment of constipation.

Inserting a Rectal Suppository

• The suppository should not be too soft or it will be difficult to insert. If necessary, before removing the foil wrapper, run the suppository under cold water or chill it in the refrigerator for about a half hour, until it is firm.

• Wearing a latex glove, unwrap the suppository and moisten it with water. Lie on your side and gently push the suppository, rounded end first, well up into the rectum with your finger.

• In children, gently insert the suppository no more than 3 inches into the rectum.

• Lie still and try to retain the suppository for at least 20 minutes so that the drug is absorbed.

VAGINAL MEDICATIONS

Use the special applicator that comes with your medicine and follow the directions carefully. To administer the medicine, lie on your back with your knees pulled up. Insert the applicator into the vagina as far as you can without forcing it, then press the plunger to release the medicine. After you withdraw the applicator, wash it with soap and warm water.

INHALERS AND SPACERS

Many people who have asthma or related respiratory disorders need to use a metered-dose inhaler (also known as a nebulizer). This pressurized container propels aerosolized medication into the mouth and down the throat where it can be delivered to the airways. The inhaler must be used properly to assure that enough of the medication is delivered to the airways, where it will exert its therapeutic effect, rather than to the sides of the mouth and throat.

Using an Inhaler Correctly

• Shake the inhaler well before use.

• Tilt the head back slightly and hold the mouthpiece a half an inch from the mouth. The bottom of the nebulizer bottle should be pointing up.

• Exhale normally. At the end of the exhale, inhale slowly over 5 seconds while firmly pressing the bottle against the mouthpiece, which releases the drug. Slow inhalation is the key to getting an effective dose. Hold your breath for 5 to 10 seconds.

• If your doctor wants you to receive more than one dose of the drug, wait a few minutes and then repeat the steps above.

A spacer—a plastic chamber or holding bag that attaches to the inhaler and acts as a reservoir to hold the mist—may make the job easier by allowing you to inhale at a comfortable rate. Follow the doctor's instructions for how much drug to take and how often, and have the doctor check your technique from time to time to be sure it is correct.

NASAL MEDICATIONS

Blow the nose gently before administering nasal medications. After use, rinse the tip of the applicator with hot water and dry with a clean tissue. To avoid spreading infection, don't share medications with others.

Administering Nose Drops

• Tilt the head back and place the recommended number of drops in each nostril. Keep the head back for several minutes to allow the medicine to spread through the nasal passages.

Administering Nasal Sprays

• Keep the head upright and squeeze bottle firmly to spray medicine into each nostril while sniffing in briskly. Hold the breath for a few seconds, then breathe out through the mouth.

LIQUID MEDICATIONS

Measure the liquid carefully. Don't use ordinary kitchen spoons to measure out a dose; instead, use the measuring device that comes with the drug, or ask your pharmacist for one.

INJECTIONS

Some drugs (for example, insulin for diabetes or an anaphylaxis medication for life-threatening allergic reactions) are best administered by injection. Injections are given intravenously (into a vein), intramuscularly (into a muscle), or subcutaneously (under the skin). If you need to give yourself or someone else home injections, go over the correct procedure with your doctor or other health educator. Don't be reluctant to ask questions, and return for periodic reviews.

A distinction is sometimes made between local and systemic drugs. Local drugs tend to exert their effects over a limited area of the body. They include topical preparations—which are applied to the skin, eyes, ears, hair, or mucous membranes (lips, nasal passages, vagina, rectum, for example)—and certain types of injections into the skin, muscles, or joints. In contrast, systemic drugs are absorbed by the bloodstream and circulated widely through many of the body's organ systems. This category includes oral preparations that are taken by mouth (such as tablets, capsules, or liquids) as well as injections into a vein. Locally acting formulations tend to cause fewer and less serious side effects (for example, a limited skin rash) than systemic drugs, though local drugs do sometimes cause widespread reactions as well.

The type of formulations can also affect how rapidly a drug is absorbed, how much of the drug is absorbed, or how quickly it can take effect. An injection of a medication directly into a vein takes effect nearly immediately and can be critical during emergency situations. At the other end of the spectrum are the controlled-release, timed-release, sustained-release, or prolonged-action preparations, including specially formulated capsules or transdermal skin patches. These are made specifically to provide slow, uniform absorption of a drug over a period of 8 hours or longer. Enteric-coated oral preparations are designed to keep the drug from being dissolved by stomach acids, lessening the likelihood of gastrointestinal side effects.

Other drug formulations include sublingual preparations (which are placed under the tongue and then rapidly absorbed), nasal and inhalant

DRUG NAMES **THAT LOOK OR SOUND ALIKE**

Marketers continue to think up new brand names for drugs. Every year, however, a certain number of these are rejected by regulators because the proposed brand name looks or sounds too similar to existing names—which may lead to errors when a drug prescription is filled. Even so, mix-ups continue to occur, in part because prescriptions are all too often scribbled in semi-legible script or quickly phoned in to a pharmacy. Review the common name-related errors below (brand names are in upper case), which are based on reports to the Food and Drug Administration (FDA). This is only a small sample—so be on guard the next time you have a prescription filled!

Accutane (for acne) ....Accupril (for hypertension)
acetazolamide (for glaucoma, ...acetohexamide (for diabetes)
    seizures, heart failure)
Altace (for hypertension).........................Artane (for Parkinson's disease)
Ambien (for insomnia)..............................Amen (for menstrual disorders)
Asacol (for bowel disease).......................Os-Cal (calcium supplement)
Ativan (for anxiety) ....Atarax (for allergies, anxiety)
Cardene (for angina)................................codeine (for pain relief)
Cardura (for hypertension, ...Coumadin (for blood clots)
    prostate enlargement)
Cardene SR (for angina) ....Cardizem SR (for heart disease)
Celebrex (for pain relief) ....Celexa (for depression)
codeine (for pain relief).............................Lodine (for pain relief)
cycloserine (for tuberculosis) ....cyclosporine (for organ transplants)
Darvon (for pain relief)..............................Diovan (for hypertension)
Levoxine (for thyroid disease) ....Lanoxin (for heart disease)
Lorabid (for infections) ....Lortab (for infections)
Luvox (for obsessive-...............................Lasix (for heart disease)
    compulsive disorder)
Naprosyn (for pain relief).........................Naprelan (for pain relief)
Ocuflox (for eye infections) ....Ocufen (for eye disorders)
penicillamine (for arthritis) ....penicillin (for infections)
pindolol (for hypertension) ....Plendil (for hypertension)
Plendil (for hypertension).........................Prinivil (for heart disease)
Prilosec (for ulcer, heartburn) ....Prozac (for depression)
Prozac (for depression).............................Proscar (for prostate enlargement)
Verelan (for heart disease) ....Virilon (for hormone disorders)
Zantac (for digestive disorders)...............Xanax (for anxiety)

preparations (breathed in through the nose or mouth), rectal suppositories, and vaginal creams or suppositories. Many additional drug preparations are available. Your doctor can advise which form of medication is best for you.

◆ *Available OTC?*
Most new drugs are available only by prescription initially and later may become available over-the-counter (OTC). Each drug profile indicates whether or not a drug is also available

OTC—that is, obtainable without a prescription in a drug store, supermarket, or other convenience store. Common OTC drugs include laxatives; diet pills; vitamins; cold medicine; aspirin or other pain, headache, or fever medicine; cough medicine; allergy relief medicine; antacids; and sleeping pills.

A prescription drug is granted OTC status by the FDA after a panel of experts determines that it can be used safely and effectively without a doctor's supervision, although all drugs carry at least a few risks.

Many medications continue as prescription drugs even after an OTC version becomes available. Typically, the OTC form has a different brand name, a lower dosage, and more limited uses. OTC drugs must be taken with the same caution as prescriptions. Always read the labels, which give proper dosing and list possible food or drug interactions.

◆ Available as Generic?

The drug profile tells you whether or not a drug is available in a generic form. A generic drug is a copycat version of a brand-name drug—it should not be confused with the generic name for a drug (see page 7). All medications have a scientific, or generic, name, but only certain drugs are available in generic versions.

Typically, a pharmaceutical company will conduct exhaustive research and testing to launch a pioneer drug, or the first version of a new drug. In return, the company usually has patents and an exclusive license to sell that new drug for a set period of time, normally about 20 years from the time testing begins. The drug is usually marketed under a brand name. However, once that license expires, other drug companies are free to make generic versions of that drug—provided the copy is as safe and effective as the original.

The FDA estimates that about three-fourths of generic drugs are made by the same manufacturers who make the brand name drug. Generic drugs are usually sold under their generic, or scientific, name, often at half the price of the brand name version. Commonly, there are many generic versions of a popular parent drug, and generics are available for both prescription and OTC drugs.

◆ Drug Class

Each drug is classified according to its drug class—a group of drugs that have similar chemical structures or similar actions on the body. For example, a drug that reduces hypertension falls into the antihypertensive class; one that kills infectious bacteria belongs in the antibiotic class. Some drugs have multiple functions and may therefore belong to more than one drug class.

In general, drugs with similar chemical structures have somewhat similar effects. If you're having a problem with one medication, an alternative from the same drug group may be an appropriate option to discuss with your doctor.

▼ USAGE INFORMATION

◆ Why It's Prescribed

The specific conditions, disorders, diseases, or symptoms for which a drug is prescribed are known as its indications. All drugs—prescription and OTC—must be approved specifically for one or more indications before they are brought to market; additional indications may later be approved by the FDA after appropriate studies have been conducted.

For OTC drugs, all indications listed on the drug's label must be approved by the FDA. Hence, you will sometimes see OTC indications referred to as "FDA approved uses" or simply "approved uses."

The situation is slightly different for prescription drugs. Once a drug has been approved for at least one indication, doctors are free to prescribe it for any purpose they deem appropriate—a common practice known as "off-label use." For example, various antibiotics that are not specifically approved for Lyme disease are often used to treat it and other infectious diseases. Indeed, about half of all prescriptions are written for off-label purposes.

Approved indications for specific drugs are included in each drug profile under the heading "Why It's Prescribed." In addition, beginning on page 19 you will find a listing of "Common Disorders and the Drugs Prescribed for Them." Here you can look up a disease or ailment and find a list of drugs that have been specifically approved by the FDA for that condition. Off-label uses are not noted in either location, because their use is unofficial. If you're taking a particular drug but don't see its indication listed, you may be following an off-label prescription. You should discuss any concerns you may have about this with your doctor or pharmacist.

◆ How It Works

This section of the drug profile briefly describes how a medicine acts on or within your body to achieve its desired therapeutic effect. Some drug actions are well understood. For many drugs, however, the precise mechanism of action is unknown.

▼ DOSAGE GUIDELINES

The first safety rule for any medicine—be it prescription or OTC—is to take the correct dose at the right intervals. You should take great care to precisely follow the dosage instructions of your doctor or pharmacist, and to read the label on the bottle. Never take more or less than the recommended dose without talking to your doctor first.

◆ Range and Frequency
The drug profile lists the usual dosage ranges for each drug. Use these figures as general guidelines, but don't be alarmed if your doctor recommends a dosage is slightly above or below the range given. The correct dosage will vary from person to person and will depend on many factors, including your age, weight, state of health, kidney and liver function, and use of other medications.

All these factors can affect how much of the drug your body absorbs, how it is distributed in your body, how long it stays there, and the amount needed for a response. Your doctor will determine the right dosage for you. If you have any questions or concerns, or suspect a dosing error, do not hesitate to contact your doctor or other health-care professional.

Note that drug dosages are often given in metric units of weight, such as grams (g); milligrams (mg, or one thousandth of a gram); or micrograms (mcg, or one millionth of a gram). In addition, dosages for some medications, including vitamins, may be given in milliequivalents (mEq), a standard chemical unit of measure. Sometimes drug dosages are allocated per pound of body weight; this method is especially useful in determining the optimal dosage for children.

◆ Onset of Effect
Many drugs exert their effects within minutes. Common analgesics such as aspirin or acetaminophen, for example, begin to relieve pain within an hour. Often, though, you must take multiple doses of a drug before levels have built up in your body sufficiently to be effective. Usually this will occur within a day or two; for certain drugs, such as some antidepressants, however, it may take several weeks for the drug to exert a noticeable effect.

◆ Duration of Effect
How long a drug exerts its effects depends on the individual medication. Some can stay in your system for days, or even much longer; others will last only a few hours. The body metabolizes different drugs at different rates. In general, the faster a medication is metabolized, the more frequently you will need to take another dose.

The drug profile indicates how long, on average, a medication may remain in your system. Various factors, including your general health, kidney or liver function, and food or drug interactions, can significantly increase or decrease a drug's duration of action.

◆ Dietary Advice
The drug profile tells you if a medication should be taken with or without food. Food can affect how much of the drug will be absorbed into your body, and how quickly.

Many drugs should be taken with a meal, especially with foods that contain some protein and fat. Food delays the emptying of stomach contents, allowing more time for a pill or capsule to be dissolved before entering the intestines, where many drugs are absorbed. In addition, some drugs can irritate the stomach's lining if taken on an empty stomach. Taking them with food, or even a glass of milk, can help minimize the likelihood of stomach upset or other gastrointestinal disturbances. Avoid taking drugs with coffee, tea, or other hot beverages, however, because heat can inactivate or alter some medications.

Other drugs should be taken on an empty stomach—which means at least an hour before or two hours after a meal. In general, such drugs are poorly absorbed if they're taken with food. They should, however, be taken with a glass of water.

Specific foods and drinks, including alcohol, can also interact with individual drugs. These effects are discussed under "Precautions" (see page 14) and "Food Interactions" (see page 18).

◆ Storage
Requirements for storing medicines should be clearly indicated on the label. In general, it is recommended that most medications be kept in a cool and dry place. This usually precludes the bathroom medicine cabinet, because bathrooms tend to be humid. Similarly, drugs should not be kept near a hot kitchen stove. A bedroom or kitchen closet, which tends to be cooler and drier, may be preferable.

Some liquid medicines, such as insulin or antibiotics for children's use, may need to be refrigerated. Unless your doctor or pharmacist tells you otherwise, though, it is not necessary to refrigerate most medications.

It's always a good idea to store drugs in their original containers. Discard the cotton at the top of pill bottles; once it is touched, it can quickly become contaminated with the bacteria on your skin. If you need to use a pill organizer, check with your doctor or pharmacist to make sure that the amount of light or moisture it lets through will not adversely affect any of your medicines.

If young children are around the house, be sure to store medicines in containers with childproof caps and well out of a child's reach. In addition, don't store medications near any dangerous substances that might be taken by mistake.

◆ Missed Dose

Everyone misses a dose of medication now and then. The drug profile tells you what to do when this occurs. For some drugs, the missed dose should be taken right away. For others, you can modify your schedule or wait until the next scheduled dose. In general, it's better not to simply double up on missed doses because you run the risk of raising the drug concentrations in your body to dangerously high levels.

Products are available that help remind you to take your medicines on a proper schedule. These items, sometimes called compliance aids, include containers with sections for daily doses, check-off calendars, electronic devices that beep when it's time for a dose, and computerized pill dispensers. If you need help in selecting one of these aids, check with your doctor or pharmacist.

◆ Stopping the Drug

Never stop taking a prescribed drug, even if you're feeling better, without consulting your doctor. For example, even a minor infection that appears to have cleared up with a few days' worth of antibiotics usually requires a full course of therapy (often 2 weeks). If you stop taking the antibiotic too soon, resistant bacteria can multiply and cause an even more serious infection. Abrupt changes in dosage of

AVOIDING **PRESCRIPTION ERRORS**

Prescription errors can—and do—occur. There are a number of easy steps you can take to help avoid these errors. First, make sure you understand the prescription fully, including what drug has been pre-scribed as well as its generic and, if applicable, brand name. Ask your doctor to write legibly and carefully check prescription refills and renewals. Many doctors use Latin abbreviations and other notations when writing out a drug prescription; below is a list of some commonly used terms. It may also be a good idea to have the doctor include the intended use of the drug (for example, by indicating that it is for diabetes or hypertension) on the prescription.

READING A PRESCRIPTION

TERM	ABBREVIATION	MEANING
ante cibum	ac	before meals
bis in die	bid	twice a day
gutta	gt	drop
hora somni	hs	at bedtime
milligrams	mg	
milliliters	ml	
oculus dexter	od	right eye
oculus sinister	os	left eye
per os	po	by mouth
post cibum	pc	after meals
pro re nata	prn	as needed
quaque 3 hora	q3h	every 3 hours
quaque die	qd	every day
quattuor in die	qid	4 times a day
ter in die	tid	3 times a day

The Brown Bag Review

Another measure to help avoid prescription errors, especially if you're taking several drugs on a regular basis, is to have an annual "brown bag review." Once a year, bring in all the medications you are taking, both prescription and over-the-counter, so that your doctor can evaluate them and, if needed, modify your regimen. In addition, keep thorough records, and clearly indicate any medications you are taking to any new doctors who may be prescribing additional drugs. Finally, check refills and renewals carefully. A refill or renewal of a generic drug may be a different color, shape, or size because the drug comes from a different manufacturer; but it can also mean an error has been made. If you have any doubts, don't hesitate to ask your doctor or pharmacist.

some drugs can also be dangerous. For example, a narcotic pain reliever may have to be reduced gradually to avoid withdrawal symptoms. Or if a hypertensive medicine is stopped suddenly, blood pressure may soar.

For all drugs, it's important that you follow through with the recommended course of therapy. Some drugs may take months to produce their full benefit. Others may need to be continued on a long-term basis. If you experience bothersome side effects or don't feel that a drug is having the intended effect, talk to your doctor or pharmacist, but don't change your medication schedule on your own.

◆ *Prolonged Use*

If you require a drug for a chronic condition, you may need to take it for extended periods, or even a lifetime. Regular checkups or periodic testing or monitoring may be required to make sure the drug is not causing any insidious adverse effects.

▼ SIDE EFFECTS

Along with their desired therapeutic actions, drugs typically exert other effects on the body, many of which are undesirable. Such side effects can occur with virtually all prescription and over-the-counter drugs, even when they're taken properly. Keep in mind, though, that only a small percentage of patients who are taking a drug actually experience significant side effects, even the relatively common ones.

The drug profile lists the side effects as serious, common, and less common. Serious side effects are those that may be life-threatening or otherwise have a significant impact on your well-being. You should seek immediate medical assistance if you experience a serious side effect from a drug. Of course, even a mild one is significant if it has a negative impact on your quality of life.

It's a good idea to call your doctor if you are concerned about any side effect, even a seemingly minor one. Write down any problems you have with your medicine so you'll remember them when you talk with your doctor or pharmacist, and don't be afraid to ask questions.

 TRAVELING **WITH YOUR MEDICATIONS**

• Make sure you bring enough medications to last your entire trip, plus an extra supply to cover unexpected travel delays. Don't pack medications in suitcases that you plan to check; the luggage might be delayed or lost. If you carry syringes or certain drugs like narcotic pain relievers, it's wise to carry a note from your doctor that clearly explains your health history and medication requirements; in some countries, these belongings may otherwise be confiscated at customs.

• Keep drugs in their original, labeled containers. Pill bottles should be stuffed with cotton to prevent damage during transit; liquid medications should be stored in self-sealing plastic bags.

• Carry extra copies of any prescriptions, in case you need to obtain additional medicine during your trip. Prescriptions should be typed, with the generic drug name included, since drugs may be known by different brand names outside of the United States.

• Be up to date on your immunizations. You may also need additional shots or medications for travel to certain exotic locales. Consult your doctor, or a doctor who specializes in travel medicine, at least six weeks prior to your trip about the need for any new vaccinations or drugs. You may also want to check beforehand about where to obtain emergency medical help while traveling.

• Be aware that a change in climate may bring on untoward drug side effects. In hot climates, for example, diuretics may cause some dizziness at first, but such side effects are usually fleeting. Other drugs, such as antihistamines, cold preparations, and tranquilizers, can decrease your ability to perspire.

• If you are crossing several time zones and are on a fixed dosage schedule (for example, for insulin injections), you may have to make dosing adjustments. Discuss these and any other concerns with your doctor before you depart.

▼ PRECAUTIONS

◆ *Over 60*

Drugs should be used with special caution by people over age 60. Physiologic changes brought on by aging—including diminishing kidney and liver function, an increase in the ratio of fat to muscle, and a decrease in the amount of water in the tissues of the body—all act to concentrate drugs and prevent them from being eliminated at a normal rate. For this reason, older adults may require lower dosages than the standard amounts usually recommended.

According to the FDA, 17 percent of all hospitalizations among older adults are caused by the side effects of prescription medications—six times more than for the general population. Drug side effects, as well as drug and food interactions and overdose, are more common in older patients in part because they are much more likely than younger people to be taking medications in the first place. The problem is compounded when multiple medicines are involved, particularly when drugs are prescribed by different doctors, who are not always aware of other medications the patient is taking. In addition, studies have shown that a surprisingly sizeable percentage of elderly patients are prescribed drugs that are contraindicated for those in their age group.

It's important to tell your doctors about all the medications you are taking—whether prescription or OTC—and to learn as much as possible about these drugs. As a general rule, don't attribute any changes in mood or any new or unusual reactions or physical changes simply to old age; they may actually be drug side effects or even dangerous interactions.

◆ *Driving and Hazardous Work*

Because some medications may cause drowsiness or confusion, they should not be used when driving, working with dangerous tools or machinery, or in other situations where a lapse in concentration could cause serious injury. If a drug makes you drowsy, talk to your doctor about scheduling doses near your bedtime, or ask about other drugs that might be substituted. Always check to see if a drug may affect alertness and concentration before driving or engaging in a potentially hazardous activity.

◆ *Alcohol*

Certain medications, including many OTC drugs, can be dangerous if they are taken with alcohol. It's important for you to know whether or not alcohol should be avoided whenever you begin taking a new drug.

Common signs of alcohol-drug interactions include excessive sleepiness, difficulty breathing, and stomach irritation. When in doubt, it is always a good idea to give up alcoholic beverages entirely while you are taking a medication. According to the FDA, "Of the 100 medicines most commonly prescribed, more than half contain at least one substance that reacts badly with alcohol."

◆ *Pregnancy*

Some drugs are known to be harmful during pregnancy and should unequivocally be avoided during that time. A few have been shown to be safe. But for most drugs, not enough studies have been conducted for researchers to know for sure if the drug is truly dangerous to the fetus.

In general, it's a good idea to minimize the use of prescription and OTC drugs during pregnancy (though certain medications, such as vitamin supplements, may be recommended by your doctor). This precaution should extend to the use of alcohol (present in some drug preparations), which most experts recommend avoiding. Your

---

BASIC MEDICINE SAFETY TIPS

1. Follow instructions carefully. It's essential that you take the correct dose at the proper time intervals, and avoid potential food and drug interactions.

2. Keep a log of your medicines and let your doctor know your drug and medical history. It's a good idea to review your medications with your primary-care doctor annually, including both prescription and OTC drugs.

3. Try to have prescriptions filled at one pharmacy. The pharmacist will get to know you and your medicines, and will be more likely to detect any possible prescription errors.

4. Store medicines properly, away from sunlight, heat, and humidity. The bathroom medicine cabinet, because of the humidity, is not a good location. A locked closet—away from the reach and sight of children—is ideal.

5. Discard outdated medicines. Prescription drugs should not be used past their expiration date. Some drugs lose their potency with time; other outdated medicines, such as the tetracycline antibiotics, may have dangerous side effects. Ask your pharmacist to label your prescription container with an expiration date, and regularly discard old medicines down the toilet.

6. Don't share prescription drugs or borrow them from others. What's good for one person may be harmful to another.

7. Don't take medicines in the dark. You could take the wrong pill by accident. Read the label carefully each time you take a drug to be sure you are getting the right medicine.

8. Keep emergency phone numbers handy. You should have the numbers of your doctor, emergency medical services, and the nearest poison control center readily available in case a medical emergency arises.

9. Don't be afraid to ask questions. Understand your medicines as thoroughly as possible: Why you are taking them, how and when they should be taken, things to look out for. People who ask questions are more satisfied with their medical care.

10. Alert your doctor to any side effects or changes in your condition. He or she may be able to adjust your dosage or give you a substitute medication.

specific medical needs—as assessed by your doctor—will determine whether a drug is absolutely necessary. Keep in mind that the benefits of many drugs, when indicated, far outweigh the slight possible risk to mother or fetus.

◆ Breast Feeding

Check with your doctor before taking any prescription or OTC medicine if you are nursing. Most drugs (including vitamins and herbal supplements) pass into breast milk to some extent, though some do so more readily than others. And while most medications have little or no apparent effect on the nursing infant, some—such as anticancer drugs—are dangerous.

The drug profile indicates if a specific drug should be avoided by nursing mothers. In general, as with pregnancy, it's a good idea to minimize the use of medications during this time. Most experts recommend avoiding or strictly limiting alcohol intake as well. For mild pain relief, ibuprofen may be preferable to aspirin or other analgesics, although most analgesics can be used relatively safely while breast feeding; check with your doctor about the best choice for you.

Of course, your medical condition may require that you take certain medications while breast feeding. Ask your doctor to help you to weigh the risks and benefits of drug therapy. In some cases, a drug regimen can be suspended during the nursing period, breast feeding can be stopped if a drug is needed for only a short time, the dosing regimen can be modified, or a substitute drug can be used.

◆ Infants and Children

Children are more sensitive than adults to many drugs. If a drug is indicated for use by children, be very attentive to adverse reactions. If you have any concerns, talk to your doctor, pediatrician, or pharmacist.

◆ Special Concerns

The drug profile notes any additional special concerns that you should be aware of. One such possibility is an allergic drug reaction, which occurs when the immune system mounts a response against a particular medication. Allergic reactions can occur with virtually any drug, though they are most common with penicillin and related antibiotics. Other common allergens include sulfa drugs, barbiturates, anticonvulsants, certain insulin preparations, and local anesthetics.

Common signs of an allergic drug reaction include a skin rash, hives, and itching. Very severe reactions, known medically as anaphylaxis, can result in swelling of the face, tongue, lips, arms, or legs; swelling can also extend to the airways, making breathing difficult—a life-threatening emergency that requires immediate medical attention.

Call the doctor if you develop any signs of an allergic reaction to a drug. Most drug allergies respond readily to treatment. Antihistamines or topical corticosteroids may be advised for skin rashes, hives, or itching. Bronchodilators can make breathing easier. Epinephrine relieves severe reactions. In some cases, a doctor may improve your tolerance to a particular drug, such as penicillin, by giving you a series of slightly increasing doses of that drug—a treatment process that is known medically as desensitization.

DRUGS AND CHILDREN: SPECIAL SAFETY MEASURES

• Keep all prescription and over-the-counter medications out of the reach of children. Some medicines, such as iron supplements, are very toxic to youngsters.

• Use child-resistant caps, and never leave containers uncapped.

• Never give medicine to children unless it is recommended for them on the label or by a doctor.

• Check with the doctor or pharmacist before giving a child more than one medicine at a time.

• Examine dose cups carefully. Cups may be marked with various standard abbreviations. Follow label directions.

• When using a dosing syringe that has a cap, discard the cap before using the syringe.

• Never guess when converting measuring units—from teaspoons or tablespoons to ounces, for example. Consult a reliable source, such as a pharmacist.

• Don't try to remember the dose used during previous illnesses; read the label each time.

• Never use medicine for purposes not mentioned on the label, unless so directed by a doctor.

• Check with the doctor before giving a child aspirin products. Never give aspirin to a child or teenager who has or is recovering from chicken pox, or has flu symptoms (nausea, vomiting, or fever). Aspirin may be associated in such patients with an increased risk of Reye's syndrome, a rare but serious illness.

FDA Consumer

Take note of the drug that caused the reaction and let doctors, dentists, and other health-care professionals know of it in the future. You should be careful to avoid taking that drug again, since the allergic reaction may be more serious with subsequent doses.

A medical alert tag, worn as a bracelet or necklace or carried as a card, may also be helpful. The tag states the medical concern and often includes a telephone number that can be dialed for a detailed medical history; you can discuss this option with your doctor.

◆ Overdose: Symptoms and What to Do

Virtually any drug can be toxic if taken in high enough doses, but the seriousness will depend on the individual and the particular drug taken. Every profile includes a discussion of the symptoms that are typical of an overdose and what to do in the event that one occurs.

Accidental poisonings are of particular concern for infants and children. Prescription diet pills, stimulants, decongestants, and antidepressants are common causes of childhood poisoning. With certain drugs, even a single tablet can be life-threatening to a small child.

Be sure to store all medications in child-resistant containers and keep them out of the reach—and sight—of children. Remember that a child-resistant container is designed so that it takes longer than 5 minutes for 80 percent of 5-year-olds to open the bottle. However, child-resistant does not mean completely child-proof!

The elderly are also at increased risk for overdose. They are more sensitive to some drugs or may forget when they took their last dose.

An intentional overdose, commonly associated with suicide attempts, is a concern in depressed patients of any age, who may have access to large quantities of potentially lethal antidepressant medications.

Most drug poisonings work fairly quickly, though some overdose effects can take weeks to appear. Signs and symptoms of an overdose vary widely and may include listlessness, rolling eyes, confusion, breathing difficulties, unusual sleepiness, or stomach upset. If a child is involved, look for open drug containers around the house, stains around the mouth, and check for a strange breath odor.

If you suspect an overdose, don't panic. Call your doctor or poison control center right away. Depending on the drug, an antidote such as ipecac syrup may be recommended. It's a good idea to keep a bottle of ipecac on hand (safely stored); it induces vomiting and helps rid the body of the drug. Some experts also recommend activated charcoal (available in drugstores, usually in liquid form) for overdose. It acts to absorb the poison, preventing it from spreading through the body. (Activated charcoal should not be given with ipecac syrup, since the charcoal will absorb it).

For both antidotes, the patient must be conscious. Unconscious victims need immediate professional attention. Neither antidote should be used until you have talked with a doctor or poison control center, because in some cases, ipecac or charcoal can make a patient worse.

▼ INTERACTIONS

Drugs can interact with other drugs or particular foods or be affected by

certain diseases. The drug profile indicates specific interactions to watch for. Effects can range from extremely mild to life-threatening. People over age 60 are especially prone to these drug interactions and should exercise special caution.

◆ Drug Interactions

Drug interactions occur when two or more medications react with one another, causing adverse effects. Some drugs can diminish the effectiveness of others; conversely, some bolster another medications' actions. Drug interactions may be felt almost immediately, or they can take days, weeks, or even months to develop.

It's important to note that the effects of drug interactions vary from person to person. Most patients who receive drugs that could interact do not develop notable adverse effects. On the other hand, a few patients do experience life-threatening reactions and will require immediate treatment.

Special care should be taken by anyone who is on multiple medications, especially if the drugs are prescribed by different doctors. In some cases, however, a doctor will knowingly prescribe two potentially interacting drugs after determining that the benefits they provide will sufficiently outweigh the drawbacks of a possible interaction between them.

Check with your doctor if you are concerned about possible drug interactions or notice unusual symptoms. Take care with OTC drugs as well; they may interact with prescription drugs or with other OTC preparations. For example, don't automatically take an OTC antacid if another drug causes stomach upset, since antacids can alter the effectiveness of certain drugs. Similarly, some vitamin or herbal supplements can interact with drugs (see box at right).

◆ Food Interactions

Certain drugs should be taken on an empty stomach, whereas others should be taken with food. For still others, it doesn't really make a great deal of difference whether you eat or don't eat when you take them. These general dietary recommendations are covered in the drug profile under "Dietary Advice" (see page 12).

Listed in this section are specific foods or drinks that can interact with a particular drug. For example, dairy products can inactivate certain antibiotics. Peculiar interactions have likewise been noted between certain drugs and specific foods such as grapefruit juice (but not orange juice).

The list of potential food interactions is long and drug specific. Pay close attention to the food or drink interactions for your medications to help assure you're not interfering with the proper course of your drug therapy.

◆ Disease Interactions

The final section of each drug profile details specific diseases that can have a significant impact on a particular medication. Kidney or liver disease, for example, can dramatically affect drug levels in your system. Many drugs are metabolized in the liver and excreted by way of the kidneys. If either of these organs is impaired, an excess of a drug may build up in your body.

Many other disorders, such as diabetes mellitus or heart disease, may also affect your course of medication. It's important to tell your doctor about all diseases or conditions that you have, even if they are not related to your immediate medical concerns.

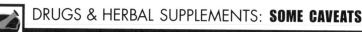

DRUGS & HERBAL SUPPLEMENTS: **SOME CAVEATS**

Drug-Herb Interactions

While there are entire databases documenting how drugs may interact with other drugs, few studies have been done on how drugs interact with herbal supplements. Furthermore, unlike prescription and OTC drugs, herbal products are not regulated by the FDA. Thus many consumers are unaware of the potentially serious risks of mixing botanicals with other pharmaceutical products.

The main drugs to worry about are known as narrow therapeutic index (NTI) agents. These drugs require precise dosages in order to be effective without being toxic. The anticoagulant drug warfarin (Coumadin) is one example: Too little is ineffective; too much can cause life-threatening bleeding episodes. Supplements such as feverfew, fish oils, garlic, pau d'arco, devil's claw, and dong quai, the enzyme papaya, and vitamins E and K can dangerously alter blood levels of anticoagulants.

Other Notable Examples

Ginkgo biloba—when taken with aspirin, acetaminophen, caffeine-containing pain relievers or with anticoagulants—may lead to bleeding complications such as hyphema (bleeding into the front chamber of the eye) or hemorrhagic stroke (bleeding into the brain).

Licorice can interfere with blood pressure medications, diuretics, hormone replacement therapy, and corticosteroids, and can cause serious complications in women who are taking oral contraceptives.

Ginseng may interact adversely with MAO inhibitors (a class of antidepressant) and digoxin (a heart drug).

St. John's wort may be hazardous to people taking selective serotonin reuptake inhibitors (SSRIs) for depression, and it may interfere with the action of warfarin, digoxin, oral contraceptives, and cyclosporine (an immunosuppressant drug taken for organ transplants).

Some supplements pose such significant risks that they should be avoided altogether. These include comfrey, coltsfoot, chaparral, ephedra (ephedrine or ma huang), sassafras, and yohimbe.

Avoiding Problems

• Tell your doctor about any supplements you take, and ask him or her or a pharmacist about risks of specific herb-drug interactions. People taking medication for such chronic conditions as diabetes, heart disease, or hypertension should be especially cautious.

• Avoid supplements if you are pregnant, trying to conceive, or are breast feeding. Do not give herbal preparations to children without first checking with their doctor.

• Discontinue herbal supplements two to three weeks prior to and following surgery. Certain supplements may promote unwanted bleeding and other complications.

• Don't take an herb and a drug for the same condition; it would be risky, for example, to use both St. John's wort and Prozac for depression. Side effects might increase.

• Don't abruptly start or stop taking herbs or drugs, as this may produce unpredictable and potentially harmful fluctuations in the blood levels of your medications.

• Stop taking supplements right away if you experience side effects.

COMMON DISORDERS AND THE DRUGS PRESCRIBED FOR THEM

As a rule, your doctor can choose from a variety of drugs to treat a particular medical condition. He or she will determine which drug or combination of drugs should be right for you based on a number of factors: the duration and severity of your illness, other medications you may be taking, your age and general health, any accompanying medical problems, and drug allergies or past experiences you've had with particular medications.

If you think that a drug is not working well or you cannot tolerate its side effects, consult your doctor about trying another medication. Do not, however, ever discontinue the drug on your own, and never borrow prescription medicines from others.

The drugs covered in this book are grouped below according to the specific diseases, disorders, symptoms, and conditions for which they are typically used. The list is not exhaustive; it is meant to be a general resource so you can explore which drugs may be useful for specific medical concerns.

Don't be alarmed if a drug you are taking is not listed under your condition. Only indications that have been approved by the Food and Drug Administration (FDA) are included here. However, it's important to note that once a drug has been FDA-approved for one indication, doctors are free to prescribe it for other purposes—a common and often effective practice known as "off-label use."

ACID INDIGESTION AND UPSET STOMACH
Famotidine
Nizatidine
Omeprazole
Ranitidine

ACNE
Tetracycline Hydrochloride
Tretinoin

AIDS (HIV INFECTION)
Indinavir
Interferon beta-1b
Saquinavir
Zidovudine (AZT)

ALCOHOL WITHDRAWAL
Diazepam

ALLERGIES AND ALLERGIC REACTIONS
Beclomethasone Inhalant and Nasal
Cetirizine
Dexamethasone Systemic
Fexofenadine
Fexofenadine/ Pseudoephedrine
Loratadine
Loratadine/Pseudoephedrine
Methylprednisolone
Mometasone Furoate Nasal
Prednisone
Promethazine Hydrochloride
Triamcinolone Inhalant and Nasal

ALZHEIMER'S DISEASE
Donepezil
Rivastigmine Tartrate
Tacrine

ANEMIA
Dexamethasone Systemic
Folic Acid
Methylprednisolone
Prednisone

ANGINA PECTORIS
Amlodipine
Atenolol
Diltiazem Hydrochloride
Isosorbide Mononitrate
Metoprolol
Nifedipine
Nitroglycerin
Propranolol Hydrochloride
Verapamil Hydrochloride

ANXIETY
Alprazolam
Buspirone Hydrochloride
Diazepam
Lorazepam

ARTHRITIS
Celecoxib
Dexamethasone Systemic
Diclofenac/Misoprostol
Ibuprofen
Methotrexate
Methylprednisolone
Nabumetone
Naproxen
Oxaprozin
Prednisone
Rofecoxib

ASTHMA
Albuterol
Beclomethasone Inhalant and Nasal
Dexamethasone Systemic
Methylprednisolone
Montelukast
Nifedipine
Prednisone
Salmeterol Xinafoate
Theophylline
Triamcinolone Inhalant
Zafirlukast

ATHLETE'S FOOT
Terbinafine Hydrochloride

ATTENTION DEFICIT HYPERACTIVITY DISORDER (ADHD)
Amphetamine/ Dextroamphetamine
Methylphenidate HCl

BEHAVIOR PROBLEMS IN CHILDREN
Haloperidol

BLEEDING, ABNORMAL UTERINE
Estradiol
Estrogens, Conjugated
Estrogens, Conjugated/Medroxyprogesterone Acetate
Medroxyprogesterone Acetate

BLOOD CLOTS AND DISORDERS
Clopidogrel Bisulfate
Warfarin

BRONCHITIS
Albuterol
Amoxicillin
Azithromycin
Cefprozil
Cefuroxime
Ciprofloxacin Systemic
Clarithromycin
Erythromycin Systemic
Ipratropium Bromide
Levofloxacin
Penicillin V
Tetracycline Hydrochloride
Theophylline
Trimethoprim/ Sulfamethoxazole

BURSITIS AND JOINT INFLAMMATION
Dexamethasone Systemic
Methylprednisolone

CANCER
Estradiol
Estrogens, Conjugated
Interferon beta-1b
Levothyroxine Sodium
Medroxyprogesterone
   Acetate
Methotrexate
Tamoxifen Citrate

CHLAMYDIA
Azithromycin
Erythromycin Systemic

CHOLESTEROL, HIGH LEVELS OF
Atorvastatin
Fluvastatin
Gemfibrozil
Lovastatin
Pravastatin
Simvastatin

COLDS AND COUGH
Codeine
Promethazine Hydrochloride

CONGESTION, NASAL AND SINUS
Loratadine
Mometasone Furoate Nasal
Promethazine Hydrochloride

CONGESTIVE HEART FAILURE
Digoxin
Enalapril Maleate
Lisinopril
Metoprolol
Nitroglycerin

CONJUNCTIVITIS (ITCHY EYES) DUE TO ALLERGIES
Cetirizine
Dexamethasone Systemic
Loratadine
Methylprednisolone
Mometasone Furoate Nasal
Prednisone
Promethazine Hydrochloride

CONTRACEPTION
Contraceptives, Oral (Combination Products)
Levonorgestrel Implants
Medroxyprogesterone
   Acetate

COUGHING
Codeine
Promethazine Hydrochloride

CUSHING'S DISEASE/SYNDROME
Dexamethasone Systemic

DEMENTIA
Tacrine

DEPRESSION
Amitriptyline Hydrochloride
Bupropion Hydrochloride
Citalopram Hydrobromide
Fluoxetine Hydrochloride
Nefazodone Hydrochloride
Paroxetine Hydrochloride
Sertraline Hydrochloride
Trazodone
Venlafaxine

DIABETES
Acarbose
Glimepiride
Glipizide
Glyburide
Insulin Glargine (rDNA origin)
Insulin (Lispro rDNA origin)
Metformin
Repaglinide
Rosiglitazone Maleate

DIZZINESS (VERTIGO)
Promethazine Hydrochloride

EAR INFECTIONS
Amoxicillin
Amoxicillin/Potassium
   Clavulanate
Cefprozil
Cefuroxime
Cephalexin
Clarithromycin
Erythromycin Systemic
Penicillin V
Tetracycline Hydrochloride
Trimethoprim/
   Sulfamethoxazole

EPILEPSY AND SEIZURES
Carbamazepine
Clonazepam
Gabapentin
Phenytoin
Valproic Acid (Valproate;
   Divalproex Sodium)

ERECTILE DYSFUNCTION
Alprostadil Injection
Sildenafil Citrate

EYE INFECTIONS AND INFLAMMATION
Dexamethasone Systemic
Fexofenadine
Fexofenadine/
   Pseudoephedrine
Loratadine
Loratadine/
   Pseudoephedrine
Methylprednisolone
Mometasone Furoate Nasal
Neomycin/Polymyxin B/
   Hydrocortisone Oph.
Prednisone
Promethazine Hydrochloride

FEVER
Ibuprofen
Naproxen

FLU
Oseltamivir Phosphate
Rimantadine Hydrochloride
Zanamavir

FLUID RETENTION
Furosemide
Hydrochlorothiazide
Hydrochlorothiazide/
   Triamterene

FUNGAL INFECTIONS
Betamethasone/Clotrimazole
Fluconazole
Terbinafine Hydrochloride

GINGIVITIS AND GUM DISEASE
Penicillin V
Tetracycline Hydrochloride

GLAUCOMA
Brimonidine Tartrate
Latanoprost

GOITER
Levothyroxine Sodium

GONORRHEA
Amoxicillin
Cefuroxime
Erythromycin Systemic

GOUT
Allopurinol
Dexamethasone Systemic
Methylprednisolone
Naproxen
Prednisone

HEADACHES— MIGRAINE, SINUS, TENSION, VASCULAR
Naratriptan Hydrochloride

Propranolol Hydrochloride
Sumatriptan Succinate
Valproic Acid (Valproate;
   Divalproex Sodium)
Zolmitriptan

HEART ATTACK PREVENTION
Atenolol
Clopidogrel Bisulfate
Metoprolol
Propranolol Hydrochloride
Warfarin

HEARTBURN
Famotidine
Nizatadine
Omeprazole
Ranitidine

HEART RHYTHM DISORDERS
Digoxin
Diltiazem Hydrochloride
Propranolol Hydrochloride
Verapamil Hydrochloride

HEPATITIS
Interferon beta-1b

HIGH BLOOD PRESSURE
Amlodipine
Atenolol
Benazepril Hydrochloride
Bisoprolol Fumarate/
   Hydrochlorothiazide
Clonidine Hydrochloride
Diltiazem Hydrochloride
Doxazosin Mesylate
Enalapril Maleate
Felodipine
Fosinopril Sodium
Furosemide
Hydrochlorothiazide
Hydrochlorothiazide/
   Triamterene
Irbesartan
Lisinopril

Lisinopril/
   Hydrochlorothiazide
Losartan Potassium
Metoprolol
Nifedipine
Propranolol Hydrochloride
Quinapril Hydrochloride
Ramipril
Terazosin
Valsartan
Verapamil Hydrochloride

HIVES
Cetirizine
Fexofenadine
Fexofenadine/
   Pseudoephedrine
Loratadine
Loratadine/
   Pseudoephedrine
Mometasone Furoate Nasal
Promethazine Hydrochloride

HYPOTHYROIDISM
Levothyroxine Sodium

IMPETIGO
Mupirocin

INFLAMMATORY BOWEL DISEASE
Dexamethasone Systemic
Methylprednisolone
Prednisone

INSOMNIA
Diazepam
Lorazepam
Temazepam
Zaleplon
Zolpidem Tartrate

JOCK ITCH
Terbinafine Hydrochloride

KIDNEY STONES
Allopurinol

LEGIONNAIRES' DISEASE
Erythromycin Systemic

LEUKEMIA
Dexamethasone Systemic
Methotrexate
Methylprednisolone
Prednisone
Tretinoin

LUNG DISEASE
Albuterol
Ipratropium Bromide
Theophylline

LUPUS
Dexamethasone Systemic
Fluticasone
Methylprednisolone

LYME DISEASE
Cefuroxime
Lyme Disease Vaccine
   (Recombinant OspA)

MALARIA
Mefloquine Hydrochloride

MELANOMA
Interferon beta-1b

MENOPAUSE
Estradiol
Estrogens, Conjugated
Estrogens, Conjugated/Med-
   roxyprogesterone Acetate

MENSTRUAL CRAMPS
Ibuprofen
Naproxen

MENSTRUAL PERIODS, REGULATION OF
Medroxyprogesterone
   Acetate

MOTION SICKNESS
Promethazine Hydrochloride

MULTIPLE SCLEROSIS
Dexamethasone Systemic
Interferon beta-1b
Methylprednisolone
Prednisone

MUSCLE SPASM
Carisoprodol
Cyclobenzaprine

NAIL FUNGUS
Terbinafine Hydrochloride

NARCOLEPSY
Amphetamine/
   Dextroamphetamine
Methylphenidate
   Hydrochloride

NASAL POLYPS
Beclomethasone Inhalant
   and Nasal
Dexamethasone Systemic
Methylprednisolone
Prednisone

NAUSEA AND VOMITING
Promethazine Hydrochloride

OBESITY
Orlistat
Sibutramine Hydrochloride
   Monohydrate

OBSESSIVE-COMPULSIVE DISORDERS
Fluoxetine Hydrochloride
Paroxetine Hydrochloride

OSTEOPOROSIS
Alendronate Sodium
Calcitonin-Salmon
Estrogens, Conjugated
Estrogens, Conjugated/Med-
   roxyprogesterone Acetate
Estradiol
Raloxifene Hydrochloride
Risedronate Sodium

PAGET'S DISEASE
Alendronate Sodium
Calcitonin-Salmon
Risedronate Sodium

PAIN RELIEVERS
Acetaminophen with-
  Codeine Phosphate
Clonidine Hydrochloride
Codeine
Hydrocodone Bitartrate/
  Acetaminophen
Ibuprofen
Naproxen
Nifedipine
Oxycodone
Oxycodone/Acetaminophen
Promethazine Hydrochloride
Propoxyphene/
  Acetaminophen
Rofecoxib
Tramadol Hydrochloride

PANIC ATTACKS
Alprazolam
Paroxetine Hydrochloride

PARKINSON'S DISEASE
Levodopa

PERTUSSIS (WHOOPING COUGH)
Erythromycin Systemic

PNEUMONIA
Amoxicillin
Amoxicillin/Potassium
  Clavulanate
Azithromycin
Cefuroxime
Cephalexin
Ciprofloxacin Systemic
Clarithromycin
Erythromycin Systemic
Levofloxacin
Tetracycline Hydrochloride
Trimethoprim/
  Sulfamethoxazole

PROSTATE ENLARGEMENT, BENIGN
Doxazosin Mesylate
Finasteride
Terazosin

PSORIASIS
Fluticasone

PSYCHOTIC DISORDERS
Haloperidol
Olanzapine
Risperidone

RHEUMATIC FEVER
Erythromycin Systemic
Penicillin V

ROCKY MOUNTAIN SPOTTED FEVER
Tetracycline Hydrochloride

RUNNY NOSE AND POSTNASAL DRIP
Cetirizine
Ipratropium Bromide
Loratadine
Mometasone Furoate Nasal
Promethazine Hydrochloride

SCHIZOPHRENIA
Olanzapine

SINUS INFECTION
Amoxicillin
Amoxicillin/Potassium Clavulanate
Clarithromycin
Erythromycin Systemic
Levofloxacin
Tetracycline Hydrochloride

SKIN IRRITATIONS, INFLAMMATION, RASHES
Betamethasone/Clotrimazole
Dexamethasone Systemic
Fluticasone
Methylprednisolone
Prednisone

SNEEZING
Fexofenadine
Fexofenadine/
  Pseudoephedrine
Loratadine
Loratadine/
  Pseudoephedrine
Mometasone Furoate Nasal
Promethazine Hydrochloride

STREP THROAT
Azithromycin
Clarithromycin
Erythromycin Systemic

SUNBURN
Fluticasone

SYPHILIS
Erythromycin Systemic
Tetracycline Hydrochloride

THRUSH
Fluconazole

THYROID HORMONE DEFICIENCY
Levothyroxine Sodium

TONSILLITIS
Cefprozil
Cefuroxime

TOURETTE'S SYNDROME
Haloperidol

TRAVELER'S DIARRHEA
Trimethoprim/
  Sulfamethoxazole

TRIGEMINAL NEURALGIA
Carbamazepine

TUBERCULOSIS
Dexamethasone Systemic
Methylprednisolone
Prednisone

TYPHOID FEVER
Ciprofloxacin Systemic

TYPHUS FEVER
Tetracycline Hydrochloride

ULCERS
Clarithromycin
Famotidine
Lansoprazole
Nizatidine
Omeprazole
Ranitidine

URINARY TRACT INFECTIONS
Amoxicillin
Amoxicillin/Potassium
  Clavulanate
Cefuroxime
Cephalexin
Ciprofloxacin Systemic
Levofloxacin
Nitrofurantoin
Tetracycline Hydrochloride
Trimethoprim/
  Sulfamethoxazole

VAGINAL IRRITATION OR INFECTION
Estradiol
Estrogens, Conjugated
Estrogens, Conjugated/Med-
  roxyprogesterone Acetate
Medroxyprogesterone
  Acetate

VOMITING
Promethazine Hydrochloride

WRINKLES
Tretinoin

YEAST INFECTIONS, VAGINAL
Fluconazole

A to Z
Drug Profiles

ACARBOSE

Available in: Tablets
Available OTC? No   **As Generic?** No
Drug Class: Antidiabetic agent

▼ USAGE INFORMATION

WHY IT'S PRESCRIBED
As an adjunct (supplemental) therapy in patients with diabetes who do not require insulin injections yet are unable to control their blood glucose levels with diet alone or with other medications.

HOW IT WORKS
Acarbose inhibits the activity of enzymes that are required to break carbohydrates down into simple sugars within the intestine. This effect delays the digestion of carbohydrates and thus reduces the rise in blood sugar that typically occurs after meals.

▼ DOSAGE GUIDELINES

RANGE AND FREQUENCY
Initially, 25 mg, 1 to 3 times a day. The dose may be increased (at 4- to 8-week intervals) to a maximum of 100 mg, 3 times daily.

ONSET OF EFFECT
Within 1 hour.

DURATION OF ACTION
Up to 2 hours.

DIETARY ADVICE
This medicine should be taken with the first bite of breakfast, lunch, and dinner. Follow your doctor's advice regarding diet, weight loss, and exercise.

STORAGE
Keep in a tightly sealed container away from heat and direct light.

MISSED DOSE
If you have finished a meal without taking the medication, skip the missed dose and resume your regular dosing schedule with the next meal. Do not double the next dose.

STOPPING THE DRUG
Take this medication as prescribed for the full treatment period.

PROLONGED USE
Since non-insulin-dependent diabetes is a chronic condition, use of acarbose will be ongoing. Blood glucose levels should be checked regularly during treatment so that the dosage may be adjusted if necessary.

▼ PRECAUTIONS

Over 60: No special precautions required.

Driving and Hazardous Work: Acarbose should not impair your ability to perform such tasks safely.

Alcohol: Drink only in moderation when taking acarbose.

Pregnancy: Consult your doctor for advice. Insulin is usually the treatment of choice for women with diabetes who are pregnant.

Breast Feeding: Trace amounts of acarbose can be found in breast milk; however, adverse effects in infants have not been documented. Consult your doctor for advice.

Infants and Children: Safety and effectiveness have not been established for patients under 18 years of age. Consult your doctor for more specific advice.

Special Concerns: You should not take acarbose if you've had an allergic reaction to this drug previously or if you are taking, or took within the past 14 days, a monoamine oxidase (MAO) inhibitor (a class of antidepressant drugs).

OVERDOSE
Symptoms: Increased gas, diarrhea, and stomach pain.

What to Do: These symptoms usually subside on their own within a short period of time. If they do not, consult your doctor for more specific advice. Symptoms of hypoglycemia should not occur when taking acarbose alone, but may occur if a patient is also taking sulfonylurea or insulin for diabetes.

▼ INTERACTIONS

DRUG INTERACTIONS
Do not take acarbose if you are taking, or took within the past 14 days, an MAO inhibitor. Consult your doctor for specific advice if you are taking any of the following drugs that may interact with acarbose: digestive enzyme preparations containing amylase or pancreatin, intestinal absorbents (such as charcoal), insulin, or sulfonylureas (oral antidiabetic agents).

FOOD INTERACTIONS
Avoid foods that contain large amounts of sugar (for example, cake, cookies, candy, acidic fruits). Closely follow the diet your doctor has prescribed.

DISEASE INTERACTIONS
Acarbose should not be taken by patients with a history of any of the following disorders: diabetic ketoacidosis, intestinal disorders (including malabsorption or obstruction), inflammatory bowel disease (for example, Crohn's disease or ulcerative colitis), liver disease, kidney disease, or gastric ulcers.

≡ SIDE EFFECTS ≡

SERIOUS
There are no serious side effects associated with acarbose.

COMMON
Feelings of bloating, gas, abdominal discomfort, diarrhea. These symptoms tend to decrease over time.

LESS COMMON
Rise in liver enzymes, causing yellowish tinge to eyes or skin (jaundice), when maximal dose is exceeded. When used in combination with sulfonylureas, may cause symptoms of low blood sugar, which include sweating, tremor, anxiety, hunger, confusion, seizures, rapid heartbeat, vision changes, dizziness, headache, loss of consciousness. Hypoglycemia must be treated by ingestion of glucose (dextrose). Sucrose (table sugar) and foods or drinks containing sugars or starches are ineffective because acarbose prevents their breakdown and absorption.

ACETAMINOPHEN WITH CODEINE PHOSPHATE

Available in: Capsules, tablets, oral solution, oral suspension
Available OTC? No **As Generic?** Yes
Drug Class: Opioid (narcotic) analgesic/antipyretic

APAP with Codeine, Capital with Codeine, Codaphen, EZ III, Margesic, Myapap and Codeine, Phenaphen with Codeine, Proval, Pyregesic-C, Ty-Deine, Ty-Pap with Codeine, Ty-Tab with Codeine, Tylagesic 3, Tylenol with Codeine

▼ USAGE INFORMATION

WHY IT'S PRESCRIBED
To relieve mild to severe pain when nonprescription pain relievers prove inadequate. A narcotic analgesic, such as codeine, in combination with acetaminophen may provide better pain relief than either medicine when it's used alone. In addition, when taken together, the two medications can often achieve better pain relief at lower doses.

HOW IT WORKS
Acetaminophen appears to interfere with the action of prostaglandins, naturally occurring substances in the body that cause inflammation and make nerves more sensitive to pain impulses. This medication also relieves fever, probably by acting on the heat-regulating center of the brain. Unlike aspirin, however, acetaminophen does not reduce inflammation. Codeine, a narcotic analgesic, is believed to relieve pain by acting on specific areas in the spinal cord and in the brain that together process pain signals from nerves throughout the body.

▼ DOSAGE GUIDELINES

RANGE AND FREQUENCY
Adults—Capsules or tablets: 1 or 2 capsules containing 15 or 30 mg of codeine with acetaminophen or 1 capsule containing 60 mg of codeine with acetaminophen, every 4 hours as needed. Oral solution or suspension: 1 tablespoon every 4 hours as needed. Children—Oral solution or suspension: Ages 3 to 6: 1 teaspoon 3 or 4 times a day as needed. Ages 7 to 12: 2 teaspoons 3 or 4 times a day as needed.

ONSET OF EFFECT
Acetaminophen: Rapid.
Codeine: Within 2 hours.

DURATION OF ACTION
Up to 4 hours.

DIETARY ADVICE
Take this medication with meals or milk to avoid stomach upset, unless doctor directs you to do otherwise.

STORAGE
Store in a tightly sealed container away from moisture, heat, and direct light. Keep liquid forms from freezing.

MISSED DOSE
If you are taking acetaminophen with codeine on a fixed schedule, take it as soon as you remember. If it is near the time for the next dose, skip the missed dose and resume your regular dosage schedule. Do not double the next dose.

STOPPING THE DRUG
You should take the medication as prescribed for the full treatment period, but you may stop taking it if you are feeling better before the scheduled end of therapy. This drug should never be stopped abruptly after long-term regular use.

PROLONGED USE
Narcotic drugs such as codeine may cause physical dependence. Taking too much acetaminophen may cause liver damage. Therapy with acetaminophen and codeine should not continue for more than 2 weeks and may actually cease to be effective before then.

▼ PRECAUTIONS

Over 60: Adverse reactions may be more likely and more severe in older patients.

Driving and Hazardous Work: Acetaminophen with codeine can cause dizziness or drowsiness; pay attention and proceed with caution.

Alcohol: Avoid alcohol. The combination of alcohol and this drug may increase the depressant effects of the medicine. Drinking alcohol-containing beverages while taking acetaminophen greatly increases your risk of developing liver damage.

Pregnancy: Use of this drug during pregnancy can cause fetal addiction and may cause breathing problems in the newborn infant if taken during or just before delivery. Consult your doctor for specific guidelines and advice and discuss the relative risks and benefits of using this drug while pregnant.

Breast Feeding: Acetaminophen with codeine passes into breast milk; avoid or discontinue nursing while taking this drug.

Infants and Children: This medicine should not be given to infants. The drug may be used by children over the age of 3, but only with extreme caution and under the careful supervision of your doctor. Children are generally prescribed the oral solution or suspension instead of the capsule or tablet.

Special Concerns: Taking a narcotic such as codeine for an extended period of time can lead to physical dependence. When discontinuing the drug after using it for an extended period, it is important to decrease the dosage gradually under the supervision of your doctor to reduce the risk of suffering from

☰ SIDE EFFECTS ☰

▼ SERIOUS ▼
See Overdose and Special Concerns.

COMMON
Dizziness, lightheadedness, nausea or vomiting, drowsiness, constipation, unusual fatigue.

LESS COMMON
Stomach pain, allergic reaction, false sense of well-being (euphoria), depression, loss of appetite, blurring or change in vision, nightmares or unusual dreams, dry mouth, general feeling of illness, headache, nervousness, insomnia.

(continued)

ACETAMINOPHEN WITH CODEINE PHOSPHATE (continued)

withdrawal symptoms. Call your doctor if you notice these symptoms after discontinuing the drug: shivering or trembling; insomnia; gooseflesh; nausea or vomiting; body aches; loss of appetite; stomach cramps; weakness; diarrhea; restlessness, nervousness, or irritability; rapid heartbeat; sneezing, runny nose, or fever; increased yawning; or increased sweating. Overuse of acetaminophen with codeine may also lead to anemia, liver problems, or central nervous system disorders. Contact your doctor as soon as possible if you experience any of the following symptoms during or after the use of this drug: bloody, dark, or cloudy urine; severe pain in the lower back or side; frequent urge to urinate; painful or difficult urination; sudden decrease in urine output; pale or black, tarry stools; yellow discoloration of the eyes or skin (jaundice); hallucinations; unusual bleeding or bruising; skin rash, hives, or itching; pinpoint red spots on skin; sore throat and fever; unusual excitability; trembling or uncontrolled muscle movements; redness, flushing, or swelling of the face.

OVERDOSE

Symptoms: Severe dizziness or drowsiness; cold, clammy skin; difficult or slow breathing or shortness of breath; severe confusion; seizures; stomach cramps or pain; diarrhea; low blood pressure; increased sweating; nausea or vomiting; constricted pupils; irregular heartbeat; severe weakness.

What to Do: Call your doctor, emergency medical services (EMS), or the nearest poison control center immediately.

▼ INTERACTIONS

DRUG INTERACTIONS
Some drugs may interact with acetaminophen and codeine. Consult your doctor for specific advice if you are taking any prescription or over-the-counter drugs, especially if they contain acetaminophen; central nervous system depressants such as antihistamines or medicine for hay fever, allergies, or colds; barbiturates; seizure medicine; muscle relaxants; anesthetics; or tranquilizers, sedatives, or sleep medications.

FOOD INTERACTIONS
No significant food interactions have been reported.

DISEASE INTERACTIONS
Consult your doctor if you have a head injury or brain disease, an underactive thyroid, an enlarged prostate, seizures, kidney or liver disease, gallbladder problems, a blood disorder, or a history of alcohol or drug abuse. Any of these medical conditions may increase the likelihood of developing side effects from acetaminophen and codeine.

ALBUTEROL

BRAND NAMES

Airet, Proventil,
Ventolin, Volmax

Available in: Inhaler, solution, capsules, tablets, syrup
Available OTC? No   **As Generic?** Yes
Drug Class: Bronchodilator/sympathomimetic

▼ USAGE INFORMATION

WHY IT'S PRESCRIBED
To dilate air passages in the lungs that have become narrowed as a result of disease or inflammation. It is used in the treatment of asthma and chronic obstructive pulmonary disease (COPD).

HOW IT WORKS
Albuterol widens constricted airways by relaxing the smooth muscles that surround the bronchial passages in the lungs.

▼ DOSAGE GUIDELINES

RANGE AND FREQUENCY
Use it when needed to relieve breathing difficulty. For bronchospasm: 1 to 2 puffs of aerosol inhaler every 4 to 6 hours; or 2.5 mg of solution delivered via nebulizer 3 to 4 times a day; or 200 micrograms (mcg) of capsules for inhalation using Rotahaler every 4 to 6 hours; or 2 to 4 mg of tablets 3 or 4 times a day, not to exceed 32 mg per day. Children may require a smaller dose. For prevention of exercise-induced asthma: 1 or 2 inhalations (at least 1 full minute apart), 15 minutes prior to exercise.

ONSET OF EFFECT
Inhalant: Within 5 minutes. Oral forms: Within 15 to 30 minutes.

DURATION OF ACTION
Inhalant: 3 to 6 hours. Oral forms: 8 hours.

DIETARY ADVICE
Albuterol can be taken on an empty stomach or with food or milk.

STORAGE
Contents of aerosol canisters are under pressure; be careful not to puncture the container. Store canister away from heat, open flame, and direct light.

MISSED DOSE
Skip the missed dose and resume your regular dosage schedule. Do not double the next dose.

STOPPING THE DRUG
It may not be necessary to finish the recommended course of therapy. Consult your doctor.

PROLONGED USE
Therapy may require months or years. Excessive use may result in temporary loss of effectiveness.

▼ PRECAUTIONS

Over 60: Adverse reactions may be more likely and more severe in older patients.

Driving and Hazardous Work: Do not drive or engage in hazardous work until you determine how the medicine affects you.

Alcohol: No special warnings.

Pregnancy: Albuterol may cause birth defects in mice when given in extremely large doses. Consult your doctor.

Breast Feeding: Albuterol may pass into breast milk; caution is advised.

Infants and Children: Not recommended for use by children under the age of 2.

Special Concerns: Tell your doctor if you have ever had any unusual or allergic reaction to albuterol. Prime the inhaler prior to the first use and in cases when it has not been used for more than four days. Prime it by releasing four test sprays before first use (and two test sprays when not used for a period of at least four days) in the air away from the face. You should wash your rotahaler (biweekly) and inhaler (weekly) to prevent drug build-up and blockage. Wash the two halves of the rotahaler or the mouthpiece of the inhaler (with the canister removed) with warm water and shake to remove excess water. Both the rotahaler and the inhaler should be air-dried thoroughly.

OVERDOSE
Symptoms: Confusion, delirium, severe anxiety, seizures, nervousness, headache, nausea, dry mouth, dizziness, insomnia, chest pain, muscle tremors, profound weakness, rapid and irregular pulse.

What to Do: Call your doctor, emergency medical services (EMS), or hospital immediately.

▼ INTERACTIONS

DRUG INTERACTIONS
Albuterol should not be used within 14 days of using an MAO inhibitor or tricyclic antidepressants. Consult your doctor if you are taking beta-blockers, loop or thiazide diuretics, antihypertensives, digitalis drugs, epinephrine, ergot, finasteride, furazolidone, guanadrel, guanethidine, maprotiline, methyldopa, any nitrate, a phenothiazine, pseudoephedrine-containing products, rauwolfia alkaloids, terazosin, other asthma medications, or thyroid hormone.

FOOD INTERACTIONS
No known food interactions.

DISEASE INTERACTIONS
Consult your doctor if you have an overactive thyroid, diabetes mellitus, a history of seizures, heart problems, high blood pressure, or blood vessel disease.

≣ SIDE EFFECTS ≣

SERIOUS
Inhaled form: May become ineffective if used too often, resulting in more-severe breathing difficulty that does not improve. Signs include persistent wheezing, coughing, or shortness of breath; confusion; bluish color to lips or fingernails; inability to speak. Ingested form: Chest pain or heaviness; irregular, racing, fluttering, or pounding heartbeat; lightheadedness; fainting; severe weakness; severe headache.

COMMON
Nervousness, tremor, dizziness, headache, insomnia.

LESS COMMON
Dryness and irritation of the nose, mouth, and throat; heartburn; nausea; muscle cramps.

ALENDRONATE SODIUM

Available in: Tablets
Available OTC? No **As Generic?** No
Drug Class: Bisphosphonate inhibitor of bone resorption

▼ USAGE INFORMATION

WHY IT'S PRESCRIBED
To prevent and treat osteoporosis in postmenopausal women; to treat osteoporosis in men by increasing bone mass. Alendronate also treats glucocorticoid-induced osteoporosis in those receiving corticosteroids in a daily dosage equivalent to 7.5 mg or greater of prednisone and who have low bone mineral density. Also used for Paget's disease, a disorder characterized by rapid breakdown and reformation of bone, which can lead to fragility and malformation of bones.

HOW IT WORKS
Healthy bones are continuously remodeled (broken down and then reformed); the minerals and other components of bones are reabsorbed by one set of cells (osteoclasts) and replaced by another set of cells to form new bone. Alendronate suppresses the activity of osteoclasts; consequently, the breakdown of bone tissue occurs more slowly than the laying down of new bone. This action preserves bone density and strength.

▼ DOSAGE GUIDELINES

RANGE AND FREQUENCY
For prevention of osteoporosis: 5 mg a day or 35 mg once a week. For treatment of osteoporosis: 10 mg a day or 70 mg once a week. For glucocorticoid-induced osteoporosis in men and women: 5 mg a day; postmenopausal women not receiving estrogen should take 10 mg a day. For Paget's disease: 40 mg a day. The dose is taken in the morning. Swallow tablets whole; do not suck or chew them. Do not lie down for 30 minutes following your dosage. The tablet must be taken with an 8 oz glass of water at least 30 minutes before any food or other drug.

ONSET OF EFFECT
Within 2 hours.

DURATION OF ACTION
24 hours to 7 days.

DIETARY ADVICE
Take alendronate at least 30 minutes before your first food or beverage of the day, with a full glass of water. Some patients may be advised to take calcium or vitamin C supplements to aid in the formation of new bone tissue.

STORAGE
Store in a tightly sealed container away from moisture, heat, and direct light.

MISSED DOSE
Take it as soon as you remember. If it is near the time for the next dose, skip the missed dose and resume your regular dosage schedule. Do not double the next dose.

STOPPING THE DRUG
The decision to stop taking the drug should be made by your doctor. In most cases, patients with Paget's disease are treated for 6 months; the drug is then stopped. Retreatment may be necessary if such patients show signs of relapse after a subsequent 6-month observation period.

PROLONGED USE
No special precautions.

▼ PRECAUTIONS

Over 60: No special problems are expected.

Driving and Hazardous Work: No special precautions.

Alcohol: Alcohol should be restricted in high-risk women because it is a risk factor for developing osteoporosis.

Pregnancy: The drug should not be given to pregnant women because animal studies have shown adverse effects in the fetus.

Breast Feeding: Alendronate may pass into breast milk. Consult your doctor for advice.

Infants and Children: Use not recommended for children.

Special Concerns: Patients taking alendronate are encouraged to engage in regular weight-bearing exercise and should avoid cigarettes and limit alcohol, which inhibit healthy bone production.

OVERDOSE
Symptoms: Severe heartburn, stomach cramps, or throat irritation might occur if an overdose of alendronate disturbs the body's normal mineral (electrolyte) balance.

What to Do: Few cases have been reported. However, if someone takes a much larger dose than prescribed, call your doctor or the nearest poison control center.

▼ INTERACTIONS

DRUG INTERACTIONS
Consult your doctor for specific advice if you are taking antacids, calcium supplements, aspirin or other non-steroidal anti-inflammatory drugs (NSAIDs), or hormone replacement therapy. Wait at least 30 minutes after taking alendronate before taking any other drugs.

FOOD INTERACTIONS
Any food eaten within 30 minutes of taking alendronate decreases its effect. Mineral water, coffee, tea, and fruit juice can interfere with the absorption of alendronate.

DISEASE INTERACTIONS
Kidney impairment or a gastrointestinal disease may increase the risk of side effects. Low blood calcium levels and vitamin D deficiency must be treated before using alendronate.

≡ SIDE EFFECTS ≡

SERIOUS
No serious side effects have been reported.

COMMON
Abdominal pain or bloating (persistent pain should be reported to your doctor), indigestion, heartburn, nausea.

LESS COMMON
Headache, constipation, diarrhea, gas, swallowing difficulty, throat irritation, abdominal swelling or tightness, muscle or bone pain, changes in taste perception.

ALLOPURINOL

BRAND NAMES

Lopurin, Purinol, Zyloprim

Available in: Tablets
Available OTC? No   **As Generic?** Yes
Drug Class: Antigout drug

▼ USAGE INFORMATION

WHY IT'S PRESCRIBED
To treat chronic gout or the excessive uric acid buildup caused by kidney disorders, by cancer, or by the use of chemotherapy drugs for cancer. Also prescribed to prevent recurrence of uric acid kidney stones. Allopurinol should not be used for treating acute gout attacks in progress.

HOW IT WORKS
Allopurinol blocks the enzyme xanthine oxidase, which is required for the production of uric acid, thus reducing blood levels of uric acid.

▼ DOSAGE GUIDELINES

RANGE AND FREQUENCY
Adults: Initially 100 mg per day, increased by 100 mg per week to a maximum of 800 mg per day. 100 mg doses are administered once a day; doses of 300 mg or more are taken in 2 or 3 evenly divided portions throughout the day.

Children ages 6 to 10: 300 mg per day for certain types of cancer. Children age 6 and under: 50 mg per day in 3 evenly divided portions.

ONSET OF EFFECT
Reduces uric acid levels in 2 to 3 days; may take 6 months for full effect to occur.

DURATION OF ACTION
1 to 2 weeks.

DIETARY ADVICE
Take it with food or milk to avoid stomach irritation. Drink 10 to 12 glasses (8 oz each) of water a day while on this medication.

STORAGE
Store in a tightly sealed container away from heat and direct light.

MISSED DOSE
Take the medicine as soon as you remember. However, if it is near the time for you to take your next dose, skip the missed dose and resume your regular dosage schedule. Do not double the next dose.

STOPPING THE DRUG
Take allopurinol as prescribed for the full treatment period, even if you begin to feel better before the scheduled end of therapy.

PROLONGED USE
Consult your doctor about the need for tests of liver function, kidney function, blood counts, and blood and urine levels of uric acid.

▼ PRECAUTIONS

Over 60: Adverse reactions may be more likely and more severe in older patients.

Driving and Hazardous Work: Allopurinol may cause drowsiness. If possible, avoid driving and hazardous work.

Alcohol: No special precautions are necessary.

Pregnancy: Caution is advised; consult your doctor about whether the benefits outweigh potential risks to the unborn child.

Breast Feeding: Allopurinol passes into breast milk; avoid or discontinue use while breast feeding.

Infants and Children: Follow your doctor's instructions carefully for children.

OVERDOSE
Symptoms: No specific symptoms have been reported.

What to Do: An overdose of allopurinol is unlikely to be life-threatening. However, if someone takes a much larger dose than prescribed, contact your doctor, poison control center, or local emergency room for instructions.

▼ INTERACTIONS

DRUG INTERACTIONS
Consult your doctor for specific advice if you are taking an antibiotic (such as amoxicillin, ampicillin, or bacampicillin), an anticoagulant drug (warfarin, dicumarol), an anticancer (chemotherapy) drug, chlorpropamide, a diuretic, or theophylline.

FOOD INTERACTIONS
None are likely, but a low-purine diet is recommended to reduce the risk of gout attacks. Foods high in purines include anchovies, sardines, legumes, poultry, sweetbreads, liver, kidneys, and other organ meats.

DISEASE INTERACTIONS
Caution is advised when taking allopurinol. Consult your doctor if you have high blood pressure, diabetes mellitus, kidney disease, or impaired iron metabolism.

≡ SIDE EFFECTS ≡

▼ SERIOUS ▼
Anemia or other blood or bone marrow disorders that may produce fatigue, bleeding, or bruising; yellowish tinge to eyes or skin (signifying hepatitis or liver damage); severe skin reactions (marked by rashes, skin ulcers, hives, intense itching); chest tightness; weakness. Call your doctor right away if such symptoms arise.

COMMON
Mild rash, drowsiness, nausea, diarrhea. The frequency of gout attacks may increase during the first weeks of use.

LESS COMMON
Headache, abdominal pain, boils on face, chills or fever, vomiting, hair loss.

ALPRAZOLAM

BRAND NAME

Xanax

Available in: Tablets, oral solution
Available OTC? No   **As Generic?** Yes
Drug Class: Benzodiazepine tranquilizer; antianxiety agent

▼ USAGE INFORMATION

WHY IT'S PRESCRIBED
To treat anxiety and panic disorder.

HOW IT WORKS
In general, alprazolam produces mild sedation by depressing activity in the central nervous system. In particular, alprazolam appears to enhance the effect of gamma-aminobutyric acid (GABA), a natural chemical that inhibits the firing of neurons and dampens the transmission of nerve signals, thus decreasing nervous excitation.

▼ DOSAGE GUIDELINES

RANGE AND FREQUENCY
Adults: Initial dose is 1.5 mg a day, taken in 3 divided doses; may be gradually increased to a maximum dose of 4 mg a day. Older adults: Initial dose is 0.5 to 0.75 mg per day, taken in 2 or 3 divided doses; may be gradu-ally increased to a maximum dose of 2 mg a day. Children: Not usually prescribed.

ONSET OF EFFECT
2 hours.

DURATION OF ACTION
Up to 6 hours.

DIETARY ADVICE
Alprazolam can be taken on an empty stomach or with food or milk.

STORAGE
Store in a tightly sealed container away from heat and direct light.

MISSED DOSE
If you miss a dose, take it if you remember within 1 hour. Otherwise, skip the missed dose and take the next one at the regular time. Do not double the next dose.

STOPPING THE DRUG
Never stop taking the drug abruptly, as this can cause withdrawal symptoms (seizures, sleep disruption, nervousness, irritability, diarrhea, abdominal cramps, muscle aches, memory impairment). Dosage should be reduced gradually as directed by your doctor.

PROLONGED USE
Short-term therapy (8 weeks or less) is typical; do not take it for a longer period unless so advised by your doctor.

▼ PRECAUTIONS

Over 60: Use with caution; side effects such as drowsiness and dizziness may be more pronounced in older patients.

Driving and Hazardous Work: Alprazolam can impair mental alertness and physical coordination. Adjust your activities accordingly.

Alcohol: Alcohol intake should be extremely moderate or stopped altogether while taking alprazolam.

Pregnancy: Use of this drug during pregnancy should be avoided if possible. Be sure to tell your doctor if you are pregnant or if you plan to become pregnant.

Breast Feeding: Alprazolam passes into breast milk; do not take it while nursing.

Infants and Children: Safety and effectiveness have not been established for children under age 18.

Special Concerns: Use of this drug can lead to psychological or physical dependence. Short-term therapy (8 weeks or less) is typical; patients should not take the drug for a longer period unless so advised by their doctor. Never take more than the prescribed daily dose.

OVERDOSE
Symptoms: Extreme drowsiness, confusion, slurred speech, slow reflexes, poor coordination, staggering gait, tremor, slowed breathing, loss of consciousness.

What to Do: Call your doctor, emergency medical services (EMS), or the nearest poison control center immediately.

▼ INTERACTIONS

DRUG INTERACTIONS
Other drugs may interact with alprazolam. Consult your doctor for specific advice if you are taking any drugs that depress the central nervous system; these include antihistamines, antidepressants (including nefazodone) or other psychiatric medications, barbiturates, sedatives, cough medicines, decongestants, and painkillers. Be sure your doctor knows about any over-the-counter medication you may take.

FOOD INTERACTIONS
None reported.

DISEASE INTERACTIONS
Consult your doctor if you have a history of alcohol or drug abuse, stroke or other brain disease, any chronic lung disease, hyperactivity, depression or other mental illness, myasthenia gravis, sleep apnea, epilepsy, porphyria, kidney disease, or liver disease.

☰ SIDE EFFECTS ☰

SERIOUS
Difficulty concentrating, outbursts of anger, other behavior problems, depression, hallucinations, low blood pressure (causing faintness or confusion), memory impairment, muscle weakness, skin rash or itching, sore throat, fever and chills, sores or ulcers in throat or mouth, unusual bruising or bleeding, extreme fatigue, yellowish tinge to eyes or skin. Call your doctor immediately.

COMMON
Drowsiness, loss of coordination, unsteady gait, dizziness, lightheadedness, slurred speech.

LESS COMMON
Change in sexual desire or ability, constipation, false sense of well-being, nausea and vomiting, urinary problems, unusual fatigue.

ALPROSTADIL INJECTION

BRAND NAMES

Caverject, Edex,
Prostin VR Pediatric

Available in: Injection
Available OTC? No **As Generic?** Yes
Drug Class: Vasodilator

▼ USAGE INFORMATION

WHY IT'S PRESCRIBED
To treat erectile dysfunction
(impotence) in men; also, to
help maintain an adequate
blood flow in infants during
heart surgery.

HOW IT WORKS
Alprostadil causes dilation
of blood vessels, thereby
increasing blood flow to
the tissues supplied by the
vessels affected by the drug.
When injected into the penis,
alprostadil causes the penile
arteries to dilate, thus promoting erection.

▼ DOSAGE GUIDELINES

RANGE AND FREQUENCY
For adult men: Injection of
0.001 to 0.04 mg, self-
administered at the base of
the penis as needed. It should
not be administered more
than once a day. For infants:
Injection of 0.005 to 0.01 mg
before surgery.

ONSET OF EFFECT
5 to 10 minutes.

DURATION OF ACTION
30 minutes to 3 hours.

DIETARY ADVICE
Diet is not significant in
alprostadil therapy.

STORAGE
Keep the liquid form of
alprostadil refrigerated, but
do not allow it to freeze.

MISSED DOSE
Not applicable; the drug is
taken only when the patient
chooses to take it.

STOPPING THE DRUG
Consult your doctor if you
wish to discontinue therapy
or if you feel alprostadil is
losing its effectiveness.

PROLONGED USE
Alprostadil should not be
used more frequently than a
physician recommends, which
is generally not more than
3 times a week, with at least
24 hours between each dose.
Patients who self-administer
alprostadil should visit their
doctor every three months
for evaluation; dosage adjustments or the decision to stop
using the drug will be made

at these times. Never increase
the dosage without consulting
your doctor.

▼ PRECAUTIONS

Over 60: Information about
use specifically in older persons is not available, though
elderly patients are more
likely to suffer from circulatory problems and thus may
be less responsive to the drug
than their younger counterparts. Your doctor may need
to adjust the dosage.

**Driving and Hazardous
Work:** No special precautions.

Alcohol: No special precautions are necessary.

Pregnancy: Not applicable;
the drug is used only in men
and infants. No problems
have been reported in women
who became pregnant by
partners using alprostadil.

Breast Feeding: Not applicable; the drug is used only by
men or in infants.

Infants and Children:
Prostin VR Pediatric should
be used for infants only in a
hospital setting.

Special Concerns: A doctor
should instruct you about
administering the injection
before you attempt to do it
yourself. Only men who have
been diagnosed with and are
being medically treated for
erectile dysfunction should
use this drug as a sexual aid.

OVERDOSE
Symptoms: Painful erection
or an erection that persists
for more than 4 hours.

What to Do: Call your doctor,
emergency medical services
(EMS), or your local hospital
right away. Prolonged erection may result in permanent
damage to the tissues of the
penis and the inability to
achieve subsequent erections.

▼ INTERACTIONS

DRUG INTERACTIONS
None reported in infants.
Adults should notify their
doctor if they are taking any
other drugs.

FOOD INTERACTIONS
No significant interactions
have been reported.

DISEASE INTERACTIONS
An adult who has a blood
coagulation defect, liver disease, sickle cell disease, or a
history of priapism (erections
lasting more than 4 hours)
should inform his physician
before using alprostadil.

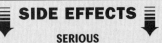

≡ SIDE EFFECTS ≡

SERIOUS
Painful or prolonged erection (lasting more than 4 hours),
usually as a result of excessive dosage. If erection does not
resolve on its own in a reasonable amount of time, seek
medical help promptly. If erection does resolve on its own,
subsequent doses should be reduced; consult your doctor
for specific guidelines.

COMMON
Pain, itching, or burning at site of injection.

LESS COMMON
Bruising or bleeding at site of injection.

AMITRIPTYLINE HYDROCHLORIDE

Available in: Tablets
Available OTC? No   **As Generic?** Yes
Drug Class: Tricyclic antidepressant; antimanic agent

▼ USAGE INFORMATION

WHY IT'S PRESCRIBED
To relieve symptoms of major depression and chronic pain.

HOW IT WORKS
Amitriptyline affects levels of certain brain chemicals (serotonin, norepinephrine, and acetylcholine) thought to be linked to mood, emotions, and mental state.

▼ DOSAGE GUIDELINES

RANGE AND FREQUENCY
Adults: To start, 25 mg, 2 to 4 times a day; may be increased to 150 mg a day. Teenagers: 10 mg, 3 times a day, and 20 mg at bedtime. Children ages 6 to 12: 10 to 30 mg a day. Older adults: To start, 25 mg a day at bedtime; may be increased to 100 mg a day.

ONSET OF EFFECT
1 to 6 weeks.

DURATION OF ACTION
Unknown.

DIETARY ADVICE
To lessen stomach upset, take with food, unless your doctor instructs otherwise. Increase intake of fiber and fluids.

STORAGE
Store in a tightly sealed container away from moisture, heat, and direct light.

MISSED DOSE
If you take a one-time daily bedtime dose, do not take the missed dose in the morning; it may cause drowsiness. Call your doctor. If you take more than 1 dose a day, take it as soon as you remember. If it is near the time for the next dose, skip the missed dose and resume your regular dosage schedule. Do not double the next dose.

STOPPING THE DRUG
Take it as prescribed for the full treatment period, even if you feel better before the scheduled end of therapy. The decision to stop taking the drug should be made in consultation with your doctor. The dosage should be gradually tapered over 5 to 7 days when stopping.

PROLONGED USE
The usual course of therapy lasts 6 months to 1 year; some patients may benefit from additional therapy.

▼ PRECAUTIONS

Over 60: Adverse reactions are more likely and more severe in older patients. Amitriptyline is generally not recommended, as there are safer alternatives for older patients. A lower dose may be warranted.

Driving and Hazardous Work: Use caution when driving and engaging in hazardous work until you determine how the medicine affects you. Drowsiness or lightheadedness can occur.

Alcohol: Avoid alcohol.

Pregnancy: Adequate human studies have not been done in pregnant women. Consult your doctor for advice.

Breast Feeding: Amitriptyline passes into breast milk; do not use it while nursing.

Infants and Children: Not prescribed for children under the age of 6.

Special Concerns: This is a potentially dangerous drug, especially if taken in excess. Tricyclic antidepressants should not be within easy reach of suicidal patients. If dry mouth occurs, use sugarless gum or candy.

OVERDOSE
Symptoms: Breathing difficulty, fever, severe fatigue, impaired concentration, mental confusion, hallucinations, dilated pupils, irregular heartbeat or palpitations, and seizures.

What to Do: Call your doctor, emergency medical services (EMS), or the nearest poison control center immediately.

▼ INTERACTIONS

DRUG INTERACTIONS
Consult your doctor for specific advice if you are taking antithyroid agents, cimetidine, cisapride, clonidine, guanadrel, guanethidine, metrizamide, appetite suppressants, isoproterenol, ephedrine, epinephrine, amphetamines, phenylephrine, antipsychotic drugs, pimozide, methyldopa, metyrosine, metoclopramide, pemoline, promethazine, trimeprazine, rauwolfia alkaloids, MAO inhibitors, or any drugs that depress the central nervous system.

FOOD INTERACTIONS
No known food interactions.

DISEASE INTERACTIONS
Consult your doctor if you have any of the following: a history of alcohol abuse, difficulty urinating, asthma, bipolar disorder, high blood pressure, stomach or intestinal problems, glaucoma, an overactive thyroid, enlarged prostate, schizophrenia, seizures, a blood disorder, or kidney, heart, or liver disease.

≣ SIDE EFFECTS ≣

SERIOUS
Confusion, heartbeat irregularities, hallucinations, seizures, extreme fatigue or drowsiness, blurred or altered vision, breathing difficulty, constipation, impaired concentration, difficult urination, fever, extreme and persistent restlessness, loss of coordination and balance, difficulty swallowing or speaking, dilated pupils, eye pain, fainting. Also trembling, shaking, weakness, and stiffness in the extremities; shuffling gait. Call your doctor immediately.

COMMON
Drowsiness, dizziness, or lightheadedness, headache, dry mouth or unpleasant taste, fatigue, heightened sensitivity to light, unusual weight gain, increased appetite, nausea.

LESS COMMON
Heartburn, insomnia, diarrhea, increased sweating, vomiting.

AMLODIPINE

Norvasc

Available in: Tablets, capsules
Available OTC? No   **As Generic?** No
Drug Class: Calcium channel blocker

▼ USAGE INFORMATION

WHY IT'S PRESCRIBED
To relieve angina (chest pain associated with heart disease) and to treat hypertension.

HOW IT WORKS
Amlodipine interferes with calcium's movement into cells of the heart muscle and cells of the smooth muscle in artery walls. This relaxes blood vessels (causing them to widen), which lowers blood pressure, increases the heart's blood supply, and decreases the heart's overall workload.

▼ DOSAGE GUIDELINES

RANGE AND FREQUENCY
2.5 to 10 mg per day in one daily dose (usually in the morning, with breakfast).

ONSET OF EFFECT
1 to 2 hours.

DURATION OF ACTION
24 hours.

DIETARY ADVICE
It can be taken with or after meals to minimize stomach irritation. Be sure to follow a low-sodium, low-fat diet if your doctor so advises.

STORAGE
Store in a tightly sealed container away from heat and direct light.

MISSED DOSE
If you miss a dose, take it as soon as you remember, unless the next dose is less than 4 hours away. In that case, skip the missed dose and go back to your regular schedule. Do not double the next dose.

STOPPING THE DRUG
Take as prescribed for the full treatment period. Do not stop taking this drug suddenly, as this may cause potentially serious health problems. If therapy is to be discontinued, dosage should be reduced gradually, according to doctor's instructions.

PROLONGED USE
In some cases amlodipine therapy may be required for years or even a lifetime. Consult your doctor about the need for medical or laboratory tests of heart activity, blood pressure, kidney function, and liver function.

▼ PRECAUTIONS

Over 60: Adverse reactions may be more likely and more severe in older patients. Smaller doses (2.5 mg per day) are generally prescribed.

Driving and Hazardous Work: Avoid driving or engaging in hazardous work until you determine how this medication affects you. Be cautious if it causes dizziness.

Alcohol: Alcohol should be used with caution because it may increase the effect of the drug and cause an excessive drop in blood pressure.

Pregnancy: Amlodipine should not be taken during the first 3 months of pregnancy and should be used in the last 6 months only if your doctor so advises.

Breast Feeding: Amlodipine should not be taken by nursing mothers.

Infants and Children: Amlodipine is not usually prescribed for patients under the age of 12.

Special Concerns: The drug should not be taken by anyone who has had a prior adverse reaction to it. When taking amlodipine, try to avoid abrupt changes in position, especially standing up too quickly after sitting or lying down; such movements may cause dizziness.

OVERDOSE

Symptoms: Severe drop in blood pressure resulting in weakness, dizziness, drowsiness, confusion, or slurred speech.

What to Do: Call your doctor, emergency medical services (EMS), or your local hospital immediately.

▼ INTERACTIONS

DRUG INTERACTIONS
Other heart drugs taken with amlodipine can cause heart rate and rhythm problems. In general, consult your doctor if you are taking any other prescription or OTC drugs.

FOOD INTERACTIONS
Avoid excessive intake of foods high in sodium.

DISEASE INTERACTIONS
Consult your doctor if you have kidney disease, liver disease, high blood pressure, or any heart disease other than coronary artery disease.

≣ SIDE EFFECTS ≣

SERIOUS
Increased angina attacks, dizziness upon arising from a sitting or lying position, shortness of breath, weakness, very slow heartbeat. Call your doctor immediately.

COMMON
Headache; flushing in the face and body; water retention causing decreased urination, swelling of the feet and ankles, weight gain.

LESS COMMON
Fatigue, dizziness, drowsiness, palpitations, nausea, abdominal pain.

AMOXICILLIN

BRAND NAMES

Amoxil, Larotid, Moxlin, Polymox, Trimox, Wymox

Available in: Capsules, oral suspension, chewable tablets, liquid drops
Available OTC? No   **As Generic?** Yes
Drug Class: Penicillin antibiotic

▼ USAGE INFORMATION

WHY IT'S PRESCRIBED
To treat bacterial infections of the ear, nose, and throat, genitourinary tract, skin and soft tissues, and the lower respiratory tract. It is used, often with other drugs, to treat uncomplicated gonorrhea. It is also prescribed preventively before surgery or dental work to patients at risk for endocarditis (infection of the interior lining of the heart). It is also used to treat some stages of Lyme disease and, along with other drugs, to treat H. pylori infection (the cause of stomach ulcers).

HOW IT WORKS
Amoxicillin blocks the formation of bacterial cell walls, rendering bacteria unable to multiply and spread.

▼ DOSAGE GUIDELINES

RANGE AND FREQUENCY
For infections—Adults: 250 to 500 mg every 8 hours

(3 doses per day). Children: 3 to 6 mg per lb of body weight every 8 hours (3 doses per day). To treat gonorrhea— 3 g in a single oral dose.

ONSET OF EFFECT
Rapid; within 2 hours.

DURATION OF ACTION
8 hours.

DIETARY ADVICE
Best taken on an empty stomach, but may be taken with food to minimize stomach irritation or diarrhea.

STORAGE
Store in a tightly sealed container away from heat and direct light. Keep any liquid form refrigerated, but do not allow it to freeze, and discard after 14 days.

MISSED DOSE
Take it as soon as you remember. If it is near the time for the next dose, skip the missed dose and resume your regular dosage schedule. Do not double the next dose.

STOPPING THE DRUG
Take as prescribed for the full treatment period, even if you begin to feel better before the scheduled end of therapy. Stopping the medication prematurely may slow your recovery or lead to a rebound infection, also known as superinfection, in which the heartier strains of bacteria survive and multiply, leading to a more serious and drug-resistant infection.

PROLONGED USE
Prolonged use of any antibiotic increases the risk of developing a superinfection; caution is advised.

▼ PRECAUTIONS

Over 60: No special problems are expected.

Driving and Hazardous Work: The use of amoxicillin should not impair your ability to perform such tasks safely.

Alcohol: No special precautions are necessary.

Pregnancy: Adequate studies of the use of this drug during pregnancy have not been done; however, no problems have been reported.

Breast Feeding: Amoxicillin passes into breast milk and may cause diarrhea, fungal infections, and allergic reactions in nursing infants; avoid use while nursing.

Infants and Children: No special problems are expected.

Special Concerns: Amoxicillin can cause false results on

some urine sugar tests for diabetics. Those who are prone to asthma, hay fever, hives, or allergies may be more likely to have an allergic reaction to a penicillin antibiotic. Oral contraceptives may not be effective while you are taking amoxicillin; use other methods of contraception to avoid unplanned pregnancy.

OVERDOSE
Symptoms: Severe nausea, vomiting, diarrhea, muscle spasticity, seizures.

What to Do: Call your doctor, emergency medical services (EMS), or the nearest poison control center immediately.

▼ INTERACTIONS

DRUG INTERACTIONS
Consult your doctor for specific advice if you are taking: aminoglycosides, ACE inhibitors, diuretics, potassium supplements or potassium-containing medications, anticoagulants or other anticlotting drugs, nonsteroidal anti-inflammatory drugs (NSAIDS), sulfinpyrazone, cholestyramine, colestipol, oral contraceptives, methotrexate, probenecid, allopurinol, or rifampin.

FOOD INTERACTIONS
No known food interactions.

DISEASE INTERACTIONS
Consult your doctor if you have a history of allergies, asthma, congestive heart failure, gastrointestinal disorders (especially colitis associated with the use of antibiotics), or impaired kidney function.

≡ SIDE EFFECTS ≡

SERIOUS
Irregular, rapid, or labored breathing, lightheadedness or sudden fainting, joint pain, fever, severe abdominal pain and cramping with watery or bloody stools, severe allergic reaction (marked by sudden swelling of the lips, tongue, face, or throat; breathing difficulty; skin rash, itching, or hives), unusual bleeding or bruising, yellowish tinge to eyes or skin. Call your doctor immediately.

COMMON
Rash, mild diarrhea, nausea, vomiting, headache, vaginal discharge and itching, pain or white patches in the mouth or on the tongue.

LESS COMMON
Diminished urine output, chills, weakness, fatigue.

AMOXICILLIN/POTASSIUM CLAVULANATE

Augmentin

Available in: Tablets, chewable tablets, oral suspension
Available OTC? No   **As Generic?** No
Drug Class: Penicillin antibiotic combination

▼ USAGE INFORMATION

WHY IT'S PRESCRIBED
To treat a variety of bacterial infections, including those of the sinuses and middle ear, skin and soft tissues, genitourinary tract, and the respiratory tract. The medication is effective only against infections caused by bacteria, not against infections caused by viruses, by fungi, or by other microorganisms.

HOW IT WORKS
Amoxicillin blocks the formation of bacterial cell walls, rendering the bacteria unable to multiply and spread. Clavulanate enhances the overall effectiveness of amoxicillin by inhibiting the activity of a specific enzyme (beta-lactamase) produced by certain drug-resistant strains of bacteria.

▼ DOSAGE GUIDELINES

RANGE AND FREQUENCY
Tablets—Adults and children more than 88 lbs: 250 to 500 mg of amoxicillin with 125 mg of clavulanate every 8 hours. Children up to 88 lbs: 6.7 to 13.3 mg of amoxicillin with 1.7 to 3.3 mg of clavulanate per 2.2 lbs (1 kg) of body weight every 8 hours. Chewable tablets and oral suspension—Adults and children more than 88 lbs: 250 to 500 mg of amoxicillin with 62.5 to 125 mg of clavulanate every 8 hours. Children up to 88 lbs: 6.7 to 13.3 mg of amoxicillin with 1.7 to 3.3 mg of clavulanate per 2.2 lbs (1 kg) of body weight every 8 hours. Newer dosage for adults: 875 mg of amoxicillin with 125 mg of clavulanate twice a day.

ONSET OF EFFECT
1 to 2 hours.

DURATION OF ACTION
6 to 8 hours.

DIETARY ADVICE
Best taken on an empty stomach, but may be taken with food to minimize stomach irritation or diarrhea.

STORAGE
Store in a tightly sealed container away from heat and direct light. Keep the liquid form refrigerated, but do not allow it to freeze.

MISSED DOSE
Take it as soon as you remember unless it is almost time for the next dose. In that case, skip the missed dose and take the next one. Do not double the next dose.

STOPPING THE DRUG
Take this medication as prescribed for the full treatment period, even if you begin to feel better before the scheduled end of therapy.

PROLONGED USE
Prolonged use can make you more susceptible to bacterial or fungal infections (such as yeast infections).

▼ PRECAUTIONS

Over 60: No special problems are expected.

Driving and Hazardous Work: Do not drive or engage in hazardous work until you determine how the medicine affects you.

Alcohol: No special warnings.

Pregnancy: Limited studies have found no evidence of birth defects. Consult your doctor if you are pregnant or plan to become pregnant.

Breast Feeding: Amoxicillin/clavulanate may pass into breast milk and cause problems in the nursing infant; avoid use while breast feeding.

Infants and Children: No special problems are expected.

Special Concerns: Those who are prone to asthma, hay fever, hives, or allergies may be more likely to have an allergic reaction to a penicillin antibiotic. If severe diarrhea occurs as a side effect of this drug, do not take antidiarrheal medications; call your doctor for advice instead. This drug can cause false results on some urine sugar tests for patients who have diabetes.

OVERDOSE
Symptoms: Severe diarrhea, nausea, unusual excitability, seizures, or vomiting.

What to Do: Call your doctor, emergency medical services (EMS), or the nearest poison control center immediately.

▼ INTERACTIONS

DRUG INTERACTIONS
Consult your doctor for advice if you are taking erythromycin, disulfiram, anticoagulants, tetracyclines, oral contraceptives, or gout drugs.

FOOD INTERACTIONS
None expected.

DISEASE INTERACTIONS
Consult your doctor if you have a history of allergies, asthma, congestive heart failure, gastrointestinal disorders (especially colitis associated with the use of antibiotics), or impaired kidney function.

≡ SIDE EFFECTS ≡

SERIOUS
Irregular, rapid, or labored breathing, lightheadedness or sudden fainting, seizures, joint pain, fever, severe abdominal pain and cramping with watery or bloody stools, severe allergic reaction (marked by sudden swelling of the lips, tongue, face, or throat; breathing difficulty; skin rash, itching, or hives), unusual bleeding or bruising, yellowish tinge to eyes or skin. Call your doctor immediately.

COMMON
Rash, mild diarrhea, nausea, vomiting, headache, vaginal discharge and itching, pain or white patches in the mouth or on the tongue.

LESS COMMON
Weakness, fatigue.

AMPHETAMINE/DEXTROAMPHETAMINE

Available in: Tablets
Available OTC? No **As Generic?** No
Drug Class: Central nervous system stimulant/amphetamine

▼ USAGE INFORMATION

WHY IT'S PRESCRIBED
To treat narcolepsy and attention-deficit hyperactivity disorder (ADHD).

HOW IT WORKS
Amphetamine and dextroamphetamine activate nerve cells in the brain and spinal cord to increase motor activity and alertness and also to lessen fatigue and drowsiness. In hyperactivity disorders and narcolepsy, amphetamines improve mental focus as well as the ability to stay awake or concentrate.

▼ DOSAGE GUIDELINES

RANGE AND FREQUENCY
For narcolepsy—Adults: 5 to 60 mg a day, 1 to 3 times a day; not to exceed 60 mg a day. Teenagers: To start, 10 mg a day. Children ages 6 to 12: To start, 5 mg a day. To treat ADHD—Children age 6 and older: To start, 5 mg, 1 or 2 times a day. Children ages 3 to 6: To start, 2.5 mg a day.

ONSET OF EFFECT
Within 30 to 45 minutes.

DURATION OF ACTION
Adults: 8 to 12 hours.
Children: 6 to 10 hours.

DIETARY ADVICE
Take it with liquid 30 to 45 minutes before meals. Avoid caffeinated beverages, acidic foods rich in vitamin C, and vitamin C tablets.

STORAGE
Store in a tightly sealed container away from moisture, heat, and direct light.

MISSED DOSE
If dosage is once daily, take your missed dose as soon as you remember, unless your bedtime is within the next 6 hours. If so, do not take the missed dose. Take your next dose at the proper time and resume your regular schedule. Do not double the next dose. If dosage is more than once daily, take your missed dose as soon as you remember, unless the time for your next scheduled dose is within the next 2 hours. If so, do not take the missed dose. Take your next dose at the proper time and resume your regular schedule. Do not double the next dose.

STOPPING THE DRUG
Take it as prescribed for the full treatment period, even if you begin to feel better before the scheduled end of therapy. The decision to stop taking the drug should be made by your doctor. The doctor may taper your dosage gradually to reduce the risk of withdrawal symptoms.

PROLONGED USE
Prolonged use may increase the risk of dependency.

▼ PRECAUTIONS

Over 60: Adverse reactions may be more likely and more severe in older patients.

Driving and Hazardous Work: Do not drive or engage in hazardous work until you determine how the medicine affects you.

Alcohol: Avoid alcohol.

Pregnancy: Amphetamines taken during pregnancy may cause premature delivery, low birth weight, and birth defects. Discuss with your doctor the relative risks and benefits of using this drug while pregnant.

Breast Feeding: Amphetamine passes into breast milk; avoid or discontinue use while nursing.

Infants and Children: Not recommended for use by children under age 3.

Special Concerns: Take only as directed and do not increase the dose on your own. Fatigue, excessive drowsiness, or depression that occurs while taking stimulants may mean an emergency situation is developing. Difficulty sleeping may be improved by taking the last scheduled dose several hours before bedtime.

OVERDOSE
Symptoms: Extreme restlessness, agitation, or bizarre behavior; panic; rapid breathing; confusion; high fever; hallucinations; seizures; coma.

What to Do: Call your doctor, emergency medical services (EMS), or the nearest poison control center immediately.

▼ INTERACTIONS

DRUG INTERACTIONS
Consult your doctor for specific advice if you are taking tricyclic antidepressants, caffeine, beta-blockers, digitalis drugs, central nervous system stimulants, meperidine, MAO inhibitors, sympathomimetic agents (such as ephedrine, phenylephrine, and diethylpropion), or thyroid hormones.

FOOD INTERACTIONS
Citrus juices and caffeine may interact with this drug.

DISEASE INTERACTIONS
Consult your doctor if you have any of the following: heart disease, advanced blood vessel disease, hyperthyroidism, high blood pressure, severe anxiety, Tourette's syndrome, glaucoma, or a history of drug abuse.

≡ SIDE EFFECTS ≡

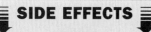

SERIOUS
Irregular heartbeat, chest pain, increased blood pressure, skin rash, uncontrollable movements of arms and legs, mental changes, unusual weakness, very high fever. Call your doctor immediately.

COMMON
Mood changes, insomnia, drowsiness, restlessness.

LESS COMMON
Blurred vision, constipation, diarrhea, loss of appetite, headache, increased sweating, stomach cramps or pain, nausea or vomiting, changes in sexual desire or decreased sexual ability.

ATENOLOL

Available in: Tablets (Injection is for hospital use only.)
Available OTC? No   **As Generic?** Yes
Drug Class: Beta-blocker

▼ USAGE INFORMATION

WHY IT'S PRESCRIBED
To treat mild to moderate high blood pressure and to treat angina; also used to prevent or control heartbeat irregularities (cardiac arrhythmias). The injectable form is used in hospitals to treat heart attack.

HOW IT WORKS
Atenolol slows the rate and force of contraction of the heart by blocking certain nerve impulses, thus reducing blood pressure. By modifying nerve impulses to the heart, the drug also helps to stabilize heart rhythm.

▼ DOSAGE GUIDELINES

RANGE AND FREQUENCY
50 to 100 mg, once a day. Smaller doses may be recommended for elderly patients or for those with impaired kidney function.

ONSET OF EFFECT
Oral: 1 to 2 hours; the full therapeutic effect may take 1 to 2 weeks. Injectable: Within 10 minutes.

DURATION OF ACTION
Up to 24 hours.

DIETARY ADVICE
Take atenolol on an empty stomach. Avoid alcohol and caffeine.

STORAGE
Store in a tightly sealed container away from heat and direct light.

MISSED DOSE
Take it as soon as you remember. If it is within 4 hours of the next scheduled dose, skip the missed dose and resume your regular schedule. Do not double the next dose.

STOPPING THE DRUG
Suddenly stopping atenolol may cause serious health problems. Slow reduction of the dose over a period of 2 to 3 weeks is advised, under doctor's careful supervision.

PROLONGED USE
Therapy with atenolol may be lifelong; prolonged use may be associated with increased risks of side effects.

▼ PRECAUTIONS

Over 60: Adverse reactions may be more likely and more severe in older patients; a reduction in dosage may be warranted.

Driving and Hazardous Work: In rare cases atenolol may impair your ability to drive or operate machinery safely or perform hazardous work. Use caution, especially soon after beginning therapy.

Alcohol: Drink in careful moderation, if at all. Alcohol may interact with the drug and cause a dangerous drop in blood pressure.

Pregnancy: Discuss with your doctor the relative risks and benefits of using this drug while pregnant.

Breast Feeding: Avoid or discontinue the use of atenolol while nursing.

Infants and Children: A proper dose will be determined by your pediatrician.

Special Concerns: Use of the drug should be considered but one element of a comprehensive therapeutic program that includes weight control, smoking cessation, regular exercise, and a healthy low-salt, low-fat diet.

OVERDOSE
Symptoms: Slow heartbeat; severe dizziness, lightheadedness or fainting; rapid or irregular heartbeat; difficulty breathing; extreme weakness; seizures; confusion; coma.

What to Do: Call your doctor, emergency medical services (EMS), or the nearest poison control center immediately.

▼ INTERACTIONS

DRUG INTERACTIONS
Consult your doctor if you are taking amphetamines, oral antidiabetic agents, asthma medication (such as aminophylline or theophylline), calcium channel blockers, clonidine, guanabenz, insulin, halothane, allergy shots, MAO inhibitors, reserpine, or other beta-blockers.

FOOD INTERACTIONS
None known.

DISEASE INTERACTIONS
Atenolol should be used with caution in people with diabetes, especially insulin-dependent diabetes, since the drug may mask symptoms of hypoglycemia. Consult your doctor for specific advice if you have allergies or asthma, heart or blood vessel disease (including congestive heart failure and peripheral vascular disease), irregular (slow) heartbeat, hyperthyroidism, myasthenia gravis, psoriasis, respiratory problems such as bronchitis or emphysema, kidney or liver disease, or a history of mental depression.

⬇ SIDE EFFECTS ⬇

SERIOUS
Depression, shortness of breath, wheezing, slow heartbeat (especially less than 50 beats per minute), chest pain or tightness, swelling of the ankles, feet, and lower legs. If you experience such symptoms, stop taking atenolol and call your doctor immediately.

COMMON
Decreased sexual ability; decreased ability to engage in usual physical activities or exercise; dizziness or lightheadedness, especially when rising suddenly from a sitting or lying position; drowsiness, fatigue, or weakness; insomnia.

LESS COMMON
Anxiety, irritability; constipation; diarrhea; dry eyes; itching; nausea or vomiting; nightmares or intensely vivid dreams; numbness, tingling, or other unusual sensations in the fingers and toes; abdominal pain; nasal congestion.

ATORVASTATIN

Available in: Tablets
Available OTC? No   **As Generic?** No
Drug Class: Antilipidemic (cholesterol-lowering agent)

▼ USAGE INFORMATION

WHY IT'S PRESCRIBED
To treat high cholesterol. Usually prescribed after the first lines of treatment—including diet changes, weight loss, and exercise—fail to reduce to acceptable levels the amounts of total and low-density lipoprotein (LDL) cholesterol in the blood.

HOW IT WORKS
Atorvastatin blocks the action of an enzyme required for the manufacture of cholesterol, thereby interfering with its formation. By lowering the amount of cholesterol in the liver cells, atorvastatin increases the formation of receptors for LDL, and thereby reduces blood levels of total and LDL cholesterol. In addition to lowering LDL cholesterol, atorvastatin also modestly reduces triglyceride levels and raises HDL (the so-called "good") cholesterol.

▼ DOSAGE GUIDELINES

RANGE AND FREQUENCY
Initial dose is 10 mg a day, taken once daily. It may be increased by your doctor as needed up to a maximum dose of 80 mg per day. Unlike other "-statin" cholesterol-lowering drugs, atorvastatin does not have to be taken in the evening to be maximally effective.

ONSET OF EFFECT
2 to 4 weeks.

DURATION OF ACTION
The effect persists for the duration of therapy.

DIETARY ADVICE
Cholesterol-lowering drugs are only one part of a total program that should include regular exercise and a healthy low-fat, low-cholesterol, and high-fiber diet.

STORAGE
Store in a tightly sealed container in a dry place away from heat and direct light.

MISSED DOSE
Take it as soon as you remember that you skipped a dose. Then take your next scheduled dose at the proper time and resume your regular dosage schedule. Do not double your next dose.

STOPPING THE DRUG
The decision to stop taking the drug should be made in consultation with your doctor. Once the medication is discontinued, blood cholesterol is likely to return to original elevated levels.

PROLONGED USE
Side effects are more likely with prolonged use. As you continue to take atorvastatin, your doctor will periodically order blood tests to evaluate liver function.

▼ PRECAUTIONS

Over 60: No special problems are expected in older patients.

Driving and Hazardous Work: The use of atorvastatin should not impair your ability to perform such tasks safely.

Alcohol: No special precautions are necessary.

Pregnancy: Should not be used during pregnancy or by women who plan to become pregnant in the near future.

Breast Feeding: This drug is not recommended for women who are nursing.

Infants and Children: Safety and effectiveness are not known; this drug is rarely used in children. Consult your pediatrician.

Special Concerns: Important elements of high cholesterol treatment include proper diet, weight loss, regular moderate exercise, and avoidance of certain medications that may increase cholesterol levels.

Because atorvastatin has potential side effects, it is important that you maintain a recommended healthy diet and cooperate with other treatments that your doctor may suggest.

OVERDOSE
Symptoms: An overdose of atorvastatin is unlikely.

What to Do: Emergency instructions not applicable.

▼ INTERACTIONS

DRUG INTERACTIONS
Consult your doctor if you are taking cyclosporine, gemfibrozil, niacin, antibiotics, especially erythromycin, or medications for fungus infections. All of these drugs may increase the risk of myositis (muscle inflammation) when taken with atorvastatin and may lead to kidney failure.

FOOD INTERACTIONS
No known food interactions.

DISEASE INTERACTIONS
Consult your doctor if you have any of the following problems: liver, kidney, or muscle disease, or a medical history involving organ transplant or recent surgery.

≡ SIDE EFFECTS ≡

SERIOUS
Fever, chest pain, unusual or unexplained muscle aches and tenderness. Call your doctor right away.

COMMON
Side effects occur in only 1% to 2% of patients. These include constipation or diarrhea, dizziness or lightheadedness, bloating or gas, heartburn, nausea, allergic reaction, stomach pain, rise in liver enzymes.

LESS COMMON
Sleeping difficulty, skin rash.

AZITHROMYCIN

Available in: Capsules, tablets, powder, injection
Available OTC? No   **As Generic?** No
Drug Class: Azalide antibiotic

▼ USAGE INFORMATION

WHY IT'S PRESCRIBED
To treat various bacterial infections, particularly of the sinuses, throat, and respiratory tract (such as bronchitis and pneumonia); infections of the ear; venereal disease due to chlamydial and chancroid infection; skin infections; and diarrhea associated with campylobacter and other bacteria that cause food poisoning. Also used to prevent and treat a tuberculosis-like disease known as Mycobacterium avium complex (MAC), which is common in people with advanced AIDS.

HOW IT WORKS
Azithromycin prevents bacterial cells from manufacturing specific proteins necessary for their survival.

▼ DOSAGE GUIDELINES

RANGE AND FREQUENCY
For bronchitis, strep throat, pneumonia, and skin infections: 500 mg (2 pills) taken in a single dose on the first day of treatment; then, 250 mg (1 pill) per day on days 2 through 5. For chlamydia and chancroid: 1,000 mg (4 pills) taken in a single one-time dose. To prevent MAC: 1,200 mg weekly. To treat MAC: 500 mg, twice a day.

ONSET OF EFFECT
Unknown.

DURATION OF ACTION
Unknown.

DIETARY ADVICE
Take capsules on an empty stomach, at least 1 hour before or 2 hours after eating. Tablets may be taken with or without food. Drink plenty of fluids (at least 2 to 3 quarts of water per day).

STORAGE
Store in a sealed container away from heat and light.

MISSED DOSE
Take it as soon as you remember. If you miss a day entirely, skip the missed dose and resume your regular dosage schedule the next day. Do not double the next dose.

STOPPING THE DRUG
It is very important to take this drug as prescribed for the full treatment period, even if you begin to feel better before the scheduled end of therapy.

PROLONGED USE
For acute infections, treatment is usually complete after 5 days with capsules, and 1 day with the powdered form. For MAC prevention and treatment, therapy may be lifelong. Prolonged use may be associated with an increased risk of side effects.

▼ PRECAUTIONS

Over 60: Adverse reactions may be more likely and more severe in this age group.

Driving and Hazardous Work: The use of the drug should not impair your ability to perform such tasks safely.

Alcohol: Avoid alcohol while taking this drug.

Pregnancy: Adequate studies of the use of azithromycin during pregnancy have not been done; consult your doctor for advice.

Breast Feeding: It is not known if azithromycin passes into breast milk; consult your doctor for advice.

Infants and Children: The safety and effectiveness of azithromycin use in patients under 16 years of age have not been established, although no special problems are expected.

Special Concerns: Before taking any antibiotic, make sure you tell your doctor about allergies that you might have. If you are allergic to erythromycin, you are likely to be allergic to azithromycin. Azithromycin is useful only against bacteria that are susceptible to its effects. Therefore, it is important to tell your doctor if your condition has not improved, or instead has worsened, within a few days of starting the drug. The particular bacteria causing your illness may be resistant to azithromycin.

OVERDOSE
Symptoms: No cases of overdose have been reported.

What to Do: Emergency instructions not applicable.

▼ INTERACTIONS

DRUG INTERACTIONS
Other drugs may interact with azithromycin. Consult your doctor for specific advice if you are taking anticoagulants (such as warfarin), anticonvulsants (such as phenytoin and carbamazepine), antihistamines (especially terfenadine), and theophylline. Antacids that contain aluminum or magnesium can interfere with the absorption of azithromycin; separate the use of azithromycin and an antacid by at least 2 hours.

FOOD INTERACTIONS
Azithromycin capsules should be taken on an empty stomach.

DISEASE INTERACTIONS
Consult your doctor if you have a medical history that includes liver disease.

≡ SIDE EFFECTS ≡

SERIOUS
Breathing difficulty, fever, hives, itching, skin rash, swelling of face, mouth, lips, throat, or tongue, sweating, yellowish discoloration of the eyes or skin. These may be signs of a rare but potentially serious allergic reaction. Seek medical assistance immediately.

COMMON
No common side effects have been reported.

LESS COMMON
Nausea and vomiting, abdominal discomfort, diarrhea (generally mild), headache, dizziness.

BECLOMETHASONE INHALANT AND NASAL

Available in: Nasal inhaler, oral inhalation
Available OTC? No **As Generic?** No
Drug Class: Respiratory corticosteroid

Beclovent, Beconase AQ
Nasal Spray, Beconase
Nasal Inhaler, Vancenase
AQ Nasal Spray,
Vancenase Nasal Inhaler,
Vanceril

▼ USAGE INFORMATION

WHY IT'S PRESCRIBED
To treat bronchial asthma; to
treat allergic rhinitis (seasonal
and perennial allergies such
as hay fever); to prevent
recurrence of nasal polyps
after they have been removed
surgically.

HOW IT WORKS
Respiratory corticosteroids
such as beclomethasone
primarily reduce or prevent
chronic inflammation of the
lining of the airways (the
underlying cause of asthma),
reduce the allergic response
to inhaled allergens, and
inhibit secretion of mucus
within airways.

▼ DOSAGE GUIDELINES

RANGE AND FREQUENCY
Adults and teenagers–Nasal
inhaler: 1 or 2 inhalations in
each nostril, 1 or 2 times a
day. Oral inhalation: 2 inhalations, 3 or 4 times a day.
For severe asthma: 12 to 16
inhalations daily (maximum of
20 inhalations per day).
Children ages 6 to 12–Nasal
inhaler: 1 inhalation in each

nostril, 1 to 3 times a day.
Oral inhalation: 1 to 2
inhalations, 3 or 4 times a
day. Maximum of 10 inhalations per day.

ONSET OF EFFECT
Within 5 to 7 days; it may
take 3 weeks for the full
effect to occur.

DURATION OF ACTION
6 hours or more.

DIETARY ADVICE
Use it before or after meals.

STORAGE
Store away from fire and
direct light.

MISSED DOSE
Take it as soon as you
remember. However, if it is
near the time for the next
dose, skip the missed dose
and resume your regular
dosage schedule. Do not
double the next dose.

STOPPING THE DRUG
Take the medication as your
doctor has prescribed for the
full treatment period, even if
you begin to feel better
before the scheduled end of
the therapy.

PROLONGED USE
Consult your doctor about the
need for periodic medical
examinations and laboratory
tests if you must take this
drug for a prolonged period.

▼ PRECAUTIONS

Over 60: No special problems are expected.

**Driving and Hazardous
Work:** The use of
beclomethasone should not
impair your ability to perform
such tasks safely.

Alcohol: No special precautions are necessary.

Pregnancy: Nasal or inhaled
steroids have not been
reported to cause birth
defects if taken during pregnancy. Before using such
drugs, tell your doctor if you
are pregnant or plan to
become pregnant.

Breast Feeding: Beclomethasone may pass into breast
milk; caution is advised. Consult your doctor for advice.

Infants and Children: It has
not been established whether
beclomethasone is safe and
effective in young children.

Special Concerns: Inhaled
steroids will not help an
asthma attack in progress.
Inhaled steroids can lower
resistance to yeast infections
of the mouth, throat, or voice
box. To prevent yeast infections, gargle or rinse your
mouth with water after each
use; do not swallow the
water. Know how to use the
inhaler effectively; read and
follow the directions that

come with the device. Before
you have surgery, tell the
doctor or dentist that you are
using a steroid.

OVERDOSE
Symptoms: No specific ones
have been reported.

What to Do: An overdose of
beclomethasone is unlikely to
be life-threatening. However,
if someone takes a much
larger dose than prescribed,
call your doctor, emergency
medical services (EMS), or
the nearest poison control
center immediately.

▼ INTERACTIONS

DRUG INTERACTIONS
Consult your doctor for specific advice if you are taking
systemic corticosteroids,
other inhaled corticosteroids,
or any drugs that suppress
the immune system.

FOOD INTERACTIONS
No known food interactions.

DISEASE INTERACTIONS
Consult your doctor if you
have any of the following:
a lung disease such as tuberculosis; an infection of the
mouth, nose, sinuses, throat,
or lungs; a herpes infection
of the eye; or any other
untreated infection.

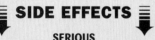

SIDE EFFECTS

SERIOUS
No serious side effects are associated with the use of
beclomethasone.

COMMON
Nasal form: Nosebleeds or bloody nasal secretions, nasal
burning or irritation, sore throat. Oral inhalation: Sore
throat, white patches in the mouth or throat, hoarseness.

LESS COMMON
Eye pain, watering eyes, gradual decrease of vision, stomach pain and digestive disturbances.

BENAZEPRIL HYDROCHLORIDE

Available in: Tablets
Available OTC? No   **As Generic?** No
Drug Class: Angiotensin-converting enzyme (ACE) inhibitor

▼ USAGE INFORMATION

WHY IT'S PRESCRIBED
To control high blood pressure; to treat congestive heart failure; to treat patients with left ventricular dysfunction (damage to the pumping chamber of the heart); and to minimize further kidney damage in diabetics with mild kidney disease.

HOW IT WORKS
Angiotensin-converting enzyme (ACE) inhibitors block an enzyme that produces angiotensin, a naturally occurring substance that causes blood vessels to constrict and stimulates the production of the adrenal hormone, aldosterone, which promotes sodium retention in the body. As a result, ACE inhibitors relax blood vessels (causing them to widen) and they also reduce sodium retention. Both of these actions lower blood pressure levels and so decrease the overall workload of the heart.

▼ DOSAGE GUIDELINES

RANGE AND FREQUENCY
If you are not also taking a diuretic, 10 mg a day to start, increased to 20 to 80 mg a day in 1 or 2 doses. If you are taking a diuretic, 5 mg per day.

ONSET OF EFFECT
60 to 90 minutes.

DURATION OF ACTION
Up to 24 hours.

DIETARY ADVICE
Take it on an empty stomach, about 1 hour before mealtime. Follow your doctor's dietary advice (such as low-salt or low-cholesterol restrictions) to improve control over high blood pressure and heart disease. Avoid high-potassium foods, unless you are also taking drugs, such as diuretics, that lower potassium levels.

STORAGE
Store in a tightly sealed container away from heat and direct light.

MISSED DOSE
Take it as soon as you remember. If it is near the time for the next dose, skip the missed dose and resume your regular dosage schedule. Do not double the next dose.

STOPPING THE DRUG
Do not stop taking this drug abruptly, as this may cause potentially serious health problems. Dosage should be reduced gradually, according to your doctor's instructions.

PROLONGED USE
See your doctor regularly for examinations and tests if you must take this drug for a prolonged period. Benazepril helps control hypertension but does not cure it. Lifelong therapy may be necessary.

▼ PRECAUTIONS

Over 60: Adverse reactions may be more likely and more severe in older patients.

Driving and Hazardous Work: Avoid such activities until you determine how the medication affects you.

Alcohol: Consume alcohol only in moderation since it may increase the effect of the drug and cause an excessive drop in blood pressure.

Pregnancy: Tell your doctor before taking this medication if you are pregnant or plan to become pregnant. Use of this drug during the last 6 months of pregnancy may cause severe defects, even death, in the fetus.

Breast Feeding: Benazepril does pass into breast milk; if possible, avoid using the drug while nursing.

Infants and Children: Benazepril is generally not prescribed for children; benefits must be weighed against risks. Consult your pediatrician.

OVERDOSE
Symptoms: None reported.

What to Do: While overdose is unlikely, call your doctor, emergency medical services (EMS), or the nearest poison control center immediately if you suspect that someone has taken a much larger dose than prescribed.

▼ INTERACTIONS

DRUG INTERACTIONS
Consult your doctor if you are taking diuretics (especially potassium-sparing diuretics), potassium supplements or drugs containing potassium (check ingredient labels), lithium, anticoagulant drugs, indomethacin or other anti-inflammatory drugs, or any over-the-counter drugs (especially cold remedies and diet pills).

FOOD INTERACTIONS
Avoid low-salt milk and salt substitutes. Many of these products contain potassium.

DISEASE INTERACTIONS
Consult your doctor if you have lupus or if you have had a prior allergic reaction to ACE inhibitors. This drug should be used with caution by patients with severe kidney disease or renal artery stenosis (narrowing of one or both of the arteries that supply blood to the kidneys).

≡ SIDE EFFECTS ≡

SERIOUS
Fever and chills, sore throat and hoarseness, sudden difficulty breathing or swallowing, swelling of the face, mouth, or extremities, impaired kidney function (ankle swelling, decreased urination), confusion, yellow discoloration of the eyes or skin (indicating liver disorder), intense itching, chest pain or palpitations, abdominal pain. Serious side effects are very rare; contact your doctor immediately.

COMMON
Dry, persistent cough.

LESS COMMON
Dizziness or fainting, skin rash, numbness or tingling in the hands, feet, or lips, unusual fatigue or muscle weakness, nausea, drowsiness, loss of taste, headache.

BETAMETHASONE/CLOTRIMAZOLE

Available in: Cream
Available OTC? No   **As Generic?** Yes
Drug Class: Topical antifungal

▼ USAGE INFORMATION

WHY IT'S PRESCRIBED
To treat fungal infections of the skin.

HOW IT WORKS
Clotrimazole prevents fungal organisms from producing the vital proteins they require for growth and function. Betamethasone dipropionate is a steroid; it interferes with the formation of natural substances within the body that are directly responsible for the process of inflammation, which produces swelling, redness, and pain. The use of these two effective medications in combination for skin infections appears to hasten recovery sooner than use of clotrimazole alone. This medication is only effective for infections caused by fungal organisms. It will not work for bacterial or viral infections.

▼ DOSAGE GUIDELINES

RANGE AND FREQUENCY
Adults and children older than 12 years of age: Apply and massage a sufficient amount of cream into the affected site twice daily for 2 to 4 weeks. This combination drug contains a high-potency topical steroid that should not be used in skin creases or with bandages (occlusive dressing) unless closely supervised by your doctor.

ONSET OF EFFECT
Clotrimazole begins killing susceptible fungi shortly after contact. The effects may not be noticeable for several days or weeks.

DURATION OF ACTION
Unknown.

DIETARY ADVICE
Drink plenty of fluids.

STORAGE
Store in a tightly sealed container away from heat and direct light. Keep away from moisture and extremes in temperature.

MISSED DOSE
Apply it as soon as you remember. If it is near the time for the next dose, skip the missed dose and resume your regular dosage schedule. Do not double the next dose or apply an excessively thick film of topical medication to try to compensate for a missed dose.

STOPPING THE DRUG
Apply as prescribed for the full treatment period, even if the fungal infection appears to be eradicated before the scheduled end of therapy. Unfortunately, it can be difficult to assess when the drug has achieved its desired effect since it suppresses redness and inflammation of the skin before the infection is completely clear; recurrence of fungal infection owing to inadequate length of therapy is a significant risk.

PROLONGED USE
Therapy with this medication should not exceed 4 weeks.

▼ PRECAUTIONS

Over 60: Adverse reactions may be more likely and more severe in older patients.

Driving and Hazardous Work: No special precautions are necessary.

Alcohol: No special precautions are necessary.

Pregnancy: Not recommended during pregnancy.

Breast Feeding: Betamethasone dipropionate/clotrimazole may pass into breast milk; caution is advised. Consult your doctor for advice.

Infants and Children: Not recommended for use by children under age 12.

Special Concerns: Avoid contact with eyes. Wash hands thoroughly after application. Tell your doctor if your condition has not improved within a few days of starting the medication. As with any other antifungal, betamethasone dipropionate/clotrimazole is useful only against organisms that are vulnerable to its effects. Therefore, it is important to tell your doctor if your condition has not improved—or has worsened—within a few days of starting betamethasone dipropionate/clotrimazole. The specific organism causing your illness may be resistant to this medication.

OVERDOSE
Symptoms: No specific ones have been reported.

What to Do: An overdose is unlikely to be life-threatening. However, if someone applies a much larger dose than prescribed or ingests the medication, call your doctor, emergency medical services (EMS), or the nearest poison control center immediately.

▼ INTERACTIONS

DRUG INTERACTIONS
No specific drug interactions have been documented.

FOOD INTERACTIONS
No known food interactions.

DISEASE INTERACTIONS
Consult your doctor if you have ever experienced an allergic reaction to any topical medication, or undesirable reactions to any steroid or steroid-containing preparation.

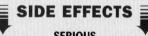

≣ SIDE EFFECTS ≣

SERIOUS
Blistering or ulceration of the skin; blistering of the lips, nose, and mouth.

COMMON
Brief burning or irritation after application; peeling.

LESS COMMON
Severe burning, itching, swelling, increased redness, or any increased discomfort developing at the application site that was not present prior to therapy; dry skin; pus or inflammation at base of hair follicles; change in skin color at site of application; acne.

BISOPROLOL FUMARATE/HYDROCHLOROTHIAZIDE

Available in: Tablets
Available OTC? No   **As Generic?** No
Drug Class: Beta-blocker/thiazide diuretic

▼ USAGE INFORMATION

WHY IT'S PRESCRIBED
To control hypertension (high blood pressure).

HOW IT WORKS
Bisoprolol, a beta-blocker, blocks certain nerve impulses to various parts of the body, which accounts for its many effects. For example, it reduces the rate and force of the heart's contractions (which helps to lower blood pressure), decreases the heart's oxygen requirement (which helps prevent angina) and helps stabilize heart rhythm. Hydrochlorothiazide (HCTZ), a diuretic, increases the excretion of salt and water in the urine. By reducing the overall amount of fluid in the body, diuretics reduce pressure within the blood vessels.

▼ DOSAGE GUIDELINES

RANGE AND FREQUENCY
Tablets contain 6.25 mg HCTZ and 2.5, 5, or 10 mg bisoprolol. Therapy is initiated with the lowest dose and may be increased at 1 week intervals to 2 tablets with 10 mg bisoprolol once a day.

ONSET OF EFFECT
Within 1 to 4 hours.

DURATION OF ACTION
Up to 24 hours.

DIETARY ADVICE
No special restrictions.

STORAGE
Store in a tightly sealed container away from moisture, heat, and direct light.

MISSED DOSE
If you miss a dose on one day, resume your regular dosage schedule the next day. Do not double the next dose.

STOPPING THE DRUG
The decision to stop taking the drug should be made in consultation with a physician. Do not stop taking this drug abruptly; your doctor will gradually decrease the dose before stopping it completely.

PROLONGED USE
Bisoprolol/hydrochlorothiazide can control high blood pressure, but cannot cure it. Lifelong therapy may be necessary. See your doctor regularly for tests and examinations if you must take this drug for a prolonged period of time.

▼ PRECAUTIONS

Over 60: Adverse reactions, especially dizziness, lightheadedness, and reduced tolerance to cold, may be more likely and more severe in older patients.

Driving and Hazardous Work: Do not drive or engage in hazardous work until you determine how the medicine affects you.

Alcohol: Drink in careful moderation if at all. Alcohol may interact with the bisoprolol component and cause a dangerous drop in blood pressure.

Pregnancy: Beta-blockers and thiazide diuretics may cause problems during pregnancy. Before taking this medication, tell your doctor if you are pregnant or plan to become pregnant.

Breast Feeding: This drug passes into breast milk; caution is advised. Consult your doctor for specific advice.

Infants and Children: Adequate studies have not been done on the use of this drug in children. No special problems are expected. Consult your pediatrician for advice.

Special Concerns: In addition to taking this medicine, follow your doctor's instructions on weight control and diet for reduction of blood pressure.

OVERDOSE
Symptoms: Slow heartbeat, severe dizziness or fainting, difficulty breathing, bluish-colored fingernails or palms of hands, seizures.

What to Do: Call your doctor, emergency medical services (EMS), or the nearest poison control center immediately.

▼ INTERACTIONS

DRUG INTERACTIONS
Do not take with other beta-blockers. Consult your doctor for specific advice if you are taking any other antihypertensive medications, insulin, oral diabetes medications, digitalis drugs, cholestyramine, colestipol, clonidine, lithium, nonsteroidal anti-inflammatory drugs, MAO inhibitors, rifampin, narcotic analgesics, or skeletal muscle relaxants.

FOOD INTERACTIONS
Avoid foods high in sodium.

DISEASE INTERACTIONS
Do not use if you have a history of bronchospasm. Consult your doctor if you have any of the following: bronchial asthma, emphysema, slow heartbeat, heart or blood vessel disease, diabetes mellitus, congestive heart failure, gout, kidney disease, liver disease, depression, parathyroid disease, or an overactive thyroid (hyperthyroidism).

≡ SIDE EFFECTS ≡

SERIOUS
Slow heartbeat, difficulty breathing, mental depression, cold hands and feet, swelling of ankles, feet, or lower legs. Call your doctor immediately.

COMMON
Dizziness or lightheadedness, decreased sexual ability, drowsiness, insomnia, fatigue, diarrhea.

LESS COMMON
Anxiety, loss of appetite, upset stomach, nervousness or excitability, constipation, numbness and tingling in the fingers and toes, stuffy nose.

BRIMONIDINE TARTRATE

BRAND NAME

Alphagan

Available in: Ophthalmic solution
Available OTC? No   **As Generic?** No
Drug Class: Antiglaucoma agent

▼ USAGE INFORMATION

WHY IT'S PRESCRIBED
To treat glaucoma.

HOW IT WORKS
Glaucoma, a sight-threatening disorder, occurs when aqueous humor (fluid inside the eye) cannot drain properly, causing increased pressure within the eyeball (intraocular pressure). Increased eye pressure can damage the optic nerve and lead to a gradually progressive loss of vision. Brimonidine decreases the production of aqueous humor and promotes its outflow, thereby reducing intraocular pressure.

▼ DOSAGE GUIDELINES

RANGE AND FREQUENCY
1 drop of brimonidine in each eye 3 times a day at 8-hour intervals.

ONSET OF EFFECT
Within 60 minutes.

DURATION OF ACTION
8 hours or more.

DIETARY ADVICE
No special restrictions.

STORAGE
Store in a tightly sealed container away from moisture, heat, and direct light. Do not allow the medication to freeze.

MISSED DOSE
Apply it as soon as you remember. If it is near the time for the next dose, skip the missed dose and resume your regular dosage schedule. Do not double the next dose.

STOPPING THE DRUG
The decision to stop using the drug should be made by your doctor.

PROLONGED USE
You should see your doctor regularly for examinations and tests as part of a glaucoma follow-up if you take this drug for a prolonged period.

▼ PRECAUTIONS

Over 60: Adverse reactions may be more likely and more severe in older patients.

Driving and Hazardous Work: Do not drive or engage in hazardous work until you determine how the drug affects your vision.

Alcohol: Use alcohol with caution.

Pregnancy: In animal studies, brimonidine caused impaired fetal circulation. Human studies have not been done. Before you take brimonidine, tell your doctor if you are pregnant or are planning to become pregnant.

Breast Feeding: Brimonidine may pass into breast milk; caution is advised. Consult your doctor for advice.

Infants and Children: The safety and effectiveness of brimonidine in children have not been established.

Special Concerns: To use the eye drops, first wash your hands. Tilt your head back. Gently apply pressure to the inside corner of the eyelid and with the index finger of the same hand, pull downward on the lower eyelid to make a space. Drop the medicine into this space and close your eye. Apply pressure for 1 or 2 minutes while keeping the eye closed without blinking. Then wash your hands again. Make sure the tip of the dropper does not touch your eye, finger, or any other surface. Bromonidine may make your eyes more sensitive to sunlight. If this occurs, wear sunglasses or avoid bright light as comfort dictates.

OVERDOSE
Symptoms: No specific ones have been reported.

What to Do: An overdose of brimonidine is unlikely to be life-threatening. However, if someone takes a much larger dose than prescribed or accidentally ingests the medicine, call your doctor, emergency medical services (EMS), or the nearest poison control center immediately.

▼ INTERACTIONS

DRUG INTERACTIONS
Consult your doctor for advice if you are taking MAO inhibitors, tricyclic antidepressants, central nervous system depressants, beta-blockers, antihypertensives, or digitalis drugs (such as digoxin).

FOOD INTERACTIONS
No known food interactions.

DISEASE INTERACTIONS
Caution is advised when taking brimonidine. Consult your doctor if you have cardiovascular disease, cerebral or coronary insufficiency, kidney disease, liver disease, depression, Raynaud's phenomenon, orthostatic hypotension, or thromboangiitis obliterans.

⬇ SIDE EFFECTS ⬇

SERIOUS
Fainting. Call your doctor immediately.

COMMON
Burning or stinging of the eyes, fatigue, dry mouth, eye discomfort, drowsiness.

LESS COMMON
Excess tear production, redness of eyes or inner lining of the eyelids, headache, swelling of eye or eyelid, eye ache or pain, blurring or other changes in vision, dizziness, mental depression, insomnia, muscle pain or weakness, nausea, increased blood pressure, vomiting, anxiety, pounding heartbeat, change in taste, crusting in corner of eye or on eyelid, discoloration of eyeball, paleness of inner lining of eyelid, dry eyes, sensitivity of eyes to light.

BUPROPION HYDROCHLORIDE

Available in: Tablets, extended-release tablets
Available OTC? No   **As Generic?** No
Drug Class: Antidepressant/smoking deterrent

▼ USAGE INFORMATION

WHY IT'S PRESCRIBED
To relieve symptoms of major depression. Bupropion is also used as a nicotine-free agent to help stop smoking. It should be used as a part of a comprehensive smoking cessation program carried out under the supervision of your doctor.

HOW IT WORKS
While the exact mechanism of action of bupropion is not known, it appears to help balance the levels of neurotransmitters (brain chemicals) that are thought to be linked to mood, emotions, and mental state. Unlike other smoking cessation medications, bupropion does not contain nicotine. It is believed that bupropion's effects on the chemistry of the brain help to curb the desire for nicotine and enhance the patient's ability to abstain from smoking.

▼ DOSAGE GUIDELINES

RANGE AND FREQUENCY
Depression (Wellbutrin)—Adults: To start, 100 mg twice a day. Dosage may be increased to 450 mg a day. No more than 150 mg should be taken within 4 hours. Older adults: To start, 75 or 100 mg twice a day. Children: Dosages must be determined by your doctor. Smoking cessation (Zyban)—Adults: For the first 3 days of treatment, 150 mg a day. Dosage may then be increased to 150 mg, 2 times a day. The doses should be taken at least 8 hours apart. Do not take more than 300 mg per day. You should not stop smoking until you have been taking Zyban for 1 week. Treatment generally lasts 7 to 12 weeks.

ONSET OF EFFECT
1 to 3 weeks.

DURATION OF ACTION
Unknown.

DIETARY ADVICE
Bupropion can be taken with food to reduce stomach irritation. The tablet should be swallowed whole, because it has a bitter taste and can produce an unpleasant numbing sensation inside of the mouth.

STORAGE
Store in a tightly sealed container away from moisture, heat, and direct light.

MISSED DOSE
Take it as soon as you remember, unless your next scheduled dose is within the next 4 hours (8 hours for smoking cessation). If so, do not take the missed dose. Take your next scheduled dose at the proper time and resume your regular dosage schedule. Do not double the next dose.

STOPPING THE DRUG
Depression: Take it as prescribed for the full treatment period, even if you begin to feel better before the scheduled end of therapy. Discontinuing the drug abruptly may produce unpleasant withdrawal symptoms. Dosage should be reduced gradually according to your doctor's instructions. The decision to stop taking the drug should be made in consultation with your doctor. Smoking cessation: If you have not made significant progress toward abstinence by the end of the seventh week of treatment, consult your doctor. Treatment should probably be discontinued. You do not need to gradually decrease the dose before stopping.

PROLONGED USE
Depression: The usual course of therapy lasts 6 months to 1 year; some patients benefit from additional therapy. Smoking cessation: Treatment generally lasts 7 to 12 weeks.

▼ PRECAUTIONS

Over 60: Dosage may be decreased because of age-related decline in liver or kidney function.

Driving and Hazardous Work: Use caution until you determine how the medication affects you. Drowsiness or lightheadedness can occur.

Alcohol: Alcohol increases the risk of seizures. It is recommended to abstain from alcohol or to drink very little while taking bupropion. If you regularly drink a lot of alcohol and then suddenly stop, this may also increase your chance of having a seizure; gradual tapering of alcohol is recommended.

Pregnancy: Bupropion has not caused birth defects in animals. Adequate human studies have not been done. The drug is not recommended while you are pregnant. Before taking it, tell your doctor if you are pregnant or plan to become pregnant.

Breast Feeding: Bupropion passes into breast milk; avoid or discontinue using the drug while nursing.

Infants and Children: Adequate studies in children have not been done. Bupropion is not recommended for use by children under age 18.

≣ SIDE EFFECTS ≣

SERIOUS
When treating depression: Hallucinations, heartbeat irregularities, confusion, skin rash, insomnia, severe headache, excitement or agitation, seizures. Call your doctor immediately. Smoking cessation: None reported.

COMMON
When treating depression: Nausea or vomiting, constipation, unusual weight loss, dry mouth, loss of appetite, dizziness, increased sweating, trembling or shaking. Smoking cessation: Dry mouth, insomnia.

LESS COMMON
When treating depression: Fever or chills, concentration difficulties, drowsiness, fatigue, change in or blurred vision, unusual feeling of euphoria, hostility or anger. Smoking cessation: Mild rash, tremor.

(continued)

Special Concerns: This is a potentially dangerous drug, especially if taken in excess. Antidepressants should not be within easy reach of suicidal patients. To prevent insomnia, take the last dose several hours before bedtime. When taking bupropion for smoking cessation, it is advised to continue smoking through the first week of treatment. Set a target date to stop smoking no later than the second week of therapy. Continuing to smoke beyond the designated date reduces your chances of successfully quitting. You may use a nicotine transdermal patch (see Nicotine) while taking Zyban, but consult your doctor before initiating such therapy. The combination of nicotine and bupropion increases the risk of hypertension; blood pressure should be monitored regularly throughout treatment. Zyban should be seen as just one small part of a comprehensive treatment program that includes counseling, social support, and regular contact with your doctor. The goal of therapy with Zyban is complete abstinence from cigarettes. Do not chew, divide, or crush the tablets or extended-release tablets.

OVERDOSE

Symptoms: Hallucinations, seizures, rapid heartbeat, chest pain, breathing difficulty, loss of consciousness. A few cases of overdose associated with treatment for smoking cessation have been reported. Some of the symptoms experienced include: vomiting, blurred vision, lightheadedness, confusion, lethargy, nausea, jitteriness, hallucinations, drowsiness, and seizures.

What to Do: Call your doctor, emergency medical services (EMS), or the nearest poison control center immediately.

▼ INTERACTIONS

DRUG INTERACTIONS

Bupropion should not be used if you are taking other medicines containing bupropion or within 14 days of taking an MAO inhibitor. Consult your doctor if you are currently taking loxapine, tricyclic antidepressants, phenothiazines, clozapine, molindone, fluoxetine, lithium, thioxanthenes, haloperidol, trazodone, maprotiline, levodopa, or theophylline.

FOOD INTERACTIONS

No known food interactions.

DISEASE INTERACTIONS

Bupropion should not be taken if you have a history of seizures, anorexia nervosa, or bulimia. Caution is advised when taking bupropion. Consult your doctor if you have any of the following: a tumor of the brain or spinal cord, heart disease, or head injury. Since the liver and kidneys work together to remove bupropion from the body, a lower dose may be prescribed for patients with impaired liver or kidney function.

BUSPIRONE HYDROCHLORIDE

Available in: Tablets
Available OTC? No   **As Generic?** No
Drug Class: Antianxiety drug

▼ USAGE INFORMATION

WHY IT'S PRESCRIBED
To treat anxiety.

HOW IT WORKS
Buspirone affects the activity of specific brain chemicals (dopamine and especially serotonin) that are profoundly linked to mood, emotions, and mental state. Unlike many other medications used to treat anxiety disorders, buspirone has no muscle relaxant or sedative effects, and does not appear to lead to physical dependence.

▼ DOSAGE GUIDELINES

RANGE AND FREQUENCY
To start, 5 mg, 3 times per day (for a total of 15 mg a day). Can be increased to 60 mg a day, taken in divided doses every 6 to 8 hours.

ONSET OF EFFECT
May take 1 to 2 weeks to attain the full therapeutic benefit of buspirone.

DURATION OF ACTION
8 hours or more.

DIETARY ADVICE
No special restrictions.

STORAGE
Store in a tightly sealed container away from moisture, heat, and direct light.

MISSED DOSE
If you miss a dose, take it as soon as you remember. If it is near the time for your next dose, skip the missed dose and resume your regular dosage schedule. Do not double the next dose.

STOPPING THE DRUG
The decision to stop taking buspirone should be made in consultation with your doctor.

PROLONGED USE
No known problems.

▼ PRECAUTIONS

Over 60: Adverse side effects and reactions may be more common and more severe in older patients.

Driving and Hazardous Work: The use of buspirone may impair your ability to drive or perform hazardous tasks safely. The danger increases if you drink alcohol or take other medications that can affect alertness, such as antihistamines, painkillers, or mind-altering drugs.

Alcohol: Avoid alcohol while using this medication.

Pregnancy: No problems are expected, but adequate studies of buspirone use during pregnancy have not been done. Consult your doctor if you are pregnant or plan to become pregnant.

Breast Feeding: Buspirone can pass into breast milk. Avoid taking it if possible or refrain from breast feeding.

Infants and Children: The safety and effectiveness of buspirone have not been established for anyone under the age of 18.

Special Concerns: Before you undergo surgery that requires anesthesia, be sure to notify the surgeon that you are taking buspirone.

OVERDOSE
Symptoms: Severe drowsiness, dizziness, nausea and vomiting, constricted (pinpoint) pupils.

What to Do: Call your doctor, emergency medical services (EMS), or the nearest poison control center immediately.

▼ INTERACTIONS

DRUG INTERACTIONS
Other drugs may interact with buspirone. Consult your doctor for specific advice if you take any of the following: antihistamines, barbiturates, MAO inhibitors, muscle relaxants, narcotics, sedatives, or other tranquilizers.

FOOD INTERACTIONS
None expected.

DISEASE INTERACTIONS
Use of buspirone may cause complications in patients with liver or kidney disease, since these organs work together to remove the medication from the body.

☰ SIDE EFFECTS ☰

SERIOUS
No serious side effects have been directly associated with the use of buspirone.

COMMON
Dizziness or lightheadedness, nausea, paradoxical increase in nervousness or excitability, restlessness, headache.

LESS COMMON
Blurred vision, impaired ability to concentrate, drowsiness, dry mouth, difficulty sleeping, muscle cramps or spasms, fatigue or weakness, ringing in the ears, dreams that are unusual, disturbing, or vivid.

CALCITONIN — SALMON

Available in: Injection, nasal spray
Available OTC? No **As Generic?** No
Drug Class: Hormone/bone resorption inhibitor

▼ USAGE INFORMATION

WHY IT'S PRESCRIBED
To treat Paget's disease, a disorder in which bone tissue is broken down and restored too rapidly, resulting in bone fragility and in some cases malformation; to prevent bone loss in women with postmenopausal osteoporosis; to treat abnormally high blood calcium levels; to treat osteoporosis resulting from hormonal disturbances, drug therapy, and immobilization; to relieve compression of nerves that may occur with Paget's disease of bone.

HOW IT WORKS
Calcitonin blocks the bone-mineral-absorbing activity of the osteoclasts (bone cells), increases calcium excretion by the kidneys, and slows bone resorption (the speed at which bone is broken down before it is replaced).

▼ DOSAGE GUIDELINES

RANGE AND FREQUENCY
Injection—For Paget's disease: 100 international units (IU) injected under the skin once a day to start. The dosage may be reduced depending on results. To prevent post-menopausal bone loss: 100 IU injected into muscle or under the skin once a day, once every other day, or 3 times a week. For excessive blood calcium: 1.8 IU per lb of body weight injected every 12 hours to start. Dose may be increased or decreased by your doctor. Nasal spray—200 IU (1 spray) a day delivered in alternating nostrils, 1 spray a day.

ONSET OF EFFECT
Within 15 minutes.

DURATION OF ACTION
8 to 24 hours.

DIETARY ADVICE
If you are using this drug to lower blood calcium, your doctor may want you to follow a low-calcium diet. An injection is best administered at bedtime.

STORAGE
Store in a tightly sealed container away from heat and direct light.

MISSED DOSE
If you take 2 doses a day: Take the missed dose if you remember within 2 hours. If not, skip the missed dose and resume your regular dosage schedule. If you take 1 dose a day: Take the missed dose if you remember it the same day, then resume your regular dosage schedule. If you remember the next day, skip the missed dose and resume your regular dosage schedule. If you take one dose every other day: Take the missed dose if you remember the same day. Otherwise, take the dose the next day, skip a day and resume your regular dosage schedule. If you take 1 dose 3 times a week: Take the missed dose the next day, set each dose back a day for the rest of the week, then resume your regular dosage schedule. In no cases should you double the next dose.

STOPPING THE DRUG
The decision to stop taking the drug should be made by your doctor.

PROLONGED USE
Development of antibodies to the medicine may diminish its effectiveness over time.

▼ PRECAUTIONS

Over 60: Fluid balance should be monitored if the drug is given to reduce blood levels of calcium.

Driving and Hazardous Work: The use of calcitonin should not impair your ability to perform such tasks safely.

Alcohol: Avoid alcohol.

Pregnancy: In animal studies, large doses of calcitonin reduced birth weight. Before you take calcitonin, tell your doctor if you are pregnant or plan to become pregnant.

Breast Feeding: Calcitonin may pass into breast milk; caution is advised. Consult your doctor for advice.

Infants and Children: Studies of calcitonin use in infants and children have not been done. Consult your doctor for specific advice.

Special Concerns: You should not take calcitonin if you have a recently healed bone fracture.

OVERDOSE
Symptoms: No specific ones have been reported.

What to Do: An overdose of calcitonin is unlikely to be life-threatening. However, if someone takes a much larger dose than prescribed, call your doctor, emergency medical services (EMS), or the nearest poison control center.

▼ INTERACTIONS

DRUG INTERACTIONS
There are no known drug interactions.

FOOD INTERACTIONS
No known food interactions.

DISEASE INTERACTIONS
Caution is advised when taking calcitonin. Consult your doctor for specific advice if you have a kidney problem or a history of allergies.

≡ SIDE EFFECTS ≡

SERIOUS
Skin rash or hives. Call your doctor immediately.

COMMON
Diarrhea, loss of appetite, nausea or vomiting, stomach pain, pain and redness at injection site, flushing or redness of face, ears, hands, or feet.

LESS COMMON
Increased output of urine, headache, dizziness, pressure in the chest, breathing difficulty, stuffy nose, nasal bleeding or crusting, tingling of hands or feet, weakness, back pain, joint pain, chills.

CARBAMAZEPINE

Available in: Oral suspension, tablets, extended-release tablets and capsules
Available OTC? No **As Generic?** Yes
Drug Class: Anticonvulsant/analgesic

▼ USAGE INFORMATION

WHY IT'S PRESCRIBED
To control certain types of seizures due to epilepsy. Also to treat facial pain in those with trigeminal neuralgia (tic douloureux).

HOW IT WORKS
Carbamazepine appears to inhibit neurons from firing repeatedly and uncontrollably (which causes seizures).

▼ DOSAGE GUIDELINES

RANGE AND FREQUENCY
Adults: 600 to 2,000 mg a day, in 3 or 4 divided doses. Children: 9 to 18 mg per lb of body weight, in 3 or 4 divided doses. Some patients require higher doses. A low dose should be used initially, then gradually increased if needed. The extended-release forms may be given twice a day.

ONSET OF EFFECT
Several hours or longer.

DURATION OF ACTION
Maximum effectiveness: 12 hours or longer; the drug's effectiveness then gradually decreases.

DIETARY ADVICE
Take with food to lessen the chance of stomach upset.

STORAGE
Store in a tightly sealed container away from moisture, heat, and direct light.

MISSED DOSE
Take the medication as soon as you remember. If it is near the time for the next dose, skip the missed dose and resume your regular dosage schedule. Do not double the next dose, unless advised to do so by your doctor. Call your doctor if you miss more than a full day's worth of the drug.

STOPPING THE DRUG
Never stop this drug abruptly; seizures may occur. Your doctor will taper the dose over many weeks.

PROLONGED USE
Therapy may last several years or longer. Some side effects may diminish after a few weeks of therapy.

▼ PRECAUTIONS

Over 60: Older patients may require lower doses to minimize side effects.

Driving and Hazardous Work: Avoid such tasks until you determine how the medication affects you.

Alcohol: May contribute to excessive drowsiness.

Pregnancy: This drug increases the risk of birth defects. However, seizures during pregnancy also increase the risks to the fetus. Discuss potential risks and benefits with your doctor. Folate supplementation is advised starting 1 to 2 months before conception and continuing throughout pregnancy. Vitamin K1 may be needed during the last 4 weeks of pregnancy.

Breast Feeding: This drug passes into breast milk, although at low levels. Consult your doctor for advice.

Infants and Children: Behavioral side effects are more likely to be seen in children.

Special Concerns: The generic form is not recommended. Do not change the brand you are taking without consulting your doctor. Your doctor may suggest you carry an ID card or bracelet saying that you take this drug.

OVERDOSE
Symptoms: Confusion, double vision, seizures, extreme drowsiness, spasms, loss of consciousness, poor muscle control, tremors, walking difficulty, abnormal heartbeat, slow or irregular breathing.

What to Do: Seek medical assistance immediately.

▼ INTERACTIONS

DRUG INTERACTIONS
Carbamazepine may interact with many drugs, including other anticonvulsants (clonazepam, ethosuximide, primidone, phenobarbital, valproic acid, and phenytoin), anticoagulants, certain anti-infectives (erythromycin, doxycycline, troleandomycin, isoniazid), oral contraceptives, cimetidine, corticosteroids, danazol, diltiazem, lithium, nicotinamide, propoxyphene, theophylline, thyroid hormones, and verapamil.

FOOD INTERACTIONS
No known food interactions.

DISEASE INTERACTIONS
Special caution is advised in those with lupus; heart, kidney, or liver disease; diabetes; or glaucoma.

≡ SIDE EFFECTS ≡

SERIOUS
Fever, sore throat, swollen glands, point-like rash, blistering or peeling, easy bruising, pallor, weakness, confusion, lethargy, or seizures may be a sign of a potentially fatal blood reaction (aplastic anemia). Call your doctor at once.

COMMON
Drowsiness, rash, itching, increased sensitivity of the skin to sunlight, dizziness, blurred vision, incoordination, nausea, vomiting, stomach pain or upset, diarrhea, constipation, loss of appetite, dry or inflamed mouth.

LESS COMMON
Impaired speech, involuntary movements of the face, limbs, or tongue, tingling or numbness in the extremities, depression, agitation, psychosis, talkativeness, abnormal eye movements, ringing in the ears, heart rhythm abnormalities, impotence, hair loss, or excessive hair growth. There are numerous additional potential side effects.

CARISOPRODOL

Available in: Tablets
Available OTC? No **As Generic?** Yes
Drug Class: Muscle relaxant

▼ USAGE INFORMATION

WHY IT'S PRESCRIBED
Skeletal muscle relaxants are used to relieve stiffness and discomfort caused by severe sprains and strains, muscle spasms, or other muscle problems. They may be prescribed in conjunction with other treatment methods, such as physical therapy.

HOW IT WORKS
Muscle relaxants such as carisoprodol depress activity in the central nervous system, which in turn interferes with the transmission of nerve impulses from the spinal cord to the muscles.

▼ DOSAGE GUIDELINES

RANGE AND FREQUENCY
Adults and teenagers: 350 mg, 3 to 4 times a day. Children ages 5 to 12: 6.25 mg per 2.2 lbs (1 kg) of body weight 4 times a day.

ONSET OF EFFECT
30 minutes.

DURATION OF ACTION
4 to 6 hours.

DIETARY ADVICE
Eat a well-balanced diet; the healing of injured tissue increases the body's protein and calorie requirements. To avoid dry mouth, maintain adequate fluid intake and suck on ice chips.

STORAGE
Store in a tightly sealed container in a dry place away from heat and direct light.

MISSED DOSE
Take it as soon as you remember. If it is within 2 hours of the next dose, skip the missed dose and resume your regular dosage schedule. Do not double the next dose.

STOPPING THE DRUG
This medication should be taken as prescribed for the full treatment period. Do not stop taking carisoprodol abruptly.

PROLONGED USE
Therapy with carisoprodol ranges from several days to weeks. Prolonged use may be associated with an increased risk of side effects.

▼ PRECAUTIONS

Over 60: Adverse reactions to medications such as carisoprodol may be more likely and more severe in older patients.

Driving and Hazardous Work: Carisoprodol may impair your ability to drive or perform hazardous work.

Alcohol: Avoid alcohol while taking this medication because it may compound the sedative effect and may cause liver damage.

Pregnancy: Adequate studies of carisoprodol during pregnancy have not been done; discuss the relative risks and benefits with your doctor.

Breast Feeding: Breast feeding is not recommended during therapy.

Infants and Children: No special problems have been documented; consult your pediatrician for advice.

Special Concerns: Carisoprodol will intensify the effect that alcohol, sedatives, and other central nervous system depressants have on the brain. It is not a substitute for other safe, nonmedical therapies for muscle stiffness, including rest, gentle guided exercise, and physical therapy.

OVERDOSE
Symptoms: Excessive drowsiness or difficulty awakening, even when being shaken or pinched; confusion; weakness; slowed breathing; coma.

What to Do: Call emergency medical services (EMS) or the nearest poison control center immediately.

▼ INTERACTIONS

DRUG INTERACTIONS
Consult your doctor for specific advice if you are taking antihistamines and decongestants, antidepressants, sleep aids, sedatives, tranquilizers, pain medication, barbiturates, or seizure medication.

FOOD INTERACTIONS
No known food interactions.

DISEASE INTERACTIONS
Caution is advised when taking carisoprodol. Consult your doctor if you have a history of any of the following medical conditions: allergies, drug abuse or dependence, kidney disease, liver disease, porphyria, epilepsy, or any other seizure disorder.

⇩ SIDE EFFECTS ⇩

SERIOUS
Fainting; palpitations or rapid heartbeat; fever; hives or severe swelling of face, lips, or tongue along with shortness of breath, chest tightness, or wheezing (indicating a potentially life-threatening allergic reaction); depression. Seek medical help immediately.

COMMON
Drowsiness, dizziness, dry mouth.

LESS COMMON
Inability to pass urine; sores on lips, ulcers in mouth; abdominal cramps or pain; clumsiness; unsteady gait; confusion; constipation; diarrhea; excitability, nervousness, restlessness, or irritability; flushing or redness of face; headache; heartburn; hiccups; muscle weakness; nausea and vomiting; trembling; insomnia or fitful sleep; burning, red eyes; stuffy nose.

CEFPROZIL

Available in: Oral suspension, tablets
Available OTC? No **As Generic?** No
Drug Class: Cephalosporin antibiotic

▼ USAGE INFORMATION

WHY IT'S PRESCRIBED
To treat a variety of bacterial infections, including those of the ear, nose, tonsils, and throat, skin and soft tissues, and the respiratory tract. The drug cefprozil is effective only against infections caused by bacteria; it is ineffective against infections caused by viruses, fungi, or other microorganisms.

HOW IT WORKS
Cefprozil prevents bacteria from forming protective cell walls that are necessary for its survival.

▼ DOSAGE GUIDELINES

RANGE AND FREQUENCY
Adults and teenagers: 250 to 500 mg every 12 to 24 hours. Children ages 2 to 12: 7.5 mg per 2.2 lbs (1 kg) of body weight every 12 hours. Children 6 months to 12 years: 15 mg per 2.2 lbs every 12 hours.

ONSET OF EFFECT
Approximately 90 minutes.

DURATION OF ACTION
Unknown.

DIETARY ADVICE
It may be taken with food to reduce stomach irritation.

STORAGE
Store in a tightly sealed container away from moisture, heat, and direct light. Keep liquid form refrigerated, but do not allow it to freeze.

MISSED DOSE
Take it as soon as you remember. This will help keep a constant level of medication in your system. If it is near the time for the next dose, skip the missed dose and resume your regular dosage schedule. Do not double the next dose.

STOPPING THE DRUG
Take it as prescribed for the full treatment period, even if you begin to feel better before the scheduled end of therapy. Stopping cefprozil prematurely may slow your recovery or lead to a rebound infection, also known as superinfection, in which the heartier strains of bacteria survive and multiply, leading to a more serious and drug-resistant infection. When taking this drug to treat a streptococcal (strep) infection, it is particularly important to take it for the entire treatment period. Serious heart and kidney problems can develop later if the drug is discontinued prematurely.

PROLONGED USE
Cefprozil is generally prescribed for short-term therapy (10 to 14 days). Use of cefprozil beyond this period increases risks of adverse effects and superinfection.

▼ PRECAUTIONS

Over 60: Adverse reactions may be more likely and more severe in older patients.

Driving and Hazardous Work: Do not drive or engage in hazardous work until you determine how the medicine affects you.

Alcohol: Avoid alcohol.

Pregnancy: Adequate studies of cephalosporin use in pregnant women have not been done. Before taking cefprozil, tell your doctor if you are pregnant or are planning to become pregnant.

Breast Feeding: Cefprozil passes into breast milk; caution is advised. Consult your doctor for specific advice.

Infants and Children: Cefprozil may be used by children 6 months and older. Consult your pediatrician for specific advice.

Special Concerns: People who are allergic to penicillin may have equally serious allergic reactions to cephalosporin antibiotics such as cefprozil. This drug is useful only against bacteria that are susceptible to its effects, not against colds, flu, or other viral infections. If your condition does not improve after a few days of taking cefprozil, or instead has worsened, tell your doctor.

OVERDOSE
Symptoms: Seizures, severe abdominal pain, bloody diarrhea, vomiting.

What to Do: Call your doctor, emergency medical services (EMS), or the nearest poison control center immediately.

▼ INTERACTIONS

DRUG INTERACTIONS
Consult your doctor for specific advice if you are getting a carbenicillin injection, or taking heparin, divalproex, anticoagulants, dipyridamole, sulfinpyrazone, pentoxifylline, plicamycin, ticarcillin, probenecid, or valproic acid.

FOOD INTERACTIONS
No known food interactions.

DISEASE INTERACTIONS
Caution is advised when taking cefprozil. Consult your doctor if you have a history of kidney disease, phenylketonuria, or colitis.

≣ SIDE EFFECTS ≣

SERIOUS
Severe allergic reaction (breathing difficulties, confusion, lightheadedness, itching, hives, swelling of the face or throat, and unusual sweating), severe stomach pain and cramps, fever, severe, sometimes bloody diarrhea. Call your doctor immediately.

COMMON
Mild diarrhea or stomach cramps, sore mouth or tongue, nausea and vomiting.

LESS COMMON
Vaginal itching or unusual discharge, decreased white blood cell count causing increased susceptibility to infection, decreased blood platelets causing increased risk of bleeding problems.

CEFUROXIME

BRAND NAMES

Ceftin, Kefurox, Zinacef

Available in: Tablets, injection, oral suspension
Available OTC? No   **As Generic?** Yes
Drug Class: Cephalosporin antibiotic

▼ USAGE INFORMATION

WHY IT'S PRESCRIBED
To treat a variety of bacterial infections, including those of the brain, ear, nose, tonsils, and throat, skin and soft tissues, genitourinary tract, respiratory tract, blood, bones, joints, and other organs. Cefuroxime also is used to treat gonorrhea and is given prior to some surgeries to prevent infection. It is effective only against susceptible infections caused by bacteria.

HOW IT WORKS
Cefuroxime prevents bacteria from forming cell walls.

▼ DOSAGE GUIDELINES

RANGE AND FREQUENCY
Adults and teenagers–
Tablets: 125 to 500 mg every 12 hours for 5 to 10 days. Injection: 750 to 1,500 mg every 6 to 8 hours into a vein or muscle. Children 3 months to 12 years–Tablets: 125 mg every 12 hours for 10 days. Injection: 16.7 to 33.3 mg per 2.2 lbs (1 kg) of body weight every 8 hours into a vein or muscle. Oral suspension: 10 to 15 mg per 2.2 lbs every 12 hours for 10 days. Gonorrhea is treated with a one-time tablet dose of 1,000 mg or a one-time injected dose of 1,500 mg into a muscle. The injected dose is divided and administered at two sites on the body, along with a single 1,000 mg oral dose of probenecid.

ONSET OF EFFECT
Into a vein: Immediate. Into a muscle: 15 to 60 minutes. Oral forms: Unknown.

DURATION OF ACTION
5 to 8 hours.

DIETARY ADVICE
Tablets can be taken without regard to meals. Take the oral suspension with food to increase the absorption of the drug by the body. Maintain normal fluid intake.

STORAGE
Store in a tightly sealed container away from moisture, heat, and direct light. Keep liquid form refrigerated, but do not allow it to freeze.

MISSED DOSE
Take it as soon as you remember. If it is near the time for the next dose, skip the missed dose and resume your regular dosage schedule. Do not double the next dose.

STOPPING THE DRUG
Take it as prescribed for the full treatment period. Stopping prematurely may slow your recovery or lead to a rebound infection, also known as superinfection, in which the heartier strains of bacteria survive and multiply, leading to a more serious and drug-resistant infection. When taking this drug to treat a streptococcal (strep) infection, it is particularly important to take it for the entire treatment period. Serious heart and kidney problems can develop later if the drug is discontinued prematurely.

PROLONGED USE
Cefuroxime is generally prescribed for short-term therapy (5 to 10 days). Using the drug beyond this period increases the risks of adverse effects and superinfection.

▼ PRECAUTIONS

Over 60: Adverse reactions may be more likely and more severe in older patients.

Driving and Hazardous Work: Do not drive or engage in hazardous work until you determine how the medicine affects you.

Alcohol: Avoid alcohol.

Pregnancy: Adequate studies of use during pregnancy have not been done. Consult your doctor for advice.

Breast Feeding: Cefuroxime passes into breast milk; caution is advised. Consult your doctor for advice.

Infants and Children: May be used by children 3 months and older. Consult your pediatrician for advice.

Special Concerns: Those who are allergic to penicillin may have equally serious allergic reactions to cephalosporin antibiotics. If your condition has not improved within a few days, or instead has worsened, tell your doctor. The tablets and the oral suspension can not be equally substituted for each other.

OVERDOSE
Symptoms: Seizures, severe abdominal pain, bloody diarrhea, vomiting.

What to Do: Seek medical assistance immediately.

▼ INTERACTIONS

DRUG INTERACTIONS
Consult your doctor if you are taking carbenicillin injection, divalproex, anticoagulants, sulfinpyrazone, dipyridamole, pentoxifylline, plicamycin, ticarcillin, probenecid, or valproic acid.

FOOD INTERACTIONS
No known food interactions.

DISEASE INTERACTIONS
Consult your doctor if you have a history of kidney disease or colitis.

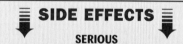

≡ SIDE EFFECTS ≡

SERIOUS
Severe allergic reaction (breathing difficulties, confusion, hives, swelling of the face or throat, and lightheadedness), severe stomach pain and cramps, fever, severe, sometimes bloody diarrhea. Call your doctor immediately.

COMMON
Mild diarrhea or stomach cramps, sore mouth or tongue, nausea and vomiting.

LESS COMMON
Vaginal itching or discharge, pain at site of injection, rash, decreased white blood cell count causing increased susceptibility to infection, decreased blood platelets causing increased risk of bleeding problems.

CELECOXIB

Available in: Capsules
Available OTC? No   **As Generic?** No
Drug Class: Nonsteroidal anti-inflammatory drug (NSAID)/COX-2 inhibitor

▼ USAGE INFORMATION

WHY IT'S PRESCRIBED
To relieve pain, inflammation, and stiffness of osteoarthritis and rheumatoid arthritis.

HOW IT WORKS
By inhibiting the activity of the enzyme cyclooxygenase-2 (COX-2), celecoxib reduces the synthesis of prostaglandins that play a role in causing arthritis pain and inflammation. It does not inhibit the activity of COX-1, the enzyme involved in the synthesis of prostaglandins that help protect against stomach ulcers and other health problems.

▼ DOSAGE GUIDELINES

RANGE AND FREQUENCY
For osteoarthritis: 200 mg a day. For rheumatoid arthritis: 100 to 200 mg twice a day. To minimize potential gastrointestinal side effects, the lowest effective dose should be used for the shortest possible time.

ONSET OF EFFECT
Within 24 to 48 hours.

DURATION OF ACTION
Unknown.

DIETARY ADVICE
Celecoxib may be taken with or without food.

STORAGE
Store in a tightly sealed container away from moisture, heat, and direct light.

MISSED DOSE
Take it as soon as you remember. If it is near the time for the next dose, skip the missed dose and resume your regular dosage schedule. Do not double the next dose.

STOPPING THE DRUG
The decision to stop taking this prescription medication should be made in consultation with your doctor.

PROLONGED USE
The risk of gastrointestinal side effects may be increased with extended use.

▼ PRECAUTIONS

Over 60: Adverse reactions may be more likely and more severe in older patients.

Driving and Hazardous Work: No special problems are expected.

Alcohol: Avoid alcohol when using this medication because it increases the risk of stomach irritation.

Pregnancy: Discuss with your doctor the relative risks and benefits of using this drug while pregnant. Do not use celecoxib during the last trimester.

Breast Feeding: Celecoxib may pass into breast milk; caution is advised. Consult your doctor for advice on whether to discontinue nursing or discontinue the drug.

Infants and Children: The safety and effectiveness of this medication have not been established for children under the age of 18.

OVERDOSE
Symptoms: No cases of overdose have been reported. Symptoms may include nausea, lethargy, drowsiness, vomiting, abdominal pain, black, tarry stools, breathing difficulty, and coma.

What to Do: If you suspect an overdose or if someone takes a much larger dose than prescribed, call your doctor, emergency medical services (EMS), or the nearest poison control center immediately.

▼ INTERACTIONS

DRUG INTERACTIONS
Do not take this drug with aspirin or any other NSAIDs without your doctor's approval. Consult your doctor if you are taking furosemide, ACE inhibitors, fluconazole, lithium, or warfarin.

FOOD INTERACTIONS
No known food interactions.

DISEASE INTERACTIONS
Celecoxib should not be taken by people who have experienced asthma, hives, or allergic-type reactions after taking aspirin or other NSAIDs. Consult your doctor if you have any of the following: bleeding problems, inflammation or ulcers of the stomach and intestines, asthma, high blood pressure, or heart failure. Use of celecoxib may cause complications in patients with liver or kidney disease, since these organs work together to remove the medication from the body.

≡ SIDE EFFECTS ≡

SERIOUS
Stomach ulcers. Black, tarry stools may signal stomach bleeding. Symptoms of liver disease (nausea, fatigue, lethargy, itching, yellowish discoloration of the eyes or skin, fluid retention). Call your doctor immediately.

COMMON
Indigestion, diarrhea, and mild abdominal pain.

LESS COMMON
Flatulence, mild swelling, sore throat, and upper respiratory tract infection.

CEPHALEXIN

Available in: Capsules, oral suspension, tablets
Available OTC? No   **As Generic?** Yes
Drug Class: Cephalosporin antibiotic

▼ USAGE INFORMATION

WHY IT'S PRESCRIBED
To treat a variety of bacterial infections, including those of the ear, nose, tonsils, and throat, bones, joints, skin and soft tissues, genitourinary tract, and respiratory tract. It is effective only against infections caused by bacteria; it is ineffective against those caused by viruses, fungi, or other microorganisms.

HOW IT WORKS
Cephalexin prevents bacteria from forming cell walls.

▼ DOSAGE GUIDELINES

RANGE AND FREQUENCY
Adults and teenagers: 250 to 500 mg every 6 to 12 hours. Children: 6.25 to 25 mg per 2.2 lbs (1 kg) of body weight every 6 hours, or 12.5 to 50 mg per kg every 12 hours.

ONSET OF EFFECT
1 hour.

DURATION OF ACTION
Unknown.

DIETARY ADVICE
Cephalexin may be taken on a full or empty stomach, but taking it with food will reduce stomach irritation.

STORAGE
Store in a tightly sealed container away from moisture, heat, and direct light. Keep liquid form refrigerated, but do not allow it to freeze.

MISSED DOSE
Take it as soon as you remember. This will help keep a constant level of medication in your system. If it is near the time for the next dose, skip the missed dose and resume your regular dosage schedule. Do not double the next dose.

STOPPING THE DRUG
Take it as prescribed for the full treatment period, even if you begin to feel better before the scheduled end of therapy. Stopping cephalexin prematurely may slow your recovery or lead to a rebound infection, also known as superinfection, in which the heartier strains of bacteria survive and multiply, leading to a more serious and drug-resistant infection. When taking this drug to treat a streptococcal (strep) infection, it is particularly important to take it for the entire treatment period. Serious heart and kidney problems can develop later if it is discontinued prematurely.

PROLONGED USE
Cephalexin is generally prescribed for short-term therapy (10 to 14 days). Further use increases the risk of adverse effects and superinfection.

▼ PRECAUTIONS

Over 60: Adverse reactions may be more likely and more severe in older patients.

Driving and Hazardous Work: Do not drive or engage in hazardous work until you determine how the medicine affects you.

Alcohol: Avoid alcohol.

Pregnancy: Adequate studies of cephalosporin use in pregnant women have not been done. Before you take cephalexin, tell your doctor if you are pregnant or plan to become pregnant.

Breast Feeding: Cephalexin passes into breast milk; caution is advised. Consult your doctor for specific advice.

Infants and Children: Adequate studies of cephalexin use in children have not been done to date. Consult your pediatrician.

Special Concerns: People who are allergic to penicillin may have equally serious allergic reactions to cephalosporin antibiotics such as cephalexin. This drug is useful only against bacteria that are susceptible to its effects, not against colds, flu, or other viral infections. If your condition has not improved within a few days of starting the medicine, or instead has worsened, tell your doctor.

OVERDOSE
Symptoms: Seizures, severe abdominal pain, bloody diarrhea, vomiting.

What to Do: Call your doctor, emergency medical services (EMS), or the nearest poison control center immediately.

▼ INTERACTIONS

DRUG INTERACTIONS
Consult your doctor for specific advice if you are taking carbenicillin injection, heparin, divalproex, anticoagulants, sulfinpyrazone, dipyridamole, pentoxifylline, plicamycin, ticarcillin, probenecid, or valproic acid.

FOOD INTERACTIONS
No known food interactions.

DISEASE INTERACTIONS
Caution is advised when taking cephalexin. Consult your doctor if you have a history of kidney disease or colitis.

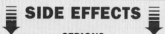

▼ SIDE EFFECTS

SERIOUS
Severe allergic reaction (breathing difficulties, confusion, hives, itching, swelling of the face or throat, unusual sweating, and lightheadedness), severe stomach pain and cramps, fever, severe, sometimes bloody diarrhea. Call your doctor immediately.

COMMON
Mild diarrhea or stomach cramps, sore mouth or tongue, nausea and vomiting.

LESS COMMON
Vaginal itching or unusual discharge, rash, decreased white blood cell count causing increased susceptibility to infection, decreased blood platelets causing increased risk of bleeding problems.

CEPHRADINE

Available in: Oral suspension, capsules
Available OTC? No **As Generic?** Yes
Drug Class: Cephalosporin antibiotic

▼ USAGE INFORMATION

WHY IT'S PRESCRIBED
To treat a variety of bacterial infections, including those of the ear, nose, tonsils, and throat, skin and soft tissues, genitourinary tract, and the respiratory tract. Cephradine is effective only against infections caused by bacteria; it is ineffective against those caused by viruses, fungi, or other microorganisms.

HOW IT WORKS
Cephradine prevents bacteria from forming cell walls.

▼ DOSAGE GUIDELINES

RANGE AND FREQUENCY
Oral suspension and capsules—Adults and teenagers: 250 to 500 mg every 6 hours, or 500 to 1,000 mg every 12 hours. Children: 6.25 to 25 mg every 6 hours.

ONSET OF EFFECT
1 hour.

DURATION OF ACTION
Unknown.

DIETARY ADVICE
Cephradine may be taken on a full or empty stomach, but taking it with food will reduce stomach irritation.

STORAGE
Store in a tightly sealed container away from moisture, heat, and direct light. Keep liquid form refrigerated, but do not allow it to freeze.

MISSED DOSE
Take it as soon as you remember. This will help keep a constant level of medication in your system. If it is near the time for the next dose, skip the missed dose and resume your regular dosage schedule. Do not double the next dose.

STOPPING THE DRUG
Take it as prescribed for the full treatment period, even if you begin to feel better before the scheduled end of therapy. Stopping cephradine prematurely may slow your recovery or lead to a rebound infection, also known as superinfection, in which the heartier strains of bacteria survive and multiply, leading to a more serious and drug-resistant infection. When taking this drug to treat a streptococcal (strep) infection, it is particularly important to take it for the entire treatment period. Serious heart and kidney problems can develop later if it is discontinued prematurely.

PROLONGED USE
Cephradine is generally prescribed for short-term therapy (10 to 14 days). Use of this antibiotic beyond this time frame increases the risk of adverse effects and superinfection.

▼ PRECAUTIONS

Over 60: Adverse reactions may be more likely and more severe in older patients.

Driving and Hazardous Work: Do not drive or engage in hazardous work until you determine how the medicine affects you.

Alcohol: Avoid alcohol.

Pregnancy: Adequate studies of cephalosporin use during pregnancy have not been done. Consult your doctor for specific advice about using the medication.

Breast Feeding: Cephradine passes into breast milk; caution is advised. Consult your doctor for specific advice.

Infants and Children: Cephradine may be used by children age 1 and older. Consult your pediatrician for specific advice about using the medication.

Special Concerns: People who are allergic to penicillin may have equally serious reactions to cephalosporin antibiotics such as cephradine. This drug is useful only against bacteria that are susceptible to its effects, not against colds, flu, or other viral infections. If your condition has not improved within a few days of starting to take cephradine, or instead has worsened, tell your doctor.

OVERDOSE
Symptoms: Seizures, severe abdominal pain, bloody diarrhea, vomiting.

What to Do: Call your doctor, emergency medical services (EMS), or the nearest poison control center immediately.

▼ INTERACTIONS

DRUG INTERACTIONS
Consult your doctor for specific advice if you are taking carbenicillin injection, heparin, divalproex, anticoagulants, sulfinpyrazone, dipyridamole, pentoxifylline, plicamycin, ticarcillin, probenecid, or valproic acid.

FOOD INTERACTIONS
No known food interactions.

DISEASE INTERACTIONS
Caution is advised when taking cephradine. Consult your doctor if you have a history of kidney disease or colitis.

≡ SIDE EFFECTS ≡

SERIOUS
Severe allergic reaction (breathing difficulties, confusion, hives, itching, swelling of the face or throat, sweating, and lightheadedness), severe stomach pain and cramps, fever, severe, sometimes bloody diarrhea. Call your doctor immediately.

COMMON
Mild diarrhea or stomach cramps, sore mouth or tongue, nausea and vomiting.

LESS COMMON
Vaginal itching or discharge.

CETIRIZINE

Available in: Tablets, syrup
Available OTC? No   **As Generic?** No
Drug Class: Histamine (H1) blocker

▼ USAGE INFORMATION

WHY IT'S PRESCRIBED
For symptomatic relief of perennial and seasonal allergies (including hay fever), itchy skin, and chronic hives.

HOW IT WORKS
Cetirizine blocks the effects of histamine, a naturally occurring substance within the body that causes swelling, itching, sneezing, watery eyes, hives, and other symptoms of allergic reaction.

▼ DOSAGE GUIDELINES

RANGE AND FREQUENCY
Adults and teenagers: 5 to 10 mg once a day. Do not increase the dose to obtain quicker relief of symptoms. A lower dose (no more than 5 mg a day) is recommended for patients with impaired kidney or liver function.

ONSET OF EFFECT
Within 20 to 40 minutes.

DURATION OF ACTION
Approximately 24 hours.

DIETARY ADVICE
Cetirizine can be taken without regard to diet.

STORAGE
Store in a tightly sealed container away from moisture, heat, and direct light. Do not allow the syrup to freeze.

MISSED DOSE
This drug is prescribed to be taken once a day. If you miss a day, skip the missed dose and resume your regular dosage schedule. Do not double the next dose.

STOPPING THE DRUG
Take it as prescribed for the full treatment period, even if you feel better before the scheduled end of therapy.

PROLONGED USE
Safety and effectiveness during prolonged use have yet to be established.

▼ PRECAUTIONS

Over 60:
The dosage may need to be reduced in elderly patients, especially for those individuals who have impaired kidney function.

Driving and Hazardous Work:
Do not drive or engage in hazardous work until you determine how the medication affects you.

Alcohol:
Avoid alcohol while taking this medication, since it can magnify side effects such as drowsiness and fatigue.

Pregnancy:
Adequate human studies of the use of this drug during pregnancy have not been done; caution is advised. Before taking cetirizine, tell your doctor if you are pregnant or if you plan to become pregnant.

Breast Feeding:
Cetirizine passes into breast milk; avoid or discontinue use of this drug while nursing.

Infants and Children:
The safety and effectiveness of cetirizine use by children under the age of 12 have not been established.

Special Concerns:
If cetirizine causes dry mouth as a side effect, use sugarless gum, sugarless sour hard candy, or ice chips for relief.

OVERDOSE

Symptoms: No cases of overdose have been reported.

What to Do: An overdose of cetirizine is unlikely to be life-threatening. However, if someone takes a much larger dose than prescribed, call your doctor, emergency medical services (EMS), or the nearest poison control center immediately.

▼ INTERACTIONS

DRUG INTERACTIONS
No significant drug interactions have been reported. Cetirizine may, however, increase the depressant effects of alcohol, sedatives, tranquilizers, painkillers, barbiturates, or other antihistamines on the central nervous system. Consult your doctor for specific advice.

FOOD INTERACTIONS
No food interactions have been reported.

DISEASE INTERACTIONS
Cetirizine blood levels may increase in patients with liver or kidney disease, since these organs work together to remove the medication from the body. Reduced doses may be required for such persons.

≡ SIDE EFFECTS ≡

SERIOUS
No serious side effects are associated with the use of cetirizine.

COMMON
Drowsiness, fatigue, headache, dry mouth.

LESS COMMON
Nausea and vomiting.

CIPROFLOXACIN SYSTEMIC

Available in: Tablets, oral suspension
Available OTC? No   **As Generic?** No
Drug Class: Fluoroquinolone antibiotic

▼ USAGE INFORMATION

WHY IT'S PRESCRIBED
To treat mild to severe bacterial infections, including those of the urinary tract, lower respiratory tract, bones and joints, and the skin. It is also used to treat certain sexually transmitted diseases (such as chancroid and gonorrhea), and diarrhea caused by a bacterial infection.

HOW IT WORKS
Ciprofloxacin inhibits the activity of a bacterial enzyme (gyrase) that is necessary for proper DNA formation and replication. This fights infection by preventing bacteria cells from reproducing.

▼ DOSAGE GUIDELINES

RANGE AND FREQUENCY
250 to 750 mg every 12 hours (2 times a day), for 5 to 14 days, depending on kidney function and the infection being treated. Gonorrhea is usually treated with a one-time dose of 250 mg.

ONSET OF EFFECT
Varies depending on the infection being treated.

DURATION OF ACTION
Unknown.

DIETARY ADVICE
Be sure to drink plenty of fluids, but avoid milk and dairy derivatives.

STORAGE
Store in a tightly sealed container away from heat and direct light.

MISSED DOSE
Take it as soon as you remember. If it is near the time for the next dose, skip the missed dose and resume your regular dosage schedule. Do not double the next dose.

STOPPING THE DRUG
Take the drug as prescribed for the full treatment period, even if you begin to feel better before the scheduled end of therapy.

PROLONGED USE
See your doctor regularly for tests and examinations if you must take this medicine for a prolonged period.

▼ PRECAUTIONS

Over 60: No special problems are expected.

Driving and Hazardous Work: Do not drive or engage in hazardous work until you determine how the medicine affects you.

Alcohol: It is advisable to abstain from alcohol when fighting an infection.

Pregnancy: In some animal tests, ciprofloxacin has caused birth defects. Adequate studies in humans have not been done. The drug should be used during pregnancy only if potential benefits clearly justify the risks. Before you take ciprofloxacin, tell your doctor if you are pregnant or plan to become pregnant.

Breast Feeding: Ciprofloxacin passes into breast milk and may cause serious side effects in the nursing infant; use of the drug is discouraged when nursing.

Infants and Children: Ciprofloxacin is not recommended for use by persons under the age of 18, as it has been shown to interfere with bone development.

Special Concerns: If ciprofloxacin causes sensitivity to sunlight, stop taking the drug and try to avoid exposure to sunlight for the next 5 days; also wear protective clothing and use a sunblock. Ciprofloxacin should not be taken by patients whose work makes it impossible to avoid exposure to sunlight. It is important to drink plenty of fluids while taking this drug.

OVERDOSE
Symptoms: No specific ones have been reported.

What to Do: If you have any reason to suspect an overdose, call your doctor, emergency medical services (EMS), or the nearest poison control center.

▼ INTERACTIONS

DRUG INTERACTIONS
Consult your doctor for specific advice if you are taking aminophylline, antacids, didanosine, iron supplements, oxtriphylline, sucralfate, theophylline, warfarin, or zinc salts. Also tell your doctor if you are taking any other prescription or over-the-counter medication.

FOOD INTERACTIONS
The effects of caffeine may be magnified by this drug. Milk and dairy products can reduce blood levels of ciprofloxacin by as much as half.

DISEASE INTERACTIONS
Caution is advised when taking ciprofloxacin. Consult your doctor if you have any other medical condition. Use of ciprofloxacin can cause complications in patients with kidney disease, since this organ works to remove the medication from the body.

☰ SIDE EFFECTS ☰

SERIOUS
Serious reactions to ciprofloxacin are rare and include seizures, mental confusion, hallucinations, agitation, nightmares, depression, shortness of breath, unusual swelling in the face or extremities, and loss of consciousness. Also skin burning, redness, blisters, rash, or itching on exposure to sunlight. Call your doctor immediately.

COMMON
Increased sensitivity to sunlight (and increased risk of sunburn) for days following therapy.

LESS COMMON
Diarrhea, nausea and vomiting, stomach pain and upset, gas, headache, dizziness, insomnia, changes in taste perception, drowsiness, itching, dry mouth, unusual body aches or pains.

CITALOPRAM HYDROBROMIDE

Available in: Tablet, oral solution
Available OTC? No **As Generic?** No
Drug Class: Selective serotonin reuptake inhibitor (SSRI) antidepressant

▼ USAGE INFORMATION

WHY IT'S PRESCRIBED
To treat symptoms of major depression.

HOW IT WORKS
Citalopram increases brain levels of serotonin, a chemical that is thought to be linked to mood, emotions, and mental state.

▼ DOSAGE GUIDELINES

RANGE AND FREQUENCY
To start, 20 mg once a day, taken in the morning or evening; dose may be gradually increased by your doctor to 40 mg a day.

ONSET OF EFFECT
Unknown.

DURATION OF ACTION
Unknown.

DIETARY ADVICE
No special restrictions.

STORAGE
Store in a tightly sealed container away from moisture, heat, and direct light.

MISSED DOSE
If you miss a dose on one day, do not double the dose the next day.

STOPPING THE DRUG
Take the drug as prescribed for the full treatment period even if you notice improvement. When it is time to stop therapy, your dosage will be tapered off gradually by your doctor.

PROLONGED USE
Usual course of therapy for depression lasts 6 months to 1 year; some patients may benefit from additional therapy with this drug.

▼ PRECAUTIONS

Over 60: Adverse reactions may be more likely and more severe in older patients. A lower dose may be warranted.

Driving and Hazardous Work: Use caution when driving or engaging in hazardous work until you determine how the medicine affects you.

Alcohol: Avoid alcohol.

Pregnancy: Citalopram should be used during pregnancy only if the potential benefit justifies the potential risk to the fetus. Before you take this medicine, tell your doctor if you are pregnant or plan to become pregnant.

Breast Feeding: Citalopram passes into breast milk; caution is advised. Consult your doctor for specific advice.

Infants and Children: The safety and effectiveness of the use of citalopram in children under age 18 have not been established.

OVERDOSE
Symptoms: Dizziness, nausea, sweating, vomiting, trembling, drowsiness, rapid heartbeat.

What to Do: Call your doctor, emergency medical services (EMS), or the nearest poison control center immediately.

▼ INTERACTIONS

DRUG INTERACTIONS
Citalopram and MAO inhibitors should not be used within 14 days of each other. Very serious side effects such as myoclonus (uncontrolled muscle spasms), hyperthermia (excessive rise in body temperature), and extreme stiffness may result. The following drugs may also interact with citalopram; consult your doctor for advice if you are taking cimetidine, warfarin, lithium, carbamazepine, antifungals (such as ketoconazole, itraconazole, and fluconazole), erythromycin antibiotics, omeprazole, tricyclic antidepressants, or any prescription or over-the-counter drugs that depress the central nervous system (this includes antihistamine medications, barbiturates, sedatives, cough medicines, and decongestants).

FOOD INTERACTIONS
No known food interactions.

DISEASE INTERACTIONS
Caution is advised when taking citalopram, especially if you have heart disease or a seizure disorder. Use of citalopram may cause complications in patients with liver or kidney disease.

≡ SIDE EFFECTS ≡

SERIOUS
Chest pain, rapid or irregular heartbeat, lightheadedness or fainting. Call your doctor immediately.

COMMON
Delayed ejaculation (males), dry mouth, increased sweating, nausea, trembling, diarrhea, drowsiness, numbness, tingling, or prickling sensations.

LESS COMMON
Fatigue, fever, loss of appetite, agitation, nasal congestion, sinus infection, erectile dysfunction.

CLARITHROMYCIN

Available in: Tablets, oral suspension
Available OTC? No   **As Generic?** No
Drug Class: Macrolide antibiotic

▼ USAGE INFORMATION

WHY IT'S PRESCRIBED
To treat various bacterial infections, including those of the sinuses, tonsils, and respiratory tract (such as bronchitis and pneumonia); ear infections; and venereal disease due to chlamydial infection. Clarithromycin may also be used to treat certain skin infections, Legionnaires' disease, Lyme disease, and peptic ulcers caused by the bacterium Helicobacter pylori. Also used to prevent and, when taken with other drugs, treat a tuberculosis-like disease known as Mycobacterium avium complex (MAC), which is common in people with advanced acquired immuno-deficiency syndrome (AIDS).

HOW IT WORKS
Clarithromycin prevents bacterial cells from manufac-turing the specific proteins that are necessary for their survival.

▼ DOSAGE GUIDELINES

RANGE AND FREQUENCY
For bacterial infections—Usual adult dose: 250 to 500 mg every 12 hours, for 7 to 14 days. Children 6 months of age or older: 3.4 mg per lb of body weight, up to 500 mg every 12 hours for 10 days. To prevent MAC—500 mg, 2 times a day. To treat MAC—500 mg, 2 times a day in combination with other medications.

ONSET OF EFFECT
Within 2 hours; full effect may take 2 to 5 days before occurring.

DURATION OF ACTION
Unknown.

DIETARY ADVICE
Clarithromycin may be taken with or without food. Drink plenty of liquids.

STORAGE
Store in a tightly sealed container away from moisture, heat, and direct light.

MISSED DOSE
Take it as soon as you remember. If it is near the time for the next dose, skip the missed dose and resume your regular dosing schedule. Do not double the next dose. If you are taking 2 doses a day, wait 5 to 6 hours before taking the next dose.

STOPPING THE DRUG
For acute infections, take it exactly as prescribed for the full treatment period, even if you feel better before the scheduled end of therapy. Therapy for prevention of MAC should be lifelong.

PROLONGED USE
You may become susceptible to infections caused by germs that are not responsive to clarithromycin. Also, severe drug-induced gastrointestinal problems may result from long-term use.

▼ PRECAUTIONS

Over 60: Older patients, especially those with kidney disease, may require a decrease in dose.

Driving and Hazardous Work: No special precautions are necessary.

Alcohol: No special precautions are necessary.

Pregnancy: Adequate studies of the use of this drug during pregnancy have not been done; discuss potential risks and benefits with your doctor.

Breast Feeding: It is not known if clarithromycin passes into breast milk; consult your doctor for advice.

Infants and Children: No special problems are expected.

OVERDOSE
Symptoms: Severe nausea, vomiting, diarrhea, abdominal discomfort.

What to Do: Call your doctor, emergency medical services (EMS), or the nearest poison control center immediately.

▼ INTERACTIONS

DRUG INTERACTIONS
This drug should not be taken by patients known to have had prior allergic reactions to erythromycins or other macrolide antibiotics. Do not take clarithromycin if you are taking astemizole, pimozide, or cisapride. Also, alert your doctor if you are taking any of the following drugs: carbamazepine, digoxin, theophylline, warfarin, rifabutin, rifampin, or zidovudine.

FOOD INTERACTIONS
No known food interactions.

DISEASE INTERACTIONS
Consult your doctor if you have a history of a blood disorder, liver disease, or any allergy.

≡ SIDE EFFECTS ≡

SERIOUS
Colitis (inflammation of the lower gastrointestinal tract, with symptoms including severe abdominal pain, watery or bloody stools, severe diarrhea, fever); liver toxicity (causing fever, nausea, vomiting, yellowish tinge to eyes or skin); allergic reaction (swelling of the lips, tongue, face, and throat, breathing difficulty, skin rash or hives); blood clotting disorders (causing unusual bleeding and bruising); confusion or change in behavior; heartbeat irregularities in patients with predisposing heart conditions. Such side effects are rare, but if they do occur, stop taking the drug and seek medical assistance immediately.

COMMON
No common side effects.

LESS COMMON
Changes in taste perception; mild abdominal pain or discomfort; mild diarrhea; mild nausea or vomiting; headache; oral thrush (fungal infections of the mouth or throat).

CLONAZEPAM

Available in: Tablets, wafer
Available OTC? No   **As Generic?** Yes
Drug Class: Benzodiazepine tranquilizer; antianxiety agent

▼ USAGE INFORMATION

WHY IT'S PRESCRIBED
To control seizures; for relief of anxiety and panic attacks.

HOW IT WORKS
In general, clonazepam produces mild sedation by depressing activity in the central nervous system (the brain and spinal cord). In particular, clonazepam appears to enhance the effect of gamma-aminobutyric acid (GABA), a natural chemical that inhibits firing of neurons and dampens transmission of nerve signals, thus decreasing nervous excitation.

▼ DOSAGE GUIDELINES

RANGE AND FREQUENCY
Adults: Initial dose of 0.5 mg, 3 times a day. Patients with seizures may require significantly higher doses. Your doctor will determine the optimal dose. Maximum dose rarely exceeds 20 mg a day.

Children: Dose is based on age and body weight.

ONSET OF EFFECT
Within 1 to 2 hours.

DURATION OF ACTION
Less than 24 hours.

DIETARY ADVICE
No special restrictions.

STORAGE
Store in a tightly sealed container away from moisture, heat, and direct light.

MISSED DOSE
Take it as soon as you remember, unless your next scheduled dose is within the next 2 hours. If so, do not take the missed dose. Take your next scheduled dose at the proper time and resume your regular dosage schedule. Do not double the next dose.

STOPPING THE DRUG
Discontinuing the drug abruptly may produce withdrawal symptoms (sleep disruption, nervousness, irritability, diarrhea, abdominal cramps, muscle aches, memory impairment). Dosage should be reduced gradually according to your doctor's instructions.

PROLONGED USE
Short-term therapy (8 weeks or less) is typical; do not take it for a longer period unless so advised by your doctor.

▼ PRECAUTIONS

Over 60: Adverse reactions are more likely and more severe in older patients.

Driving and Hazardous Work: Clonazepam can impair mental alertness and physical coordination. Adjust your activities accordingly.

Alcohol: Alcohol must be avoided while taking this medication.

Pregnancy: Taking clonazepam during pregnancy is not recommended.

Breast Feeding: Clonazepam passes into breast milk and may be harmful to the infant; do not take it while nursing.

Infants and Children: This drug is rarely prescribed for young patients.

Special Concerns: Clonazepam use can lead to psychological or physical dependence. Never take more than the prescribed daily dose.

OVERDOSE
Symptoms: Extreme drowsiness, confusion, slurred speech, slow reflexes, poor coordination, staggering gait, tremor, slowed breathing, loss of consciousness.

What to Do: Call your doctor, emergency medical services (EMS), or the nearest poison control center immediately.

▼ INTERACTIONS

DRUG INTERACTIONS
Other drugs may interact with clonazepam. Consult your doctor for specific advice if you are taking any drugs that depress the central nervous system; these include antihistamines, antidepressants or other psychiatric medications, barbiturates, sedatives, cough medicines, decongestants, and painkillers. Be sure your doctor knows about any over-the-counter medication you may take.

FOOD INTERACTIONS
None reported.

DISEASE INTERACTIONS
Caution is advised when taking clonazepam. Consult your doctor if you have a history of alcohol or drug abuse, stroke or other brain disease, any chronic lung disease, hyperactivity, depression or other mental illness, sleep apnea, myasthenia gravis, epilepsy, porphyria, kidney disease, or liver disease.

≡ SIDE EFFECTS ≡

▼ SERIOUS ▼
Difficulty concentrating, outbursts of anger, other behavior problems, depression, hallucinations, low blood pressure (causing faintness or confusion), memory impairment, muscle weakness, skin rash or itching, sore throat, fever and chills, sores or ulcers in throat or mouth, unusual bruising or bleeding, extreme fatigue, yellowish tinge to eyes or skin. Call your doctor immediately.

COMMON
Drowsiness, loss of coordination, unsteady gait, dizziness, lightheadedness, slurred speech.

LESS COMMON
Change in sexual desire or ability, constipation, false sense of well-being, nausea and vomiting, urinary problems, unusual fatigue.

CLONIDINE HYDROCHLORIDE

Available in: Tablets, skin patch
Available OTC? No   **As Generic?** Yes
Drug Class: Centrally acting antihypertensive

▼ USAGE INFORMATION

WHY IT'S PRESCRIBED
To treat high blood pressure (hypertension).

HOW IT WORKS
Clonidine acts upon certain areas of the central nervous system (the brain and spinal cord) that regulate the activity of the heart and the smooth muscle tissue surrounding the arteries. It causes the blood vessels to relax and widen, which lowers blood pressure.

▼ DOSAGE GUIDELINES

RANGE AND FREQUENCY
Tablets—Adults: Initial dose is 0.1 mg, 2 times per day. Your doctor may increase this to 0.3 mg, 2 times per day. Most patients achieve adequate blood pressure control with 1 mg or less per day; maximum daily dose is 2.4 mg. Children: Pediatrician will determine proper dosage. Skin patch—The starting dose is one TTS-1 patch per week. Doses above two TTS-3 patches per week are usually not effective. The patch should be applied to a hair-less area of skin, ideally on the chest or on the upper arm. The skin must be free of rashes, blisters, or any form of skin disease.

ONSET OF EFFECT
Tablets: 30 to 60 minutes. Skin patch: 2 to 3 days.

DURATION OF ACTION
Tablets: Up to 8 hours. Skin patch: 7 days per patch, if patch is left in place as directed; otherwise, up to 8 hours from the time the patch is removed.

DIETARY ADVICE
Follow a healthy diet (low-salt, low-fat, low-cholesterol) as advised by your doctor to help control blood pressure and prevent heart disease.

STORAGE
Store in a tightly sealed container away from moisture, heat, and direct light.

MISSED DOSE
Take your missed dose as soon as you remember, unless the time for your next scheduled dose is within the next 2 hours. If so, do not take the missed dose. Take your next dose at the proper time and resume your regular dosage schedule. Do not take a double dose. If you miss more than 1 day of clonidine, inform your doctor.

STOPPING THE DRUG
Stopping clonidine abruptly can lead to a dangerous increase in blood pressure. Do not stop taking clonidine on your own, even if you are feeling better. Your doctor will gradually decrease your dose if necessary.

PROLONGED USE
Long-term use may be necessary and may lead to an increased risk of side effects.

▼ PRECAUTIONS

Over 60: Adverse reactions may be more likely and more severe in older patients.

Driving and Hazardous Work: This medication may cause drowsiness and dizziness; avoid potentially dangerous activities until you know how it affects you.

Alcohol: Avoid alcohol while taking this drug.

Pregnancy: Clonidine use is not recommended during pregnancy.

Breast Feeding: Clonidine passes into breast milk; consult your doctor for advice.

Infants and Children: This drug is not recommended for young patients.

Special Concerns: Blood pressure may rise significantly after missing a few doses.

Signs of dangerously high blood pressure are chest pain, dizziness, headache, blurred vision, confusion, restlessness, trembling of hands and fingers, anxiety, stomach pains, nausea, and vomiting. Make sure you have enough clonidine to last through weekends, vacations, or extended trips. Apply each skin patch to a different area of the chest or upper arm.

OVERDOSE
Symptoms: Low blood pressure, slow heartbeat, difficulty breathing, severe dizziness, confusion, weakness or faintness, tiny, constricted pupils.

What to Do: Call your doctor, emergency medical services (EMS), or the nearest poison control center immediately.

▼ INTERACTIONS

DRUG INTERACTIONS
Consult your doctor if you are taking beta-blockers or tricyclic antidepressants.

FOOD INTERACTIONS
No known food interactions.

DISEASE INTERACTIONS
Tell your doctor if you have any of the following problems: heart or blood vessel disease, including strokes and cardiac arrhythmias; skin disease, such as scleroderma (a concern with the skin patch only); kidney disease; mental depression; Raynaud's syndrome; or systemic lupus erythematosus.

≡ SIDE EFFECTS ≡

SERIOUS
Serious side effects are less likely when clonidine is used as directed.

COMMON
Dry mouth, reduced saliva, drowsiness, dizziness, constipation. Also itching or skin irritation (with skin patch only).

LESS COMMON
Mental depression, swelling of feet and lower legs, pale or cold fingertips and toes, vivid dreams or nightmares. Also darkening of skin (skin patch only).

CLOPIDOGREL BISULFATE

Available in: Tablets
Available OTC? No   **As Generic?** No
Drug Class: Antiplatelet drug

▼ USAGE INFORMATION

WHY IT'S PRESCRIBED
To reduce the risk of recurrence of heart attack or stroke in patients diagnosed with severe arterial disease (atherosclerosis).

HOW IT WORKS
Heart attacks and strokes occur when a blood clot that forms in a narrowed portion of an artery blocks blood flow and thus cuts off the supply of oxygen and nutrients to the tissue that lies beyond the site of the clot. Clopidogrel can prevent heart attacks and strokes by preventing the aggregation (clumping) of platelets, a type of blood cell that initiates clot formation.

▼ DOSAGE GUIDELINES

RANGE AND FREQUENCY
75 mg once a day.

ONSET OF EFFECT
2 hours or more.

DURATION OF ACTION
Unknown.

DIETARY ADVICE
Clopidogrel can be taken with or without food.

STORAGE
Store in a tightly sealed container away from moisture, heat, and direct light.

MISSED DOSE
If you miss a dose on one day, do not double up on the dose the next day. Instead, resume your regular dosage schedule.

STOPPING THE DRUG
Take it as prescribed for the full treatment period.

PROLONGED USE
Side effects are more likely with prolonged use.

≡ SIDE EFFECTS ≡

▼ SERIOUS ▼
Gastrointestinal bleeding, fainting, palpitations, extreme fatigue, shortness of breath, chest pain. Call your doctor immediately. In rare instances the drug can block production of white blood cells (a major component of the immune system), leading to potentially severe infections. Seek medical attention promptly at the first signs of infection, especially a high fever.

COMMON
Stomach pain, indigestion, diarrhea, skin rash, itching, flu-like symptoms, body aches or pain, headache, dizziness, joint pain, back pain, increased risk of upper respiratory infection.

LESS COMMON
General weakness, hernia, leg cramps, tingling and numbness in the limbs, vomiting, gout, arthritis, anxiety, insomnia, anemia, dermatitis and skin eruptions, bladder infection, cataract, conjunctivitis.

▼ PRECAUTIONS

Over 60: No special problems are expected.

Driving and Hazardous Work: The use of this drug should not impair your ability to perform such tasks safely.

Alcohol: No special precautions are necessary.

Pregnancy: Adequate human studies have not been done. Before taking clopidogrel, be sure to tell your doctor if you are pregnant or are planning to become pregnant.

Breast Feeding: Clopidogrel passes into breast milk; extreme caution is advised. Consult your doctor for specific advice.

Infants and Children: The safety and effectiveness of clopidogrel use in infants and children have not been established.

Special Concerns: Before you schedule surgery, tell the surgeon or dentist that you are taking this drug.

OVERDOSE
Symptoms: No overdose symptoms have been reported.

What to Do: If a greatly excessive dose is taken, call your doctor, emergency medical services (EMS), or the nearest poison control center.

▼ INTERACTIONS

DRUG INTERACTIONS
Consult your doctor for specific advice if you are taking any of the following drugs that may interact with clopidogrel: aspirin or any other nonsteroidal anti-inflammatory drugs (NSAIDs), phenytoin, tamoxifen, tolbutamide, torsemide, fluvastatin, or warfarin.

FOOD INTERACTIONS
No known food interactions.

DISEASE INTERACTIONS
This drug should not be used if you have a peptic ulcer or a history of brain hemorrhage. Caution is advised when taking clopidogrel. Consult your doctor if you have a history of bleeding problems or if you develop bleeding problems while taking this drug. Use of clopidogrel may cause complications in patients with liver disease, since the liver inactivates the drug.

CODEINE

Available in: Tablets, oral solution
Available OTC? No **As Generic?** Yes
Drug Class: Opioid (narcotic) analgesic

▼ USAGE INFORMATION

WHY IT'S PRESCRIBED
To treat mild to moderate pain or to control a severe cough.

HOW IT WORKS
Narcotics such as codeine relieve pain by acting on specific areas of the spinal cord and brain that process pain signals from nerves throughout the body. Codeine dulls the cough reflex, which is why it may be used to treat certain coughs.

▼ DOSAGE GUIDELINES

RANGE AND FREQUENCY
Adults—For pain: 15 to 60 mg every 3 to 6 hours as needed. Usual dose is 30 mg. For cough: 10 to 20 mg every 3 to 6 hours as needed. Children—Oral solution: For pain: 0.5 mg per 2.2 lbs (1 kg) of body weight every 4 to 6 hours as needed. For cough: Age 2: 3 mg every 4 to 6 hours. Take no more than 12 mg a day. Age 3: 3.5 mg every 4 to 6 hours. Take no more than 14 mg a day. Age 4: 4 mg every 4 to 6 hours. Take no more than 16 mg a day. Age 5: 4.5 mg every 4 to 6 hours. Take no more than 18 mg a day. Ages 6 to 12: 5 to 10 mg every 4 to 6 hours. Take no more than 60 mg per day.

ONSET OF EFFECT
30 to 45 minutes.

DURATION OF ACTION
4 to 6 hours.

DIETARY ADVICE
Codeine is constipating; make sure your diet contains adequate amounts of fiber and vegetables.

STORAGE
Store in a tightly sealed container away from moisture, heat, and direct light.

MISSED DOSE
Take it as soon as you remember. If it is near the time for the next dose, skip the missed dose and resume your regular dosage schedule. Do not double the next dose.

STOPPING THE DRUG
You should take the drug as prescribed for the full treatment period, but you may stop taking the drug if you are feeling better before the scheduled end of therapy.

PROLONGED USE
Therapy varies, depending on the cause of the pain. Some patients require long-term narcotic therapy. Side effects may be more likely with prolonged use.

▼ PRECAUTIONS

Over 60: Adverse reactions may be more likely and more severe in older patients.

Driving and Hazardous Work: The use of codeine may impair your ability to perform such tasks safely.

Alcohol: Avoid alcohol.

Pregnancy: Adequate human studies have not been completed. Before taking codeine, tell your physician if you are pregnant or plan to become pregnant.

Breast Feeding: Codeine passes into breast milk; caution is advised. Consult your doctor for specific advice.

Infants and Children: Adverse reactions may be more likely and more severe in children.

Special Concerns: Codeine can cause physical dependence. Some patients may experience withdrawal symptoms when the medication is discontinued. These may include body aches, abdominal pain, stomach cramps, diarrhea, runny nose, gooseflesh, nervousness, agitation, sweating, yawning, loss of appetite, shivering, insomnia, dilated pupils, and weakness. Do not exceed recommended doses or increase the dose on your own.

OVERDOSE
Symptoms: Confusion; sleepiness; slurred speech; unconsciousness; small, pinpoint pupils; cold, clammy skin; slow breathing; seizures; severe drowsiness, weakness, or dizziness.

What to Do: Call your doctor, emergency medical services (EMS), or the nearest poison control center immediately.

▼ INTERACTIONS

DRUG INTERACTIONS
Consult your doctor for specific advice if you are taking carbamazepine or other medicine for seizures, barbiturates, sedatives, cough medicines, decongestants, antidepressants, other prescription pain medications, MAO inhibitors, naltrexone, rifampin, or zidovudine.

FOOD INTERACTIONS
None known.

DISEASE INTERACTIONS
Consult your doctor if you have any of the following: emotional illness; brain disorders or head injury; seizures; lung disease; prostate problems or other problems with urination; gallstones; colitis; heart, kidney, liver, or thyroid disease; or a history of alcohol or drug abuse.

≣ SIDE EFFECTS ≣

SERIOUS
Serious side effects of codeine are indistinguishable from those of overdose: Confusion; sleepiness; slurred speech; unconsciousness; small, pinpoint pupils; cold, clammy skin; slow breathing; seizures; severe drowsiness, weakness, or dizziness.

COMMON
Mild dizziness or lightheadedness, nausea or vomiting, constipation, drowsiness, itching.

LESS COMMON
Headache, sweating, false sense of well-being (euphoria).

CONTRACEPTIVES, ORAL (COMBINATION PRODUCTS)

Available in: Tablets
Available OTC? No   **As Generic?** Yes
Drug Class: Hormones, estrogen with progestins

▼ USAGE INFORMATION

WHY IT'S PRESCRIBED
To prevent pregnancy.

HOW IT WORKS
Such products stop a woman's egg from fully developing each month.

▼ DOSAGE GUIDELINES

RANGE AND FREQUENCY
For 21-day cycle: 1 tablet a day for 21 days. Skip 7 days; repeat the cycle. For 28-day cycle: 1 tablet a day for 28 days. Repeat cycle. Each package of pills has 21 active tablets only, or 21 active tablets and 7 placebos. When taking placebos or no tablets, menstruation should occur.

ONSET OF EFFECT
At least 7 days.

DURATION OF ACTION
As long as tablets are taken.

DIETARY ADVICE
Take it with food if stomach upset occurs.

STORAGE
Store in a tightly sealed container away from heat and direct light.

MISSED DOSE
If you miss the first tablet of a new cycle or 1 tablet during the cycle, take the missed tablet as soon as you remember and take the next tablet at the usual time. If you miss 2 tablets in a row in the first or second week, take 2 tablets the day you remember and 2 the next day, then resume normal dosage schedule and use another birth control method until the next cycle begins. If you miss 2 tablets during the third week or 3 tablets at any time, begin a new cycle on its scheduled starting day, but use another birth control method for 7 days into the new cycle.

STOPPING THE DRUG
You may stop at any time you choose after completing a full 21-day cycle of tablets.

PROLONGED USE
See your doctor at least every 6 months.

▼ PRECAUTIONS

Over 60: Generally not used by older persons.

Driving and Hazardous Work: No special precautions are necessary.

Alcohol: No special precautions are necessary.

Pregnancy: Discontinue use if you become pregnant or suspect that you might be pregnant.

Breast Feeding: Oral contraceptive hormones pass into breast milk; avoid or discontinue use while nursing.

Infants and Children: No special problems have been found in teenagers who use oral contraception.

Special Concerns: Limit your exposure to sunlight until you determine how this medication affects you. Smoking can reduce the effectiveness of oral contraceptives and can increase the risk of potentially dangerous blood clots.

OVERDOSE
Symptoms: Unexplained vaginal bleeding.

What to Do: An overdose is unlikely to be life-threatening. However, if someone takes a much larger dose than prescribed, call your doctor, emergency medical services (EMS), or the nearest poison control center immediately.

▼ INTERACTIONS

DRUG INTERACTIONS
Consult your doctor for advice if you are taking: amiodarone, anabolic steroids, corticosteroids, androgens, anti-infectives, barbiturates, carbamazepine, carmustine, dantrolene, daunorubicin, disulfiram, divalproex, estrogens, etretinate, gold salts, griseofulvin, hydroxychloroquine, mercaptopurine, methotrexate, naltrexone, phenothiazines, phenylbutazone, phenytoin, plicamycin, primidone, rifabutin, rifampin, troleandomycin, theophylline, cyclosporine, or ritonavir.

FOOD INTERACTIONS
No known food interactions.

DISEASE INTERACTIONS
Consult your doctor if you have any of the following: endometriosis, fibroid tumors of the uterus, heart or circulation disease, a history of stroke, breast disease, cancer, gallbladder disease, diabetes, high blood cholesterol, liver disease, mental depression, epilepsy, or migraines.

≡ SIDE EFFECTS ≡

SERIOUS
Sudden, severe, or continuing stomach pain; sudden or severe headache or migraine; loss of coordination; loss of or change in vision; pains in chest, groin, or leg; sudden slurring of speech; weakness, numbness, or pain in an arm or leg; changes in uterine bleeding pattern; prolonged bleeding at menses; vaginal infection. Call your doctor immediately.

COMMON
Abdominal cramps or bloating; acne; breast pain, tenderness, or swelling; dizziness; nausea; swelling of ankles or feet; unusual fatigue; vomiting; absence of normal menstruation. Call your doctor if you do not have your period at the end of the cycle and before you start a new cycle.

LESS COMMON
Blotchy spots on skin, gain or loss of hair, increased sensitivity to sunlight, changes in sexual interest.

CYCLOBENZAPRINE

Available in: Tablets
Available OTC? No   **As Generic?** Yes
Drug Class: Muscle relaxant

▼ USAGE INFORMATION

WHY IT'S PRESCRIBED
To relieve painful, temporary muscle stiffness and spasms. It is not used for stiffness and spasms due to serious, chronic illnesses of the nervous system and muscles, such as spinal cord injury or cerebral palsy.

HOW IT WORKS
Cyclobenzaprine appears to work by decreasing nerve impulses from the brain and spinal cord that lead to tensing or tightening of muscles.

▼ DOSAGE GUIDELINES

RANGE AND FREQUENCY
Adults and teenagers 15 years of age and older: Usual dose is 10 mg, 3 times a day, which may be increased by your doctor to a maximum total dose of no more than 60 mg per day. Children and teenagers up to 15 years of age: Consult pediatrician.

ONSET OF EFFECT
Within 1 hour. The maximum effect may require 1 to 2 weeks of therapy.

DURATION OF ACTION
12 to 24 hours following a single dose.

DIETARY ADVICE
Dry mouth is a common complaint with muscle relaxants; maintain adequate fluid intake and suck on ice chips if desired.

STORAGE
Store in a tightly sealed container away from heat and direct light. Keep it away from moisture and extremes in temperature.

MISSED DOSE
Take it as soon as you remember. If it is near the time for the next dose, skip the missed dose and resume your regular dosage schedule. Do not double the next dose.

STOPPING THE DRUG
You should take it as prescribed for the full treatment period, but you may stop if you are feeling better before the scheduled end of therapy.

PROLONGED USE
Therapy with cyclobenzaprine is usually completed within 14 to 21 days. Do not take cyclobenzaprine for a longer period without your doctor's approval. Muscle pain and stiffness that does not improve within 14 to 21 days may require a more thorough evaluation.

▼ PRECAUTIONS

Over 60: Adverse reactions may be more likely and more severe in older patients.

Driving and Hazardous Work: The use of cyclobenzaprine may impair your ability to perform such tasks safely; use caution.

Alcohol: Avoid alcohol.

Pregnancy: Adequate studies of cyclobenzaprine use during pregnancy have not been done; discuss the relative risks and benefits of taking the drug with your doctor.

Breast Feeding: Cyclobenzaprine may pass into breast milk; caution is advised. Consult your doctor for advice.

Infants and Children: Cyclobenzaprine is not recommended for use by children under the age of 15.

Special Concerns: Cyclobenzaprine is not meant to be used as the only treatment for sore or stiff muscles. It should be accompanied by bed rest, physical therapy, and other measures to relieve discomfort, such as the application of heat or ice packs (as suggested by your physician).

OVERDOSE
Symptoms: Severe mental confusion, agitation, impaired concentration, difficulty walking or standing, dilated pupils, severe drowsiness, coma.

What to Do: Call emergency medical services (EMS), your doctor, or the nearest poison control center immediately.

▼ INTERACTIONS

DRUG INTERACTIONS
Consult your doctor for specific advice if you are taking sedatives, tranquilizers, or other medications that cause drowsiness (including alcohol); tricyclic antidepressants; or MAO inhibitors.

FOOD INTERACTIONS
No known food interactions.

DISEASE INTERACTIONS
Consult your doctor if you have a history of any of the following conditions: glaucoma, difficult urination, prostate problems, heart disease, or overactive thyroid.

▬ SIDE EFFECTS ▬

SERIOUS
Unusual heartbeat (racing, pounding, or fluttering), confusion, seizures, hallucinations.

COMMON
Drowsiness, dry mouth, dizziness.

LESS COMMON
Fatigue or excessive tiredness, weakness, nausea, heartburn, constipation, unpleasant bitter or metallic taste in mouth, vision problems, headache, restlessness, nervousness, difficulty urinating, unusual bleeding or bruising.

DEXAMETHASONE SYSTEMIC

Available in: Elixir, oral solution, tablets, injection
Available OTC? No   **As Generic?** Yes
Drug Class: Corticosteroid

▼ USAGE INFORMATION

WHY IT'S PRESCRIBED
To treat numerous conditions that involve inflammation (a response by body tissues, producing redness, warmth, swelling, and pain). Such conditions include arthritis, allergic reactions, asthma, some skin diseases, multiple sclerosis flare-ups, and other autoimmune diseases. Also prescribed to treat deficiency of natural steroid hormones.

HOW IT WORKS
This hormone mimics the effects of the body's natural corticosteroids. It depresses the synthesis, release, and activity of inflammation-producing body chemicals. It also suppresses the activity of the immune system.

▼ DOSAGE GUIDELINES

RANGE AND FREQUENCY
Adults and teenagers—Oral dosage: 25 to 300 mg a day, depending on condition, in 1 or several doses. Injection: 20 to 300 mg once a day, depending on condition. Children—Consult your doctor.

ONSET OF EFFECT
Within 2 hours of oral form, 1 hour of injection.

DURATION OF ACTION
More than 2 days for oral form; 6 days after injection.

DIETARY ADVICE
It can be taken with food or milk to minimize any stomach upset. Your doctor may recommend a low-salt, high-potassium, high-protein diet.

STORAGE
Store in a tightly sealed container away from moisture, heat, and direct light.

MISSED DOSE
Take it as soon as you remember. If you take several doses a day and it is close to the next dose, double the next dose. If you take 1 dose a day and you do not remember until the next day, skip the missed dose and do not double the next dose.

STOPPING THE DRUG
With long-term therapy, do not stop taking the drug abruptly; the dosage should be decreased gradually.

PROLONGED USE
See your doctor regularly for tests and examinations. Long-term use of the drug may lead to cataracts, diabetes, hypertension, or osteoporosis.

▼ PRECAUTIONS

Over 60: Adverse reactions may be more likely and more severe in older patients.

Driving and Hazardous Work: Do not drive or engage in hazardous work until you determine how the medicine affects you.

Alcohol: May cause stomach problems; avoid it unless your physician approves occasional moderate drinking.

Pregnancy: Overuse during pregnancy can retard the child's growth and cause other developmental problems. Consult your physician.

Breast Feeding: Do not use while nursing.

Infants and Children: Dexamethasone may retard the normal growth and development of bone and other tissues. Consult your doctor.

Special Concerns: Avoid immunizations with live vaccines if possible. Remember that this drug can lower your resistance to infection. Those undergoing long-term therapy should wear a medical-alert bracelet. Call your doctor if you develop a fever.

OVERDOSE
Symptoms: Fever, muscle or joint pain, nausea, dizziness, fainting, difficulty breathing. Prolonged overuse: Moon-face, obesity, unusual hair growth, acne, loss of sexual function, muscle wasting.

What to Do: Call your doctor, emergency medical services (EMS), or the nearest poison control center immediately.

▼ INTERACTIONS

DRUG INTERACTIONS
Consult your doctor for specific advice if you are taking aminoglutethimide, antacids, barbiturates, carbamazepine, griseofulvin, mitotane, phenylbutazone, phenytoin, primidone, rifampin, injectable amphotericin B, oral antidiabetes agents, insulin, digitalis drugs, diuretics, or medications containing potassium or sodium.

FOOD INTERACTIONS
Avoid excess sodium.

DISEASE INTERACTIONS
Consult your doctor if you have a history of bone disease, chicken pox, measles, gastrointestinal disorders, diabetes, recent serious infection, tuberculosis, glaucoma, heart disease, hypertension, liver or kidney disorders, high blood cholesterol, overactive or underactive thyroid, myasthenia gravis, or lupus.

≡ SIDE EFFECTS ≡

SERIOUS
Vision problems, frequent urination, increased thirst, rectal bleeding, blistering skin, confusion, hallucinations, paranoia, euphoria, depression, mood swings, redness and swelling at injection site. Call your doctor immediately.

COMMON
Increased appetite, indigestion, nervousness, insomnia, greater susceptibility to infections, increased blood pressure, slow healing of wounds, weight gain, easy bruising, fluid retention.

LESS COMMON
Change in skin color, dizziness, headache, increased sweating, unusual growth of body or facial hair, increased blood sugar, peptic ulcers, adrenal insufficiency, muscle weakness, cataracts, glaucoma, osteoporosis.

DIAZEPAM

BRAND NAMES

Di-Tran, Diastat, Diazepam Intensol, Diazepm, T-Quil, Valium, Valrelease, Vazepam, X-O'Spaz, Zetran

Available in: Tablets, capsules, injection, rectal gel
Available OTC? No **As Generic?** Yes
Drug Class: Benzodiazepine tranquilizer; antianxiety agent/muscle relaxant

▼ USAGE INFORMATION

WHY IT'S PRESCRIBED
To treat anxiety, panic attacks, and muscle spasms; also used in acute treatment of seizures.

HOW IT WORKS
Diazepam generally produces mild sedation by depressing activity in the central nervous system. This medication appears to enhance the effect of gamma-aminobutyric acid (GABA), a natural chemical produced by the body that inhibits the firing of neurons and dampens the transmission of nerve signals, thus decreasing nervous excitation.

▼ DOSAGE GUIDELINES

RANGE AND FREQUENCY
For anxiety–Adults: 2 to 10 mg, 4 times a day. Children: 1 to 2.5 mg, 3 or 4 times a day. For muscle spasms–2 to 10 mg, 2 to 4 times a day. For treatment of seizures–Injection and rectal gel: Your doctor will determine the correct dosage.

ONSET OF EFFECT
30 minutes.

DURATION OF ACTION
Up to 48 hours.

DIETARY ADVICE
No special restrictions.

STORAGE
Store in a tightly sealed container away from moisture, heat, and direct light.

MISSED DOSE
Take the missed dose if you remember within 2 hours. If more than 2 hours, skip the missed dose and return to your regular schedule. Do not double the next dose.

STOPPING THE DRUG
Discontinuing the drug abruptly may produce withdrawal symptoms (seizures, sleep disruption, nervousness, irritability, diarrhea, abdominal cramps, muscle aches, memory impairment). Dosage should be reduced gradually according to your physician's instructions.

PROLONGED USE
Diazepam may slowly lose its effectiveness with prolonged use. You should see your doctor for periodic evaluation if you must take it for an extended time.

▼ PRECAUTIONS

Over 60: Dosage is often reduced because adverse reactions are more likely and may be more severe in older patients.

Driving and Hazardous Work: Diazepam can impair mental alertness and physical coordination. Adjust your activities accordingly.

Alcohol: Alcohol intake should be extremely moderate or stopped altogether while taking this drug.

Pregnancy: Use during pregnancy should be avoided if possible. Be sure to tell your doctor if you are pregnant or plan to become pregnant.

Breast Feeding: Diazepam passes into breast milk; do not take it while nursing.

Infants and Children: Diazepam should be used by children only under close medical supervision.

Special Concerns: Diazepam use can lead to psychological or physical dependence. Never take more than the prescribed daily dose. Your physician will teach you how to determine when it is appropriate and how to properly administer the rectal gel.

OVERDOSE
Symptoms: Extreme drowsiness, confusion, slurred speech, slow reflexes, poor coordination, staggering gait, tremor, slowed breathing, loss of consciousness.

What to Do: Call your doctor, emergency medical services (EMS), or the nearest poison control center immediately.

▼ INTERACTIONS

DRUG INTERACTIONS
Other drugs may interact with diazepam. Consult your doctor for advice if you are taking any drugs that depress the central nervous system; these include antihistamines, antidepressants or other psychiatric medications, barbiturates, sedatives, cough medicines, decongestants, and painkillers. Be sure your doctor knows about any over-the-counter drug you may take.

FOOD INTERACTIONS
None reported.

DISEASE INTERACTIONS
Do not take diazepam if you have acute narrow angle glaucoma. Consult your doctor if you have a history of alcohol or drug abuse, stroke or other brain disease, any chronic lung disease, hyperactivity, depression or other mental illness, myasthenia gravis, sleep apnea, epilepsy, porphyria, kidney disease, or liver disease.

≡ SIDE EFFECTS ≡

SERIOUS
Difficulty concentrating, outbursts of anger, other behavior problems, depression, hallucinations, low blood pressure (causing faintness or confusion), memory impairment, muscle weakness, skin rash or itching, sore throat, fever and chills, sores or ulcers in throat or mouth, unusual bruising or bleeding, extreme fatigue, yellowish tinge to eyes or skin. Call your doctor immediately.

COMMON
Drowsiness, loss of coordination, unsteady gait, dizziness, lightheadedness, slurred speech.

LESS COMMON
Change in sexual desire or ability, constipation, false sense of well-being, nausea and vomiting, urinary problems, unusual fatigue.

DICLOFENAC/MISOPROSTOL

Available in: Tablets
Available OTC? No   **As Generic?** No
Drug Class: Antirheumatic

▼ USAGE INFORMATION

WHY IT'S PRESCRIBED
To relieve the symptoms of osteoarthritis or rheumatoid arthritis in patients at high risk of developing peptic ulcers as a result of NSAID therapy.

HOW IT WORKS
Diclofenac, a nonsteroidal anti-inflammatory drug (NSAID), works by interfering with the formation of prosta-glandins, substances that cause pain and inflammation. Ongoing NSAID therapy can irritate and damage the stomach lining, increasing the risk of peptic ulcers. Misoprostol, a synthetic prostaglandin, helps prevent ulcers and pro-motes healing by increasing the production of protective mucus and inhibiting the secretion of stomach acid.

▼ DOSAGE GUIDELINES

RANGE AND FREQUENCY
Osteoarthritis: 1 tablet of Arthrotec 50 (50 mg diclofenac/200 micrograms [mcg] misoprostol), 3 times a day. Rheumatoid arthritis: 1 tablet of Arthrotec 75 (75 mg diclofenac/200 mcg misoprostol), 3 to 4 times a day. Different doses may be warranted in some patients.

ONSET OF EFFECT
Unknown.

DURATION OF ACTION
Unknown.

DIETARY ADVICE
The drug should be taken with food to minimize stomach upset and diarrhea.

STORAGE
Store in a tightly sealed container away from moisture, heat, and direct light.

MISSED DOSE
Take it as soon as you remember you missed a dose. If it is near the time for the next dose, skip the missed dose and resume your regular dosage schedule. Do not double the next dose.

STOPPING THE DRUG
Take it as prescribed for the full treatment period.

PROLONGED USE
Side effects are more likely with prolonged use; regular follow-up visits with your doctor are important. To minimize the risk of an adverse effect, take the lowest effective dose for the shortest possible duration (misoprostol is generally not prescribed for longer than 4 weeks).

▼ PRECAUTIONS

Over 60: No special problems are expected.

Driving and Hazardous Work: Do not drive or engage in hazardous work until you determine how the medicine affects you.

Alcohol: Avoid alcohol, as it may increase the risk of stomach irritation.

Pregnancy: This drug combination should not be used during pregnancy. The misoprostol component can cause miscarriage and induce abortion. Before the drug can be prescribed, female patients are required to have had a negative pregnancy test within the previous 2 weeks. Therapy then begins only on the second or third day of the following menstrual period. An effective method of birth control should be used while taking this drug. If you suspect you are pregnant, stop taking the drug immediately and consult your doctor.

Breast Feeding: Avoid use while nursing.

Infants and Children: Not recommended for use by children under 18.

OVERDOSE
Symptoms: Nausea, vomiting, severe headache, confusion, seizures, tremors, sleepiness, difficulty breathing, stomach pain, severe diarrhea, fever, palpitations, dizziness or fainting, slow heartbeat.

What to Do: Call your doctor, emergency medical services (EMS), or the nearest poison control center immediately.

▼ INTERACTIONS

DRUG INTERACTIONS
The following drugs may interact with this drug: aspirin, digoxin, blood pressure medication, warfarin, methotrexate, cyclosporine, oral diabetes drugs, lithium, antacids, diuretics, or any over-the-counter drugs. Consult your doctor. To minimize the risk of diarrhea, avoid the use of magnesium-containing antacids.

FOOD INTERACTIONS
No known food interactions.

DISEASE INTERACTIONS
You should not take this drug if you have ever experienced breathing difficulty, hives, swelling of the face, tongue, or throat, or any other allergic reactions after taking aspirin or other NSAIDs. Caution is advised if you have a history of high blood pressure or asthma. Use of this drug combination may cause complications in patients with liver or kidney disease, since these organs work together to remove the medications from the body.

≡ SIDE EFFECTS ≡
▼ ▼

SERIOUS
Irregular heartbeat, fainting, coma, seizures, yellowish tinge to eyes or skin, or pain or tenderness in the upper-right abdomen. Call your doctor immediately.

COMMON
Stomach pain or upset, diarrhea, indigestion, nausea, gas.

LESS COMMON
Fatigue, fever, tremor, dizziness, loss of appetite, breathing difficulty, persistent but unproductive urge to urinate or defecate, hemorrhoids, breast pain, painful menstruation, menstrual irregularities, hives, impotence, unexpected changes in weight, muscle and joint pain, mental depression, sleeping difficulty, nightmares or unusually vivid dreams, hallucinations, irritability, nervousness, bruising, skin rash, blurred or abnormal vision.

DIGOXIN

Available in: Tablets, capsules, elixir
Available OTC? No   **As Generic?** Yes
Drug Class: Digitalis drug (cardiac glycoside)

▼ USAGE INFORMATION

WHY IT'S PRESCRIBED
To treat congestive heart failure and atrial arrhythmias (irregularities in the rhythm of the heartbeat).

HOW IT WORKS
Digitalis drugs such as digoxin enhance and strengthen the force of the heart's contractions, and help to regulate the rate and the rhythm of the heartbeat.

▼ DOSAGE GUIDELINES

RANGE AND FREQUENCY
Adults: Initial dose is 0.5 mg. Maintenance dosage, starting the next day, ranges from 0.125 to 0.25 mg a day (rarely more) taken once a day. Periodic blood tests are necessary to determine the proper dose. Children: Consult your doctor.

ONSET OF EFFECT
30 minutes to 2 hours.

DURATION OF ACTION
3 to 4 days.

DIETARY ADVICE
Take it on an empty stomach, at the same time every day. Taking digoxin with food can decrease the absorption rate and the peak concentration.

STORAGE
Store in a tightly sealed container away from moisture, heat, and direct light.

MISSED DOSE
Take it as soon as you remember. If it is within 12 hours of the next scheduled dose, skip the missed dose and resume your regular dosage schedule. Do not double the next dose.

STOPPING THE DRUG
Do not stop taking it unless a doctor advises otherwise. Abrupt discontinuation can cause serious heart problems. Most patients take digoxin for an extended period or for the rest of their lives.

PROLONGED USE
Prolonged use requires a doctor's supervision and periodic assessments of the continued need to take the drug. Blood levels of digoxin must be measured at regular intervals to ensure proper dosing.

▼ PRECAUTIONS

Over 60: Underweight or frail older persons may require a lower maintenance dose.

Driving and Hazardous Work: Digoxin may cause drowsiness or vision changes. Do not drive or engage in hazardous work until you determine how it affects you.

Alcohol: No interactions are expected.

Pregnancy: Human studies have not been done. In animal studies, no birth defects have been reported. Digoxin should be used during pregnancy only if your doctor decides it is clearly needed.

Breast Feeding: Digoxin passes into breast milk. The nursing infant should be monitored carefully. Stop using the drug or discontinue breast feeding if adverse effects develop.

Infants and Children: The dosage for infants and children must be determined by your pediatrician.

Special Concerns: You should carry a card that says you are taking digoxin. Do not take over-the-counter antacids or cold or allergy remedies without consulting your doctor. Digoxin causes impotence and enlarged breasts in a third of the men who take it. Mental changes induced by the drug may be mistaken for psychosis or senility.

OVERDOSE
Symptoms: Heart palpitations, abdominal pain, diarrhea, nausea, vomiting, very slow pulse.

What to Do: Call your doctor, emergency medical services (EMS), or the nearest poison control center immediately.

▼ INTERACTIONS

DRUG INTERACTIONS
Numerous drugs interact with digoxin and may alter blood levels of the drug, leading to toxicity. Consult your doctor for specific advice if you are taking any medications, especially antiarrhythmic drugs, such as quinidine or procainamide, airway-opening drugs (bronchodilators), antacids, antibiotics such as neomycin or tetracycline, anticholinergic drugs such as atropine, cholesterol-lowering drugs, diuretics (water pills), steroids, indomethacin, or any other heart drug.

FOOD INTERACTIONS
Ask your doctor about the advisability of eating high-potassium foods.

DISEASE INTERACTIONS
Tell your doctor if you have any other medical condition, especially lung disease, kidney disease, or poor thyroid function.

≡ SIDE EFFECTS ≡

▼ SERIOUS
Heartbeat irregularities causing dizziness, palpitations, shortness of breath, sweating, or fainting. Other serious side effects include hallucinations, confusion, and mental changes; extreme drowsiness; visual disturbances such as double vision or seeing colored halos around objects; weakness, fatigue, blurred vision; nausea; or agitation. Call your doctor immediately.

COMMON
Erectile dysfunction, male breast enlargement. Notify your doctor if such symptoms occur.

LESS COMMON
Headache, vertigo, numbness or tingling sensation, overall feeling of illness, sensitivity of eyes to light, diarrhea, vomiting. Call your doctor if such symptoms persist.

DILTIAZEM HYDROCHLORIDE

Available in: Tablets, extended-release capsules, injection
Available OTC? No   **As Generic?** Yes
Drug Class: Calcium channel blocker

▼ USAGE INFORMATION

WHY IT'S PRESCRIBED
To relieve and control angina (chest pain associated with heart disease), to reduce high blood pressure, and to correct heartbeat irregularities (cardiac arrhythmia).

HOW IT WORKS
Diltiazem interferes with the movement of calcium into heart muscle cells and the smooth muscle cells in the walls of the arteries. This action relaxes blood vessels (causing them to widen), which lowers blood pressure, increases the blood supply to the heart, and decreases the heart's overall workload.

▼ DOSAGE GUIDELINES

RANGE AND FREQUENCY
Tablets (for chest pain)—30 mg, 3 or 4 times a day to start, increased to 40 to 60 mg, 3 or 4 times a day. Extended-release capsules (for high blood pressure)—120 to 240 mg a day taken in 1 or 2 divided doses. (For heartbeat irregularities, diltiazem is administered by injection by a health care professional.)

ONSET OF EFFECT
Tablets: 30 to 60 minutes. Extended-release capsules: 2 to 3 hours.

DURATION OF ACTION
Tablets: 6 to 8 hours. Extended-release capsules: 10 to 14 hours.

DIETARY ADVICE
Diltiazem is best taken before meals or at bedtime.

STORAGE
Store tablets and capsules in a tightly sealed container away from heat, moisture, and direct light.

MISSED DOSE
Take it as soon as you remember. However, if it is near the time for the next dose, skip the missed dose and resume your regular dosage schedule. Do not double the next dose.

STOPPING THE DRUG
Do not stop taking this drug suddenly, as this may cause potentially serious health problems. If therapy is to be discontinued, dosage should be reduced gradually, according to doctor's instructions.

PROLONGED USE
No unusual side effects are expected with prolonged use.

▼ PRECAUTIONS

Over 60: Weakness, dizziness, and fainting are more likely in older persons.

Driving and Hazardous Work: Diltiazem can cause dizziness or drowsiness. Do not drive or engage in hazardous work until you determine how the medicine affects you.

Alcohol: Use alcohol with caution because it may increase the effect of the drug and cause an excessive drop in blood pressure.

Pregnancy: Birth defects have occurred in animal studies. Adequate human studies have not been done. Avoid this drug during the first 3 months of pregnancy and take it during the last 6 months only if your doctor says it is clearly needed.

Breast Feeding: Diltiazem passes into breast milk; avoid or discontinue use while breast feeding.

Infants and Children: Usually not prescribed; the safety and effectiveness of diltiazem for children under the age of 12 have not been established.

Special Concerns: It is important to brush and floss your teeth and see your dentist regularly, since using diltiazem may promote dental problems. This medication may make you sensitive to sunlight.

OVERDOSE
Symptoms: Heart block causing unusual shortness of breath; fatigue, excessive dizziness, fainting.

What to Do: Call your doctor, emergency medical services (EMS) or the nearest poison control center immediately.

▼ INTERACTIONS

DRUG INTERACTIONS
Consult your doctor for specific advice if you are taking aspirin, beta-blockers, digitalis preparations, carbamazepine, cyclosporine, digoxin, lithium, oral diabetes agents, phenytoin, rifampin, cimetidine, fluvoxamine, or ranitidine.

FOOD INTERACTIONS
Avoid excessive salt intake.

DISEASE INTERACTIONS
Consult your doctor if you have any of the following: kidney disease, liver disease, high blood pressure, or any kind of heart or blood vessel disease.

≡ SIDE EFFECTS ≡

SERIOUS
Irregular or slow heartbeat, shortness of breath, and fatigue caused by heart failure. Call a doctor immediately.

COMMON
Headache, drowsiness, swelling of feet and ankles, constipation, nausea, sudden weight gain, fatigue.

LESS COMMON
Dizziness, weakness, depression, nervousness, insomnia, confusion, slow pulse, vomiting, diarrhea, excessive urination, itch, sensitivity to sunlight, yellowish tinge to eyes or skin due to liver failure, skin rash, overgrowth of the gums.

DONEPEZIL

Available in: Tablets
Available OTC? No   **As Generic?** No
Drug Class: Acetylcholinesterase inhibitor

▼ USAGE INFORMATION

WHY IT'S PRESCRIBED
To treat mild to moderate Alzheimer's disease.

HOW IT WORKS
Donepezil prevents the breakdown of acetylcholine, a brain chemical crucial to memory. Acetylcholine deficiency is thought to result in memory loss associated with Alzheimer's disease.

▼ DOSAGE GUIDELINES

RANGE AND FREQUENCY
To start, 5 mg at bedtime. The dose may be increased after 4 to 6 weeks to 10 mg at bedtime.

ONSET OF EFFECT
Unknown.

DURATION OF ACTION
Unknown.

DIETARY ADVICE
No special restrictions.

STORAGE
Store in a tightly sealed container away from moisture, heat, and direct light.

MISSED DOSE
Skip the missed dose and resume your regular dosage schedule. Do not double the next dose.

STOPPING THE DRUG
The decision to stop taking the drug should be made by your doctor.

PROLONGED USE
No problems are expected with long-term use.

▼ PRECAUTIONS

Over 60: No special problems are expected.

Driving and Hazardous Work: Do not drive or engage in hazardous work until you determine how the medicine affects you.

Alcohol: Avoid alcohol while using this medication.

Pregnancy: In some animal studies, large doses of donepezil were shown to cause problems. Before you take donepezil, tell your doctor if you are pregnant or plan to become pregnant.

Breast Feeding: It is not known whether donepezil passes into breast milk; caution is advised. Consult your doctor for specific advice.

Infants and Children: Donepezil is not intended for use in children.

Special Concerns: Before you have any surgery or dental or emergency treatment, tell the doctor or dentist in charge that you are taking donepezil. Donepezil will not cure Alzheimer's disease and will not stop the disease from getting worse, but it will improve cognitive ability of some patients.

OVERDOSE
Symptoms: Seizures, severe nausea, slow heartbeat, increased muscle weakness, vomiting, greatly increased sweating, greatly increased watering of the mouth, weak pulse, irregular breathing, enlargement of the pupils of the eyes.

What to Do: Call your doctor, emergency medical services (EMS), or the nearest poison control center immediately.

▼ INTERACTIONS

DRUG INTERACTIONS
The following drugs may interact with donepezil. Consult your doctor for specific advice if you are taking carbamazepine, dexamethasone, ketoconazole, phenobarbital, phenytoin, quinidine, or rifampin. Also tell your doctor if you are taking any other prescription or over-the-counter medication.

FOOD INTERACTIONS
No known food interactions.

DISEASE INTERACTIONS
Caution is advised when taking donepezil. Consult your doctor if you have any of the following conditions: asthma, chronic obstructive pulmonary disease, urinary difficulties, heart disease, liver disease, a seizure disorder, stomach ulcers, or a blockage of the urinary tract.

≣ SIDE EFFECTS ≣

SERIOUS
No serious side effects are associated with the use of donepezil.

COMMON
Nausea, vomiting, diarrhea, headache, dizziness, fatigue, insomnia.

LESS COMMON
Vivid or unusual dreams, drowsiness, depression, loss of appetite, unusual bleeding or bruising, fainting, muscle cramps, frequent urination, joint pain, stiffness, or swelling.

DOXAZOSIN MESYLATE

Available in: Tablets
Available OTC? No   **As Generic?** No
Drug Class: Antihypertensive; BPH therapy agent

▼ USAGE INFORMATION

WHY IT'S PRESCRIBED
To treat mild to moderate high blood pressure; to ease urinary tract symptoms due to benign prostatic hyperplasia (BPH)–that is, noncancerous enlargement of the prostate gland, which is extremely common among men over the age of 50. Note: Findings from a major clinical trial indicate that doxazosin is associated with an unacceptably high incidence of cardiovascular complications. The American Academy of Cardiology has since recommended that physicians reconsider the use of doxazosin in the treatment of their hypertensive patients on a case-by-case basis.

HOW IT WORKS
For high blood pressure, the drug relaxes and widens blood vessels so blood passes through them more easily. For prostate enlargement, it relaxes muscles in the prostate and the opening of the bladder. Note that doxazosin will not shrink the prostate; symptoms may worsen and surgery may eventually be required.

▼ DOSAGE GUIDELINES

RANGE AND FREQUENCY
For high blood pressure, initial dose is 1 mg taken once a day. It can be increased gradually to a maximum of 16 mg a day. For prostate enlargement, initial dose is 1 mg taken once a day, which may be gradually increased to a maximum of 12 mg a day.

ONSET OF EFFECT
For high blood pressure: 1 to 2 hours. For prostate enlargement: 1 to 2 weeks.

DURATION OF ACTION
For high blood pressure: 24 hours. For prostate enlargement: Unknown.

DIETARY ADVICE
No special restrictions.

STORAGE
Store in a tightly sealed container in a dry place away from heat and direct light.

MISSED DOSE
Take it as soon as you remember. If it is near the time for the next dose, skip the missed dose and resume your regular dosage schedule. Do not double the next dose.

STOPPING THE DRUG
Take it as prescribed for the full treatment period, even if you feel better before the scheduled end of therapy.

PROLONGED USE
Consult your doctor about the need for follow-up medical examinations and laboratory studies if you must take doxazosin for a prolonged period.

▼ PRECAUTIONS

Over 60: Adverse reactions may be more likely and more severe in older patients. Dose should be increased slowly in patients over 60.

Driving and Hazardous Work: Do not drive or engage in hazardous work until you determine how the medicine affects you.

Alcohol: Alcohol should be avoided while taking this medicine because it may cause an excessive drop in blood pressure.

Pregnancy: In animal studies, very high doses of doxazosin damaged the fetus. Before taking this medicine, tell your doctor if you are pregnant or plan to become pregnant.

Breast Feeding: Doxazosin may pass into breast milk; caution is advised. Consult your doctor for advice.

Infants and Children: This drug is not recommended for use by children.

Special Concerns: The first dose is likely to cause dizziness or lightheadedness. Take the drug at night and get out of bed slowly the next day. Be cautious while exercising and during hot weather. Tell your doctor whether you will have surgery requiring general anesthesia, including dental surgery, within the next 2 months.

OVERDOSE
Symptoms: Cold, sweaty skin, rapid pulse, weakness, loss of consciousness.

What to Do: Call your doctor, emergency medical services (EMS), or the nearest poison control center immediately.

▼ INTERACTIONS

DRUG INTERACTIONS
Consult your doctor for specific advice if you are taking amphetamines, other antihypertensive drugs, nonsteroidal anti-inflammatory drugs (NSAIDs), estrogen, or sympathomimetic drugs.

FOOD INTERACTIONS
No known food interactions.

DISEASE INTERACTIONS
Use of doxazosin may cause complications in patients with liver or kidney disease, since these organs work together to remove the medication from the body. Also, consult your doctor if you have coronary artery disease, impaired blood circulation to the brain, or mental depression.

≣ SIDE EFFECTS ≣

SERIOUS
Irregular heartbeat. Call your doctor immediately. Another serious but rare side effect is priapism, a condition characterized by a prolonged or painful erection (lasting more than 4 hours).

COMMON
Dizziness, drowsiness.

LESS COMMON
Headache, weakness, palpitations, rapid pulse, pain and tingling sensations in the fingers or toes, diarrhea or constipation, runny nose, rash or itchy skin, muscle or joint pain, headache, mental depression.

ENALAPRIL MALEATE

Available in: Tablets
Available OTC? No   **As Generic?** No
Drug Class: Angiotensin-converting enzyme (ACE) inhibitor

▼ USAGE INFORMATION

WHY IT'S PRESCRIBED
To control high blood pressure; to treat congestive heart failure; to treat patients with left ventricular dysfunction (damage to the pumping chamber of the heart); and to minimize further kidney damage in diabetic patients with mild kidney disease.

HOW IT WORKS
Angiotensin-converting enzyme (ACE) inhibitors block an enzyme that produces angiotensin, a naturally occurring substance that causes blood vessels to constrict and stimulates production of the adrenal hormone, aldosterone, which promotes sodium retention in the body. As a result, ACE inhibitor medications relax blood vessels (causing them to widen) and reduce sodium retention, which in turn lowers blood pressure and so decreases the workload of the heart.

▼ DOSAGE GUIDELINES

RANGE AND FREQUENCY
Adults: 2.5 to 40 mg a day, taken 1 or 2 times a day. Children ages 1 month to 16 years (for high blood pressure): To start, 0.08 mg per kg (2.2 lbs) once a day, up to 5 mg a day. Your doctor may gradually raise the dose up to 40 mg a day.

ONSET OF EFFECT
Within 1 hour.

DURATION OF ACTION
Up to 24 hours.

DIETARY ADVICE
Take on an empty stomach, about 1 hour before mealtime. Follow your doctor's dietary advice (such as low-salt or low-cholesterol restrictions) to improve control over hypertension and heart disease. Avoid high-potassium foods like bananas and citrus fruits and juices, unless you are also taking drugs, such as diuretics, that lower potassium levels.

STORAGE
Keep in a tightly sealed container in a cool, dry place.

MISSED DOSE
Take it as soon as you remember. If it is near the time for the next dose, skip the missed dose and resume your regular dosage schedule. Do not double the next dose.

STOPPING THE DRUG
Do not stop taking this drug abruptly, as this may cause potentially serious health problems. Dosage should be reduced gradually, according to your doctor's instructions.

PROLONGED USE
See your doctor regularly for exams and tests if you must take this drug for a prolonged period. Enalapril helps control high blood pressure but does not cure it. Lifelong therapy may be necessary.

▼ PRECAUTIONS

Over 60: Smaller doses may be warranted.

Driving and Hazardous Work: Do not drive or engage in hazardous work until you determine how the medicine affects you.

Alcohol: Consume alcoholic beverages only in moderation since they may increase the effect of the medicine and cause an excessive drop in blood pressure.

Pregnancy: Enalapril use is not recommended, especially during the final 6 months of pregnancy. If you become pregnant, notify your doctor as soon as possible.

Breast Feeding: Although trace amounts of enalapril can be found in breast milk, adverse effects in infants have not been documented. Consult your doctor.

Infants and Children: Consult your pediatrician for specific advice.

OVERDOSE
Symptoms: No specific ones have been reported.

What to Do: While overdose is unlikely, call your doctor, emergency medical services (EMS), or the nearest poison control center immediately if you suspect that someone has taken a much larger dose than prescribed.

▼ INTERACTIONS

DRUG INTERACTIONS
Consult your doctor if you are taking diuretics (especially potassium-sparing diuretics), potassium supplements or drugs containing potassium, lithium, anticoagulants, anti-inflammatory drugs, or over-the-counter drugs (especially cold remedies and diet pills).

FOOD INTERACTIONS
Avoid low-salt milk and salt substitutes. Many of these products contain potassium.

DISEASE INTERACTIONS
Consult your doctor if you have lupus or if you have had a prior allergic reaction to ACE inhibitors. This drug should be used with caution by patients with severe kidney disease or renal artery stenosis (narrowing of one or both of the arteries that supply blood to the kidneys).

≡ SIDE EFFECTS ≡

SERIOUS
Fever and chills, sore throat and hoarseness, sudden difficulty breathing or swallowing, swelling of the face, mouth, or extremities, impaired kidney function (ankle swelling, decreased urination), confusion, yellow discoloration of the eyes or skin (indicating liver disorder), intense itching, chest pain or palpitations, abdominal pain. Serious side effects are very rare; contact your doctor immediately.

COMMON
Dry, persistent cough.

LESS COMMON
Dizziness or fainting, skin rash, numbness or tingling in the hands, feet, or lips, unusual fatigue or muscle weakness, nausea, drowsiness, loss of taste, headache, unusual dreams.

ERYTHROMYCIN SYSTEMIC

Available in: Capsules, tablets, oral suspension, injection
Available OTC? No   **As Generic?** Yes
Drug Class: Erythromycin antibiotic

▼ USAGE INFORMATION

WHY IT'S PRESCRIBED
To treat bacterial infections, including throat infections, pneumonia, Legionnaires' disease, chlamydia and diphtheria. It is also prescribed to prevent strep infections that may damage heart valves in susceptible patients (for example, those with a history of rheumatic fever or heart valve replacement) who are allergic to penicillin.

HOW IT WORKS
Erythromycin prevents bacterial cells from manufacturing specific proteins necessary for their survival.

▼ DOSAGE GUIDELINES

RANGE AND FREQUENCY
To treat infections–Adults and teenagers: 250 to 800 mg, 2 to 4 times a day. Children: 3.4 to 12.5 mg per lb of body weight, 2 to 4 times a day. To prevent strep infections–Adults and teenagers: 1 to 1.6 g before dental

appointment or surgery; 500 to 800 mg, 6 hours later. Children: 1.7 to 11.4 mg per lb of body weight before dental appointment or surgery; 4.5 mg per lb of body weight 6 hours later.

ONSET OF EFFECT
Immediate after injection; unknown for oral forms.

DURATION OF ACTION
Unknown.

DIETARY ADVICE
This drug is best taken on an empty stomach, at least 1 hour before or 2 hours after meals, with a full glass of water. If it causes stomach upset, it can be taken with food or milk.

STORAGE
Store in a tightly sealed container away from heat and direct light. Refrigerate liquid form but do not freeze.

MISSED DOSE
Take it as soon as you remember. If it is near the time for the next dose, skip

the missed dose and resume your regular dosage schedule. Do not double the next dose.

STOPPING THE DRUG
Take it as prescribed for the full treatment period.

PROLONGED USE
You should see your doctor regularly for tests and examinations, including those to evaluate liver function, if this medicine is taken for a prolonged period.

▼ PRECAUTIONS

Over 60: Older patients may be at higher risk of experiencing hearing loss as a side effect of the drug.

Driving and Hazardous Work: No special precautions are necessary.

Alcohol: No special warnings.

Pregnancy: Erythromycin has been shown to cause liver damage in some pregnant women. It has not been shown to cause birth defects or other problems in babies. Before taking erythromycin, tell your doctor if you are pregnant or if you plan to become pregnant.

Breast Feeding: Erythromycin passes into breast milk; caution is advised. Consult your doctor for specific advice.

Infants and Children: No special problems expected.

Special Concerns: Consult your doctor if your symptoms do not improve, or instead become worse, after a few days of therapy.

▼ OVERDOSE

Symptoms: Severe nausea, vomiting, abdominal pain, diarrhea, dizziness, loss of hearing.

What to Do: Call your doctor, emergency medical services (EMS), or the nearest poison control center immediately.

▼ INTERACTIONS

DRUG INTERACTIONS
Do not use erythromycin if you are taking astemizole or cisapride. Consult your doctor for specific advice if you are taking acetaminophen, amiodarone, anabolic steroids, androgens, antibiotics, azithromycin, carbamazepine, carmustine, chloramphenicol, chloroquine, clarithromycin, cyclosporine, dantrolene, daunorubicin, disulfiram, divalproex, estrogens, etretinate, gold salts, hydroxychloroquine, lincomycin, methotrexate, mercaptopurine, methyldopa, naltrexone, oral contraceptives, phenothiazines, phenytoin, plicamycin, theophylline, valproic acid, warfarin, tacrolimus, disopyramide, lovastatin, or bromocriptine.

FOOD INTERACTIONS
No known food interactions.

DISEASE INTERACTIONS
Use of this medication is not advised for patients who have a previous history of heart rhythm disorders, kidney disease, liver disease, or hearing problems. Consult your doctor.

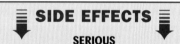

SIDE EFFECTS

SERIOUS
Fever, nausea, skin reddening or itching, severe stomach pain, yellow discoloration of the eyes or skin, fainting, slow or irregular heartbeat in patients with predisposing heart conditions, breathing difficulty, persistent or severe diarrhea, abdominal pain, temporary deafness. Also pain, swelling, or redness at injection site. Although serious side effects are rare, call your doctor immediately.

COMMON
Stomach cramps and abdominal discomfort, diarrhea, nausea, vomiting.

LESS COMMON
Soreness of mouth or tongue, vaginal itching or discharge.

ESTRADIOL

Available in: Tablets, skin patch, vaginal cream, injection
Available OTC? No   **As Generic?** Yes
Drug Class: Female sex hormone

▼ USAGE INFORMATION

WHY IT'S PRESCRIBED
To provide estrogen when the body does not produce enough; to treat carefully selected cases of advanced breast cancer; to reduce risk of osteoporosis after menopause; to ease unpleasant symptoms of menopause, including vaginal dryness; to prevent breast engorgement following childbirth; to ease symptoms of advanced prostate cancer.

HOW IT WORKS
In women, estradiol replaces deficient natural levels of estrogen in the body. In men, the hormone inhibits growth of cells in the prostate gland.

▼ DOSAGE GUIDELINES

RANGE AND FREQUENCY
To treat breast cancer: 10 mg, 3 times a day. For postmenopausal vaginal dryness or prevention of osteoporosis: 1 to 2 mg a day of oral form, or 10 to 20 mg injected every 4 weeks, or 1 Estraderm, Alora, or Vivelle patch (0.05 mg) 2 times a week or 1 Climara patch weekly. A progestin should also be taken for 10 to 14 days in each month of use, except in women who have had a hysterectomy. To relieve postmenopausal vaginal dryness using intravaginal estrogen creams: To start, ½ to 1 applicatorful daily and tapered to 1 applicatorful 1 to 3 times weekly. To treat menopausal symptoms: 1 to 5 mg injected every 3 to 4 weeks. To prevent breast engorgement after childbirth: 10 to 25 mg injected in a muscle at the time of delivery. To treat prostate cancer: 1 to 2 mg, 3 times daily.

ONSET OF EFFECT
Within 1 hour.

DURATION OF ACTION
Up to 24 hours.

DIETARY ADVICE
No special restrictions.

STORAGE
Keep in a tightly sealed container away from heat and direct light.

MISSED DOSE
Take the missed dose as soon as you remember. If it is near time for the next dose, skip the missed dose and resume your regular dosage schedule. Do not double the next dose.

STOPPING THE DRUG
The decision to stop taking the drug should be made in consultation with your doctor.

PROLONGED USE
May increase the risk of endometrial cancer and perhaps breast cancer. Consult your doctor about periodic examinations and other measures to help prevent these diseases.

▼ PRECAUTIONS

Over 60: No special problems are expected.

Driving and Hazardous Work: Do not drive or engage in hazardous work until you determine how the medicine affects you.

Alcohol: No special warnings.

Pregnancy: Not recommended during pregnancy; estrogens have been shown to cause birth defects in animals and humans.

Breast Feeding: Do not use estradiol while nursing.

Infants and Children: Not recommended for use by young patients in whom bone growth is not complete.

Special Concerns: Swelling or bleeding of gums may occur; see your dentist regularly. Do not apply a patch to the same site more than once a week.

OVERDOSE
Symptoms: Nausea, unexpected vaginal bleeding.

What to Do: An overdose is unlikely to occur. However, if someone takes a much larger dose than prescribed, seek immediate medical assistance.

▼ INTERACTIONS

DRUG INTERACTIONS
Consult your doctor for specific advice if you are taking acetaminophen, amiodarone, anticonvulsants, anti-infective drugs, antithyroid agents, carmustine, chloroquine, dantrolene, daunorubicin, gold salts, divalproex, etretinate, hydroxychloroquine, mercaptopurine, methotrexate, oral contraceptives, methyldopa, naltrexone, phenothiazines, plicamycin, steroids, bromocriptine or cyclosporine.

FOOD INTERACTIONS
No known food interactions.

DISEASE INTERACTIONS
You should not take estradiol if you have blood clot disorders, breast cancer, any hormone-dependent cancer, or abnormal genital bleeding.

≡ SIDE EFFECTS ≡

SERIOUS
For men being treated for prostate cancer: Sudden or severe headache, loss of coordination, sudden changes in vision, pains in chest, groin, or leg, shortness of breath, slurring of speech, weakness or numbness in arm or leg. For women: Breast pain or enlargement, swelling of legs and feet, rapid weight gain. Call your doctor immediately.

COMMON
Abdominal bloating, stomach cramps, loss of appetite, skin irritation at site of patch.

LESS COMMON
Diarrhea, dizziness, headaches, discomfort when wearing contact lenses, decreased sexual desire in men, increased sexual desire in women, vomiting.

ESTROGENS, CONJUGATED

Available in: Tablets, injection, vaginal cream
Available OTC? No   **As Generic?** Yes
Drug Class: Female sex hormone

▼ USAGE INFORMATION

WHY IT'S PRESCRIBED
To provide estrogen after menopause, when the body produces too little; to treat carefully selected cases of advanced breast cancer; to reduce risk of osteoporosis after menopause; to ease unpleasant symptoms of menopause, including vaginal dryness; to prevent breast engorgement following childbirth; or to ease symptoms of advanced prostate cancer.

HOW IT WORKS
In women, conjugated estrogens replace deficient natural levels of estrogen in the body. In men, estrogens inhibit growth of cells in the prostate gland.

▼ DOSAGE GUIDELINES

RANGE AND FREQUENCY
Usual adult dose is taken in cycles, with no dosing on certain days of the month. Women must also take a progestin 10 to 14 days in each month of use, except those who have had a hysterectomy (these women may take estrogen daily). To treat breast cancer in men or postmenopausal women: 10 mg, 3 times a day for 3 months or more. To prevent bone loss from osteoporosis: 0.3 to 1.25 mg a day. To ease symptoms of menopause: 0.625 to 1.25 mg a day. To treat prostate cancer: 1.25 to 2.5 mg a day.

ONSET OF EFFECT
Unknown.

DURATION OF ACTION
Unknown.

DIETARY ADVICE
Conjugated estrogens may be taken with food to reduce stomach upset.

STORAGE
Store in a tightly sealed container away from moisture, heat, and direct light. Keep it away from extremes in temperature. Keep the liquid form refrigerated, but do not allow the medication to freeze.

MISSED DOSE
Take it as soon as you remember. If it is near the time for the next dose, skip the missed dose and resume your regular dosage schedule. Do not double the next dose.

STOPPING THE DRUG
The decision to stop taking the drug should be made by your doctor.

PROLONGED USE
Prolonged use of estrogens has been reported to increase the risk of endometrial cancer and perhaps of breast cancer. Consult your doctor about the need for periodic examinations and other measures to screen for these diseases.

▼ PRECAUTIONS

Over 60: No special problems are expected.

Driving and Hazardous Work: Use of this hormone should not impair your ability to perform such tasks safely.

Alcohol: No special warnings.

Pregnancy: Do not use if you are pregnant. Estrogen use in pregnant women has been associated with birth defects.

Breast Feeding: Talk to your doctor about whether the benefits of the therapy outweigh the potential harm to the nursing infant.

Infants and Children: Should be used with caution by children, as the drug may interfere with bone growth.

OVERDOSE
Symptoms: Nausea, unexpected vaginal bleeding.

What to Do: An overdose of estrogen is unlikely to be life-threatening. However, if someone takes a much larger dose than prescribed, call your doctor, emergency medical services (EMS), or the nearest poison control center immediately.

▼ INTERACTIONS

DRUG INTERACTIONS
Other drugs may interact with estrogens. Consult a doctor if you are taking anticoagulants, anticonvulsants, antidiabetic drugs, thyroid hormones, tricyclic antidepressants, barbiturates, tranquilizers, cyclosporine, corticosteroids, corticotropin, tamoxifen, rifampin, carbamazepine, or bromocriptine.

FOOD INTERACTIONS
Calcium supplements used with estrogen may increase calcium absorption. Vitamin C may increase the effects of estrogen.

DISEASE INTERACTIONS
You should not take conjugated estrogens if you have thrombophlebitis, thromboembolitis, breast cancer, any hormone-dependent cancer, or abnormal genital bleeding. Consult your doctor if you have any of the following: a history of liver disease, heart attack, stroke, a blood clotting disorder, gallbladder disease or gallstones, or if you smoke tobacco heavily.

≡ SIDE EFFECTS ≡

SERIOUS
Women: Breast pain or enlargement; swelling of legs and feet; rapid weight gain. Men being treated for prostate cancer: Sudden or severe headache; loss of coordination; sudden changes in vision; pains in chest, groin, or leg; sudden shortness of breath; slurred speech; weakness or numbness in arm or leg. Call your doctor immediately.

COMMON
Abdominal bloating or cramps, loss of appetite, breast tenderness.

LESS COMMON
Diarrhea, dizziness, headaches, discomfort when wearing contact lenses, decreased sexual desire in men, increased sexual desire in women, vomiting.

ESTROGENS, CONJUGATED/ MEDROXYPROGESTERONE ACETATE

Available in: Tablets
Available OTC? No **As Generic?** No
Drug Class: Female sex hormones

▼ USAGE INFORMATION

WHY IT'S PRESCRIBED
To provide estrogen after menopause, when the body produces too little; to reduce the risk of osteoporosis; to ease unpleasant symptoms of menopause, including hot flashes and vaginal dryness; and to treat atrophy (wasting) of the vulva or vagina. Estrogen also protects women from developing coronary artery disease.

HOW IT WORKS
Estrogen protects against osteoporosis by diminishing the loss of bone that results from estrogen deficiency. Conjugated estrogens replace deficient levels of natural estrogen in women. When given alone to menopausal women, estrogen increases the risk of excessive growth of the uterine lining, which can lead to endometrial cancer. Medroxyprogesterone (a type of progestin) given in conjunction with estrogen nearly eliminates this risk.

▼ DOSAGE GUIDELINES

RANGE AND FREQUENCY
1 tablet, taken once a day. Prempro contains 0.625 mg of estrogen (Premarin) and 2.5 mg of medroxyprogesterone (MPA). Premphase contains 0.625 mg Premarin and 5 mg of MPA.

ONSET OF EFFECT
Unknown.

DURATION OF ACTION
As long as the medication is taken.

DIETARY ADVICE
Take it with food to reduce stomach upset.

STORAGE
Store in a sealed container away from moisture, heat, and direct light. Keep it away from temperature extremes.

MISSED DOSE
If you miss a dose on one day, do not double the dose the next day. Resume your regular dosage schedule.

STOPPING THE DRUG
The decision to stop taking this hormone combination should be made in consultation with your doctor.

PROLONGED USE
You should be reevaluated at 3-month to 6-month intervals by your doctor to determine whether or not continued treatment is necessary.

▼ PRECAUTIONS

Over 60: No special problems are expected.

Driving and Hazardous Work: Use of this hormone combination should not impair your ability to perform such tasks safely.

Alcohol: No special warnings.

Pregnancy: Do not use this hormone combination if you are or are planning to become pregnant. Estrogen use in pregnant women has been associated with birth defects in the fetus.

Breast Feeding: Do not use this hormone combination if you are nursing.

Infants and Children: Not recommended for use by children.

Special Concerns: When this hormone combination is being used in the management or prevention of osteoporosis, regular weight-bearing exercise and good nutrition are important.

OVERDOSE
Symptoms: No serious ill effects have been reported following an overdose. However, nausea, vomiting, and withdrawal bleeding may occur when extremely large doses are ingested.

What to Do: An overdose is unlikely. However, if someone takes a much larger dose than prescribed, seek medical attention.

▼ INTERACTIONS

DRUG INTERACTIONS
Other drugs may interact with this hormone combination. Consult your doctor if you are taking anticoagulants, anticonvulsants, antidiabetic drugs, thyroid hormones, tricyclic antidepressants, barbiturates, tranquilizers, cyclosporine, corticosteroids, corticotropin, tamoxifen, rifampin, carbamazepine, or bromocriptine.

FOOD INTERACTIONS
Estrogen may increase calcium absorption from calcium supplements. Vitamin C may increase the effects of estrogen.

DISEASE INTERACTIONS
You should not take this hormone combination drug if you have thrombophlebitis, breast cancer, any hormone-dependent cancer, or abnormal vaginal bleeding. Consult a doctor if you have a history of any of the following: liver disease, heart attack, diabetes mellitus, stroke, a blood clotting disorder, thromboembolic disease, gallbladder disease or gallstones, liver disease, or if you are a heavy smoker of cigarettes.

≡ SIDE EFFECTS ≡

SERIOUS
The most serious side effect is a modest increase in the incidence of breast cancer among women taking estrogen, especially for a long time (10 years or longer). Other side effects requiring your doctor's attention include swelling of legs and feet, rapid weight gain, abnormal menstrual bleeding, mental depression, and skin rash.

COMMON
Nausea, breast tenderness, headache, abdominal pain.

LESS COMMON
Change in appetite, vomiting, stomach cramps or bloating, change in blood pressure, dizziness, nervousness, insomnia, sleepiness, increase or decrease in weight, fatigue, backache.

FAMOTIDINE

BRAND NAMES

Pepcid, Pepcid AC, Pepcid RPD

Available in: Tablets, powder for suspension, orally disintegrating and chewable tablets
Available OTC? Yes   **As Generic?** No
Drug Class: Histamine (H2) blocker

▼ USAGE INFORMATION

WHY IT'S PRESCRIBED
To treat heartburn, ulcers of the stomach and duodenum, conditions that cause excess production of stomach acid (such as Zollinger-Ellison syndrome), and gastroesophageal reflux (backwash of stomach acid into the esophagus, resulting in heartburn). Chewable tablets are taken for prevention or treatment of heartburn.

HOW IT WORKS
Famotidine blocks the action of histamine (a compound produced in the body's cells), which in turn decreases the stomach's secretion of hydrochloric acid. Once the production of stomach acid is decreased, the body is better able to heal itself.

▼ DOSAGE GUIDELINES

RANGE AND FREQUENCY
To prevent heartburn: 10 mg, 1 hour before meals. For excess stomach acid: 20 to 160 mg every 6 hours. For acid reflux disease: 20 mg twice a day for up to 6 weeks. For stomach ulcers: 40 mg once a day for 8 weeks. For duodenal ulcers: To start, 40 mg once a day at bedtime or 20 mg twice a day; later, 20 mg once a day. Chewable tablets—For treatment of heartburn: Chew one tablet. For prevention of heartburn: Chew one tablet 15 to 60 minutes before eating.

ONSET OF EFFECT
Prescription form: Within 30 minutes. The lower dosage in the nonprescription form may take 45 minutes to relieve heartburn.

DURATION OF ACTION
Up to 12 hours.

DIETARY ADVICE
Take it after meals or with milk to minimize stomach irritation. Avoid foods that cause stomach irritation. Take chewable tablet with a glass of water.

STORAGE
Store tablets in a tightly sealed container away from heat, moisture, and direct light. After powder vials are reconstituted, store the medicine in the refrigerator, but keep it from freezing. Discard after 30 days.

MISSED DOSE
Take it as soon as you remember. If it is near the time for the next dose, skip the missed dose and resume your regular dosage schedule. Do not double the next dose.

STOPPING THE DRUG
The decision to stop taking the prescription drug should be made in consultation with your doctor.

PROLONGED USE
Do not take the prescription drug for more than 8 weeks unless your doctor orders it. Do not take the over-the-counter drug for more than 2 weeks unless otherwise instructed by your doctor.

▼ PRECAUTIONS

Over 60: Adverse reactions may be more likely and more severe in older patients.

Driving and Hazardous Work: Do not drive or engage in hazardous work until you determine how the medicine affects you.

Alcohol: Avoid alcohol while taking this drug; it may slow recovery. Also, this drug increases blood alcohol levels.

Pregnancy: Risks vary, depending on the patient and the dosage prescribed. Consult your physician for advice.

Breast Feeding: Famotidine passes into breast milk; you should avoid or discontinue use while breast feeding.

Infants and Children: Famotidine is not generally prescribed for infants and children.

Special Concerns: If necessary, famotidine may be given with antacids. Avoid cigarette smoking because it may increase secretion of stomach acid and thus worsen your condition.

OVERDOSE
Symptoms: Confusion, slurred speech, rapid heartbeat, difficulty breathing, delirium.

What to Do: Call your doctor, emergency medical services (EMS), or the nearest poison control center immediately.

▼ INTERACTIONS

DRUG INTERACTIONS
None reported.

FOOD INTERACTIONS
Carbonated drinks, citrus fruits and juices, caffeine-containing beverages, and other acidic foods or liquids may irritate the stomach or interfere with the therapeutic action of famotidine.

DISEASE INTERACTIONS
Patients with kidney disease should use famotidine in smaller, limited doses and only under careful supervision of a physician.

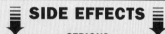 SIDE EFFECTS

SERIOUS
Irregular heart rhythm (palpitations), slowed heartbeat, severe blood problems resulting in unusual bleeding, bruising, fever, chills, and increased susceptibility to infection. Call your doctor immediately.

COMMON
Headache, fatigue, drowsiness, dizziness, nausea, vomiting, abdominal pain, diarrhea, constipation.

LESS COMMON
Blurred vision, decreased sexual desire or function, temporary hair loss, hallucinations, depression, insomnia, skin rash, hives, or redness.

FELODIPINE

Available in: Tablets, extended-release tablets
Available OTC? No   **As Generic?** No
Drug Class: Calcium channel blocker

▼ USAGE INFORMATION

WHY IT'S PRESCRIBED
To control high blood pressure (hypertension).

HOW IT WORKS
Felodipine interferes with the movement of calcium into heart muscle cells and the smooth muscle cells in the walls of the arteries. This action relaxes blood vessels (causing them to widen), which lowers blood pressure, increases the blood supply to the heart, and decreases the heart's overall workload.

▼ DOSAGE GUIDELINES

RANGE AND FREQUENCY
To start, 5 to 10 mg once a day. The dose may be increased to a maximum of 20 mg once a day. For patients over 65, starting dose is 2.5 mg per day, to a maximum of 10 mg per day.

ONSET OF EFFECT
Within 2 to 5 hours.

DURATION OF ACTION
24 hours.

DIETARY ADVICE
Felodipine should be taken either on an empty stomach or with a light meal. Do not crush or chew tablets.

STORAGE
Store in a tightly sealed container away from moisture, heat, and direct light.

MISSED DOSE
Take it as soon as you remember. However, if it is near the time for the next dose, skip the missed dose and resume your regular dosage schedule. Do not double the next dose.

STOPPING THE DRUG
Do not stop taking felodipine suddenly, as this may cause potentially serious health problems. If therapy is to be discontinued, the dosage should be reduced gradually, according to your doctor's instructions.

PROLONGED USE
Consult your doctor about the need for medical examinations or laboratory tests to check liver function, kidney function, and heart function.

▼ PRECAUTIONS

Over 60: Older patients are prescribed lower starting doses, which may be gradually increased until the doctor determines the appropriate individual maintenance dose.

Driving and Hazardous Work: Do not drive or engage in hazardous work until you determine how felodipine affects you.

Alcohol: Avoid alcohol while taking this medication as it may cause an excessive drop in blood pressure.

Pregnancy: Consult your physician to determine whether the benefits of felodipine outweigh its possible risks while pregnant.

Breast Feeding: Felodipine may pass into breast milk; caution is advised. Consult your doctor for advice.

Infants and Children: Felodipine is generally not prescribed for children.

Special Concerns: Tell all your health care providers that you are taking felodipine and carry a note that says you take this medicine. Felodipine can cause erectile dysfunction in some men. Nicotine can reduce the effectiveness of the medicine. Hot environments can also exaggerate the drug's blood-pressure-lowering effect.

OVERDOSE
Symptoms: Weakness, light-headedness, rapid pulse, shortness of breath, tremors, flushed skin, fainting, and slurred speech.

What to Do: Call your doctor, emergency medical services (EMS), or the nearest poison control center immediately.

▼ INTERACTIONS

DRUG INTERACTIONS
Consult your doctor for advice if you are taking anti-convulsants, beta-blockers, digitalis drugs, carbamazepine, cyclosporine, digoxin, disopyramide, magnesium, phenobarbital, phenytoin, quinidine, rifampin, cimetidine, or erythromycin.

FOOD INTERACTIONS
Grapefruit juice should be avoided because it can amplify the effect of the drug and cause a serious drop in blood pressure. Avoid excessive salt intake.

DISEASE INTERACTIONS
Caution is advised when taking felodipine. Consult your doctor if you have any of the following: congestive heart failure, a history of heart attack or stroke, heart rhythm disturbances, or impaired liver or kidney function.

≡ SIDE EFFECTS ≡

▼ SERIOUS ▼
Irregular or slow heartbeat, low blood pressure (causing dizziness or faintness).

COMMON
Flushing or skin rash; headache; swelling of the lower legs or feet.

LESS COMMON
Dizziness, numbness or tingling sensation, chest pain, palpitations, weakness, runny nose, rapid pulse, sore throat, abdominal discomfort, nausea, constipation or diarrhea, cough, muscle cramps, back pain, overgrowth of the gums.

FEXOFENADINE

Available in: Capsules
Available OTC? No   **As Generic?** No
Drug Class: Antihistamine

▼ USAGE INFORMATION

WHY IT'S PRESCRIBED
To prevent or relieve symptoms of hay fever and other allergies, and to treat itchy skin and hives.

HOW IT WORKS
Fexofenadine blocks the effects of histamine, a naturally occurring substance within the body that causes swelling, itching, sneezing, watery eyes, hives, and other symptoms of allergic reaction.

▼ DOSAGE GUIDELINES

RANGE AND FREQUENCY
For adults and children age 12 and over: 60 mg, 2 times a day. For patients with decreased kidney function, a starting dose of 60 mg once a day is recommended. Children under age 12: Safety and effectiveness of fexofenadine in this age group have not been established.

ONSET OF EFFECT
Within 1 to 2 hours.

DURATION OF ACTION
12 hours or longer.

DIETARY ADVICE
This drug can be taken without regard to food or drink.

STORAGE
Store in a tightly sealed container in a dry place away from heat and direct light at room temperature.

MISSED DOSE
Take it as soon as you remember. If it is near the time for the next dose, skip the missed dose and resume your regular dosage schedule. Do not double the next dose.

STOPPING THE DRUG
You should take it as prescribed for the full treatment period, but you may stop if you are feeling better before the scheduled end of therapy. Fexofenadine can be used as needed to relieve symptoms of hay fever or other allergies.

PROLONGED USE
Tolerance, or decreased responsiveness to the drug, generally does not develop with prolonged use of fexofenadine; if it does, consult your physician. No special problems are expected with long-term use.

≡ SIDE EFFECTS ≡

SERIOUS
No serious side effects are associated with the use of fexofenadine.

COMMON
No common side effects are associated with the use of fexofenadine.

LESS COMMON
Drowsiness, fatigue, stomach upset, painful menstrual bleeding.

▼ PRECAUTIONS

Over 60: No special problems are expected.

Driving and Hazardous Work: In rare cases fexofenadine may cause drowsiness and fatigue. Do not drive or engage in hazardous work until you determine how the medicine affects you.

Alcohol: No special precautions are necessary.

Pregnancy: Adequate and well-controlled studies in humans have not been done. Consult your doctor about taking fexofenadine if you are pregnant or are planning to become pregnant.

Breast Feeding: Fexofenadine may pass into breast milk; caution is advised. Consult your doctor for specific advice about the use of fexofenadine while nursing.

Infants and Children: Side effects are not expected to be any different in children ages 12 to 18 than those in patients 18 and older. The safety and effectiveness of fexofenadine for children up to 12 years of age have not been established.

OVERDOSE
Symptoms: Extreme drowsiness or fatigue.

What to Do: An overdose of fexofenadine is unlikely to be life-threatening. However, if someone takes a much larger dose than prescribed, call your doctor, emergency medical services (EMS), or local poison control right away.

▼ INTERACTIONS

DRUG INTERACTIONS
There are no known interactions between fexofenadine and other drugs.

FOOD INTERACTIONS
No known food interactions.

DISEASE INTERACTIONS
Consult your physician before taking if you have impaired kidney function .

FEXOFENADINE/PSEUDOEPHEDRINE

Available in: Extended-release tablets
Available OTC? No   **As Generic?** No
Drug Class: Antihistamine/decongestant

▼ USAGE INFORMATION

WHY IT'S PRESCRIBED
To prevent or relieve symptoms of seasonal allergies such as hay fever.

HOW IT WORKS
Fexofenadine blocks the effects of histamine, a naturally occurring substance within the body that causes swelling, itching, sneezing, watery eyes, hives, and other symptoms of allergic reaction. Pseudoephedrine narrows and constricts blood vessels to decrease the blood flow to swollen nasal passages and other tissues, which in turn reduces nasal secretions, shrinks swollen nasal mucous membranes, and improves airflow in nasal passages.

▼ DOSAGE GUIDELINES

RANGE AND FREQUENCY
Adults and teenagers: 1 tablet (60 mg fexofenadine/120 mg pseudoephedrine) twice a day.

ONSET OF EFFECT
Within 1 to 2 hours.

DURATION OF ACTION
12 hours or longer.

DIETARY ADVICE
This medication should be taken at least 1 hour before or 2 hours after a meal. Taking it with food delays the onset of the drug's effects. The tablet should be swallowed whole.

STORAGE
Store in a tightly sealed container away from moisture, heat, and direct light.

MISSED DOSE
Take it as soon as you remember. If it is near the time for the next dose, skip the missed dose and resume your regular dosage schedule. Do not double the next dose.

STOPPING THE DRUG
You may stop taking it before the scheduled end of therapy if you are feeling better.

PROLONGED USE
Consult your doctor about taking this drug for more than 5 to 7 days.

▼ PRECAUTIONS

Over 60: Adverse reactions may be more likely and more severe in older patients.

≣ SIDE EFFECTS ≣

SERIOUS
Palpitations, shortness of breath, breathing difficulty. Stop taking the medication and call your doctor right away.

COMMON
Headache, insomnia, nausea.

LESS COMMON
Dry mouth, indigestion, throat irritation, dizziness, agitation, back pain, anxiety, nervousness, stomach pain, upper respiratory infection.

Driving and Hazardous Work: Do not drive or engage in hazardous work until you determine how the medicine affects you.

Alcohol: No special warnings.

Pregnancy: Adequate human studies have not been done. Before taking this drug, tell your doctor if you are pregnant or are planning to become pregnant. Discuss with your doctor the relative risks and benefits of using this drug while pregnant.

Breast Feeding: The pseudoephedrine component of this drug passes into breast milk; avoid or discontinue taking this drug while breast feeding.

Infants and Children: Not recommended for use by children under age 12.

Special Concerns: If your symptoms do not improve within 7 days, check with your doctor. To help prevent insomnia, take the last dose of the day at least 2 hours before your bedtime.

OVERDOSE
Symptoms: No cases of overdose have been reported.

What to Do: An overdose is unlikely; however, if you have reason to suspect an overdose has occurred, call emergency medical services (EMS) to receive evaluation and treatment.

▼ INTERACTIONS

DRUG INTERACTIONS
This drug and MAO inhibitors should not be used within 14 days of each other. Consult your doctor for advice if you are taking antihypertensives or digitalis drugs.

FOOD INTERACTIONS
No known food interactions.

DISEASE INTERACTIONS
You should not take this medication if you have a history of narrow-angle glaucoma, urinary retention, severe high blood pressure, or severe coronary artery disease. Caution is advised if you have mild to moderate high blood pressure, diabetes mellitus, a history of angina or heart attack, an overactive thyroid gland, impaired kidney function, or an enlarged prostate.

FINASTERIDE

Available in: Tablets
Available OTC? No   **As Generic?** No
Drug Class: 5-alpha reductase inhibitor

▼ USAGE INFORMATION

WHY IT'S PRESCRIBED
To treat benign prostatic hyperplasia (BPH)—that is, noncancerous enlargement of the prostate gland, which is extremely common among men over 50. Also used to treat male pattern hair loss.

HOW IT WORKS
Finasteride halts or reverses enlargement of the prostate by blocking the action of the enzyme 5-alpha reductase, which the body needs to produce dihydrotestosterone (DHT), a chemical involved in the mechanism that enlarges the prostate. DHT is also integral to the process of male pattern hair loss; by decreasing DHT concentrations in the scalp, finasteride may slow or reverse this process.

▼ DOSAGE GUIDELINES

RANGE AND FREQUENCY
For BPH: 5 mg once a day.
For male pattern hair loss: 1 mg once a day.

ONSET OF EFFECT
Unknown.

DURATION OF ACTION
For BPH: 24 hours for a single dose; up to 2 weeks after standard therapy is ended. For hair loss: New hair that results from finasteride treatments will likely regress following discontinuation of the medication.

DIETARY ADVICE
Finasteride can be taken without regard to diet. If you have trouble swallowing the tablet whole, you can crush it and take it with liquid or food.

STORAGE
Store in a tightly sealed container away from moisture, heat, and direct light.

MISSED DOSE
If you miss a dose on one day, do not double the dose the next day.

STOPPING THE DRUG
The decision to stop taking the drug should be made by your doctor.

PROLONGED USE
If you take this drug for a prolonged period for BPH, see your doctor regularly so that changes in prostate size can be monitored. For hair loss, continued use is usually recommended to sustain the drug's benefits.

▼ PRECAUTIONS

Over 60: No special problems are expected.

Driving and Hazardous Work: The use of finasteride should not impair your ability to perform such tasks safely.

Alcohol: No special precautions are necessary.

Pregnancy: Although finasteride is not prescribed for women, those who are pregnant or planning to become pregnant should not handle the medication, especially if it is crushed or broken, because it can have an adverse effect on a male fetus. Men who take finasteride should use a barrier method of birth control (such as a condom), which prevents the female sexual partner from being exposed to small quantities of the drug present in semen.

Breast Feeding: Women who are nursing should avoid contact with finasteride or the sperm of a man who is taking the drug.

Infants and Children: Finasteride is not prescribed for children.

Special Concerns: Before taking this medicine for BPH, you should have a digital rectal examination and other tests for prostate cancer. Note that finasteride may affect the results of the prostate-specific antigen (PSA) test for prostate cancer; be sure any doctor you see for treatment, including your dentist, knows that you are taking this drug.

OVERDOSE
Symptoms: No specific ones have been reported.

What to Do: An overdose of finasteride is unlikely to be life-threatening. However, if someone takes a much larger dose than prescribed, call your doctor, emergency medical services (EMS), or the nearest poison control center.

▼ INTERACTIONS

DRUG INTERACTIONS
Consult your doctor for specific advice if you are taking amantadine, amphetamines, antihistamines, antidepressants, antidyskinetics (medications for Parkinson's disease or similar conditions), antipsychotics, appetite suppressants, anticholinergics (drugs for stomach spasms or cramps), bronchodilators, decongestants, ephedrine, phenylpropanolamine, or pseudoephedrine.

FOOD INTERACTIONS
No known food interactions.

DISEASE INTERACTIONS
Caution is advised when taking finasteride. Before you start, consult your doctor if you have liver disease, which may magnify the effects of the medication.

≣ SIDE EFFECTS ≣

SERIOUS
No serious side effects are associated with the use of finasteride.

COMMON
No common side effects are associated with the use of finasteride.

LESS COMMON
Reduced sex drive, erectile dysfunction (impotence), decreased quantity of ejaculate. It should be noted that this decrease is not a sign of reduced fertility.

FLUCONAZOLE

BRAND NAME
Diflucan

Available in: Tablets, oral suspension, injection
Available OTC? No   **As Generic?** No
Drug Class: Antifungal

▼ USAGE INFORMATION

WHY IT'S PRESCRIBED
To treat fungal infections of the mouth and throat (thrush), of the vagina (yeast infection), or throughout the body, as well as meningitis (inflammation of the protective membranes surrounding the brain). Often used to treat AIDS-related fungal infections. May also be used to prevent recurring fungal infections in susceptible patients weakened by AIDS or by chemotherapy or radiation treatment.

HOW IT WORKS
Fluconazole prevents fungal organisms from manufacturing vital substances required for their growth and function. This drug is effective only for infections caused by fungal organisms. It will not work for bacterial or viral infections.

▼ DOSAGE GUIDELINES

RANGE AND FREQUENCY
Adults and teenagers—For fungal infections: 200 to 400 mg on the first day, then 100 to 400 mg once a day, using oral forms or injection.

Injections are into a vein. For vaginal yeast infection: 1 dose of 150 mg, tablet or oral suspension.

ONSET OF EFFECT
Oral forms: Unknown.
Injection: Immediate.

DURATION OF ACTION
Unknown.

DIETARY ADVICE
Swallow tablets with liquid. Oral suspension should be shaken and carefully measured out before you take it. This drug can be taken without regard to diet.

STORAGE
Store in a tightly sealed container away from moisture, heat, and direct light. Keep any liquid form of the drug refrigerated, but do not allow it to freeze.

MISSED DOSE
Take it as soon as you remember. This will help keep a constant level of medication in your system. If it is near the time for the next dose, skip the missed dose and resume your regular dosage schedule. Do not double the next dose.

STOPPING THE DRUG
Take it as prescribed for the full treatment period, even if you begin to feel better before the scheduled end of therapy. The decision to stop taking the drug should be made by your doctor. Gradual reduction of the dose may be necessary if you have been taking this medicine for a long time.

PROLONGED USE
Notify your doctor if your condition does not improve, or instead becomes worse, within a few weeks.

▼ PRECAUTIONS

Over 60: Dosage may need to be reduced in older patients who have impaired kidney function.

Driving and Hazardous Work: The use of fluconazole should not impair your ability to perform such tasks safely.

Alcohol: No special precautions are necessary.

Pregnancy: Adequate studies of fluconazole use during pregnancy have not been done. Consult your doctor for specific advice if you are currently pregnant or plan to become pregnant.

Breast Feeding: Fluconazole may pass into breast milk; caution is advised. Consult your doctor for advice.

Infants and Children: Fluconazole is not generally prescribed for children under 14.

Special Concerns: A doctor should monitor your kidney function while you take fluconazole. Tell any doctor or dentist whom you consult that you are taking this medicine. Be sure to shake the oral suspension well before taking it.

OVERDOSE
Symptoms: An overdose with fluconazole is unlikely.

What to Do: Emergency instructions not applicable.

▼ INTERACTIONS

DRUG INTERACTIONS
Do not take cisapride with fluconazole. Other drugs may interact with fluconazole. Consult your doctor for specific advice if you are taking oral antidiabetic medications, cyclosporine, rifampin, phenytoin, rifabutin, tacrolimus, astemizole, or warfarin.

FOOD INTERACTIONS
No food interactions have been reported.

DISEASE INTERACTIONS
Caution is advised when taking fluconazole. Consult your doctor if you have a history of alcohol abuse (and associated liver problems), or any type of liver or kidney disease, since these organs work together to remove the medication from the body.

▼ SIDE EFFECTS ▼

SERIOUS
Skin rash or itching, fever or chills. Call your doctor right away.

COMMON
No common side effects have been reported with the use of fluconazole.

LESS COMMON
Diarrhea, nausea, vomiting, constipation, dizziness, headache, redness or flushing of skin.

FLUOXETINE HYDROCHLORIDE

Prozac, Sarafem

Available in: Capsules, oral solution
Available OTC? No   **As Generic?** No
Drug Class: Selective serotonin reuptake inhibitor (SSRI) antidepressant

▼ USAGE INFORMATION

WHY IT'S PRESCRIBED
To treat major depression, obsessive-compulsive disorder (OCD), panic disorder, chronic pain, and premenstrual dysphoric disorder (PMDD).

HOW IT WORKS
Fluoxetine affects levels of serotonin, a brain chemical that is thought to be linked to mood, emotions, and mental state.

▼ DOSAGE GUIDELINES

RANGE AND FREQUENCY
To start, 20 mg a day, taken in the morning. Your doctor may increase the dose gradually to a maximum of 80 mg a day. Older adults: To start, 10 to 20 mg a day. This dosage may be increased gradually by your doctor to reach a maximum of 40 to 60 mg a day.

ONSET OF EFFECT
1 to 4 weeks.

DURATION OF ACTION
Unknown.

DIETARY ADVICE
Taking the drug with liquid or food can lessen stomach irritation. Capsules may be opened and mixed with food or juice to aid swallowing.

STORAGE
Store in a tightly sealed container away from moisture, heat, and direct light. Keep the liquid form refrigerated, but do not allow it to freeze.

MISSED DOSE
Take it as soon as you remember. If it is near the time for the next dose, skip the missed dose and resume your regular dosage schedule. Do not double the next dose.

STOPPING THE DRUG
Take it as prescribed for the full treatment period, even if you begin to feel better before the scheduled end of therapy. Discontinuing the drug abruptly may produce unpleasant withdrawal symptoms. Dosage should be reduced gradually according to your doctor's specific instructions.

PROLONGED USE
The usual course of therapy lasts 6 months to 1 year; some patients may benefit from additional therapy. For obsessive-compulsive disorder, the usual course of therapy lasts 1 year or more.

▼ PRECAUTIONS

Over 60: Adverse reactions may be more likely and more severe in older patients, since their metabolism is slower. A lower dose may be warranted.

Driving and Hazardous Work: Use caution when driving or engaging in hazardous work until you determine how the medicine affects you.

Alcohol: Avoid alcohol.

Pregnancy: Fluoxetine should be used during pregnancy only if the potential benefit justifies the potential risk to the fetus. Before you take this medicine, tell your doctor if you are pregnant or plan to become pregnant.

Breast Feeding: Fluoxetine may pass into breast milk; caution is advised. Consult your doctor for advice.

Infants and Children: Not recommended for use by children under age 12.

Special Concerns: Take it at least 6 hours before bedtime to prevent insomnia, unless the drug causes drowsiness.

OVERDOSE
Symptoms: Agitation, excitement, severe nausea and vomiting, seizures.

What to Do: Call your doctor, emergency medical services (EMS), or the nearest poison control center immediately.

▼ INTERACTIONS

DRUG INTERACTIONS
Fluoxetine should not be used within 5 weeks of taking MAO inhibitors or thioridazine. The following drugs may interact with fluoxetine. Be sure to consult your doctor for specific advice if you are taking nortriptyline, caffeine, oral anticoagulants, central nervous system depressants, digitalis preparations, lithium, loratadine, dextromethorphan, ketorolac, buspirone, phenytoin, trazodone, tryptophan, sumatriptan, naratriptan, or zolmitriptan.

FOOD INTERACTIONS
No known food interactions.

DISEASE INTERACTIONS
Use of fluoxetine may cause complications in patients with liver or kidney disease, since these organs work together to remove the medication from the body. Use of the drug may make diabetes or seizures worse.

▤ SIDE EFFECTS ▤

SERIOUS
Agitation, shaking, difficulty breathing, rash, hives, itching, joint or muscle pain, chills or fever. If such symptoms occur, call your doctor immediately.

COMMON
Nervousness, drowsiness, anxiety, insomnia, headache, diarrhea, excessive sweating, nausea, decreased appetite, decreased initiative.

LESS COMMON
Nasal congestion, unusual or vivid dreams, cough, increased appetite, chest pain, constipation, vision disturbances, abdominal pain, stomach gas, constipation, vomiting, frequent urination, difficulty concentrating, sexual dysfunction, heartbeat irregularities, trembling, fatigue, dizziness, change in taste, flushing of the skin on the face and neck, dry mouth, menstrual pain.

FLUTICASONE

Available in: Oral inhalation, nasal spray
Available OTC? No **As Generic?** No
Drug Class: Respiratory corticosteroid

▼ USAGE INFORMATION

WHY IT'S PRESCRIBED
To preventively treat bronchial asthma, and to treat allergic rhinitis (seasonal or perennial allergies such as hay fever).

HOW IT WORKS
Respiratory corticosteroids such as fluticasone primarily reduce or prevent inflammation of the lining of airways (the underlying cause of asthma), reduce the allergic response to inhaled allergens, and inhibit the secretion of mucus within the airways.

▼ DOSAGE GUIDELINES

RANGE AND FREQUENCY
For asthma—Oral inhalation: 88 to 220 micrograms (mcg) a day, 2 times per day; not to exceed 440 mcg a day. For patients previously treated with oral corticosteroids: 880 mcg, 2 times a day. Dosage may gradually be reduced after 1 week of therapy. For allergic rhinitis—Nasal spray: Adults: 2 sprays (50 micrograms each) in each nostril once per day, or 1 spray in each nostril twice a day

(in the morning and at night). Children ages 4 to 17: One spray in each nostril once a day. Dose, if needed, may be increased to 2 sprays in each nostril once a day. Maximum daily dose should not exceed 200 micrograms. After relief is achieved, the dose may be reduced to 1 spray per day.

ONSET OF EFFECT
Usually within 1 week; it may take 3 weeks for the full effect to occur.

DURATION OF ACTION
Unknown.

DIETARY ADVICE
No special restrictions.

STORAGE
Store inhaler in a dry place away from heat and light.

MISSED DOSE
Take it as soon as you remember. If it is near the time for the next dose, skip the missed dose and resume your regular dosage schedule. Do not double the next dose.

STOPPING THE DRUG
If you have been using fluticasone for a long period, do

not stop taking it suddenly. Consult your doctor about how to stop.

PROLONGED USE
Consult your doctor about the need for regular medical tests and examinations if you must take this drug for a prolonged period of time.

▼ PRECAUTIONS

Over 60: No special problems are expected.

Driving and Hazardous Work: The use of fluticasone should not impair your ability to perform such tasks safely.

Alcohol: No special precautions are necessary.

Pregnancy: Well-controlled studies of fluticasone use during pregnancy have not been done; it is generally not recommended unless the benefits clearly outweigh the risks. Consult your doctor.

Breast Feeding: Fluticasone may pass into breast milk; caution is advised. Consult your doctor for advice.

Infants and Children: Safety and effectiveness have not been established for children under age 4.

Special Concerns: Inhaled steroids will not help an asthma attack in progress. Inhaled steroids can lower resistance to yeast infections of the mouth, throat, or voice box. To prevent yeast infections, gargle or rinse your mouth with water after each use; do not swallow the water. Know how to use the

spray properly; read and follow the directions that come with the device. Before you have surgery, tell the doctor or dentist that you are using a steroid.

OVERDOSE
Symptoms: No cases of overdose have been reported.

What to Do: An overdose of fluticasone is unlikely. If you have any reason to suspect an overdose, contact your doctor or seek medical assistance right away.

▼ INTERACTIONS

DRUG INTERACTIONS
Consult your doctor for specific advice if you are taking systemic corticosteroids, other inhaled corticosteroids, or drugs that suppress the immune system.

FOOD INTERACTIONS
No known food interactions.

DISEASE INTERACTIONS
Caution is advised when taking fluticasone. Consult your doctor if you have any of the following: a lung disease such as tuberculosis; a herpes infection of the eye; nasal ulcers or recent nose surgery or injury; or any bacterial, viral, or fungal infection. If you are exposed to chicken pox or measles, tell your doctor at once.

≡ SIDE EFFECTS ≡

SERIOUS
No serious side effects are associated with the use of fluticasone.

COMMON
Oral inhalation: Sore throat, white patches in mouth or throat, hoarseness. Nasal spray: Nosebleeds or bloody nasal secretions, nasal burning or irritation, sore throat.

LESS COMMON
Eye pain, watering eyes, gradual decrease of vision, stomach pain and digestive disturbances.

FLUVASTATIN

BRAND NAME

Lescol

Available in: Capsules
Available OTC? No **As Generic?** No
Drug Class: Antilipidemic (cholesterol-lowering agent)

▼ USAGE INFORMATION

WHY IT'S PRESCRIBED
To treat high cholesterol. Usually prescribed after first lines of treatment—including diet, weight loss, and exercise—fail to reduce total and low-density lipoprotein (LDL) cholesterol to acceptable levels.

HOW IT WORKS
Fluvastatin blocks the action of an enzyme required for the manufacture of cholesterol, thereby interfering with its formation. By lowering the amount of cholesterol in the liver cells, fluvastatin then increases the formation of receptors for LDL, and thereby reduces blood levels of total and LDL cholesterol. In addition to lowering LDL cholesterol, fluvastatin also modestly reduces triglyceride levels and raises levels of HDL (the so-called "good" cholesterol).

▼ DOSAGE GUIDELINES

RANGE AND FREQUENCY
Initial dose is 20 mg, taken once a day in the evening.

Dose may be increased by your doctor to 40 mg, taken once a day in the evening.

ONSET OF EFFECT
Within 2 to 4 weeks after starting therapy.

DURATION OF ACTION
The effect persists for the duration of therapy.

DIETARY ADVICE
Cholesterol-lowering drugs are only one part of a total lifestyle program that should include regular exercise and a healthy diet. The American Heart Association publishes a "Healthy Heart" diet, which is widely recommended for reducing cholesterol levels.

STORAGE
Store in a tightly sealed container away from heat and direct light. Keep away from moisture and extremes in temperature.

MISSED DOSE
Take it as soon as you remember. Take your next dose at the proper time and resume your regular dosage schedule. Do not double the next dose.

STOPPING THE DRUG
The decision to stop taking the drug should be made in consultation with your doctor. Once the medication is discontinued, blood cholesterol is likely to return to original elevated levels.

PROLONGED USE
Side effects are more likely with prolonged use. As you continue with fluvastatin, your doctor will periodically order blood tests to evaluate liver function.

▼ PRECAUTIONS

Over 60: No special problems are expected in older patients.

Driving and Hazardous Work: The use of fluvastatin should not impair your ability to perform such tasks safely.

Alcohol: No special precautions are necessary.

Pregnancy: Should not be used during pregnancy or by women who plan to become pregnant in the near future.

Breast Feeding: Fluvastatin passes into breast milk and is not recommended while breast feeding.

Infants and Children: Rarely used in children.

Special Concerns: Important elements for treating high cholesterol include proper diet, weight loss, regular moderate exercise, and the avoidance of certain medications that may increase your cholesterol levels. Because fluvastatin has potential side

effects, it is important that you maintain a recommended healthy diet and cooperate with other treatments your physician may suggest.

OVERDOSE
Symptoms: An overdose of fluvastatin is unlikely.

What to Do: Emergency instructions not applicable.

▼ INTERACTIONS

DRUG INTERACTIONS
Consult your doctor if you are taking cyclosporine, gemfibrozil, niacin, antibiotics, especially erythromycin, or medications for fungus infections. All of these drugs may increase the risk of myositis (muscle inflammation) when taken with fluvastatin and may lead to kidney failure.

FOOD INTERACTIONS
No known food interactions.

DISEASE INTERACTIONS
Consult your doctor if you have any of the following problems: liver, kidney, or muscle disease, or a medical history involving organ transplant or recent surgery.

≣ SIDE EFFECTS ≣

SERIOUS
Fever, unusual or unexplained muscle aches and tenderness. Call your doctor right away.

COMMON
Side effects occur in only 1% to 2% of patients. These include constipation or diarrhea, dizziness or lightheadedness, bloating or gas, heartburn, nausea, skin rash, stomach pain, rise in liver enzymes.

LESS COMMON
Sleeping difficulty.

FOLIC ACID (FOLACIN; FOLATE)

BRAND NAME

Folvite

Available in: Tablets, injectable form (for use in hospitals)
Available OTC? Yes   **As Generic?** Yes
Drug Class: Vitamin

▼ USAGE INFORMATION

WHY IT'S PRESCRIBED
The vitamin folic acid (also known as folacin and folate) is prescribed for treatment or prevention of certain types of anemia that result from folic acid deficiency. Such deficiencies may occur due to insufficient intake of folic acid (the result of a poor diet or malnutrition), an inability to absorb the vitamin (as occurs in gastrointestinal disease), impaired ability to utilize the vitamin (due to excessive alcohol intake or phenytoin use), or as a result of medical conditions requiring increased amounts of folic acid (as may occur with pregnancy, breast feeding, hemodialysis, hemolytic anemia, and bone marrow failure).

HOW IT WORKS
Folic acid, which is one of the B vitamins, enhances chemical reactions that contribute to the production of red blood cells, the manufacture of DNA needed for cell replication, and the metabolism of amino acids (compounds necessary for the manufacture of proteins).

▼ DOSAGE GUIDELINES

RANGE AND FREQUENCY
For severe deficiency–Adults and children, regardless of age: 1 mg daily. For daily supplementation following correction of a severe deficiency–Adults and adolescents: 1 mg, once daily. During pregnancy: 400 micrograms (mcg), once daily. While breast feeding: 260 to 280 mcg, once daily. Children, newborn to 3 years of age: 25 to 50 mcg, once daily; child 4 to 6 years of age: 75 mcg, once daily; child 7 to 10 years of age: 100 mcg, once daily.

ONSET OF EFFECT
Folic acid is used immediately by the body for a number of vital chemical functions.

DURATION OF ACTION
Folic acid is required by your body on a daily basis throughout a lifetime.

DIETARY ADVICE
Maintain your usual food and fluid intake. Increase fluids if you have a fever or diarrhea, in hot weather, or during exercise. Follow your doctor's dietary advice (such as low-fat, low-salt, or low-cholesterol restrictions) to improve control over high blood pressure and heart disease.

STORAGE
Store in a tightly sealed container away from heat and direct light. Keep container away from moisture and extremes in temperature.

MISSED DOSE
Take it as soon as you remember. If it is near the time for the next dose, skip the missed dose and resume your regular dosage schedule. Do not double the next dose.

STOPPING THE DRUG
The decision to stop taking the drug should be made by your doctor.

PROLONGED USE
Therapy with folacin may require weeks or months.

▼ PRECAUTIONS

Over 60: No special problems are expected in older individuals.

Driving and Hazardous Work: The use of folic acid should not impair your ability to perform such tasks safely.

Alcohol: Alcohol impairs the body's utilization of folic acid; avoid it completely if you are taking folic acid.

Pregnancy: Folic acid supplementation is recommended during pregnancy.

Breast Feeding: Folic acid supplementation is recommended while nursing.

Infants and Children: Folic acid may be used regardless of age.

Special Concerns: Folic acid ingestion can mask vitamin B12 deficiency and lead to irreversible neurological damage; therefore, folic acid should be taken only upon the recommendation of your doctor. Folic acid deficiency should not occur and supplementation is not necessary in healthy individuals who consume a normal balanced diet.

OVERDOSE
Symptoms: No specific ones have been reported.

What to Do: A folic acid overdose is not life-threatening. No emergency procedures are warranted.

▼ INTERACTIONS

DRUG INTERACTIONS
Consult your doctor for advice if you are taking pain relievers, antibiotics, anticonvulsants, epoetin, estrogens, oral contraceptives, methotrexate, pyrimethamine, triamterene, sulfasalazine, or zinc supplements.

FOOD INTERACTIONS
No known food interactions.

DISEASE INTERACTIONS
Consult your doctor if you have pernicious anemia.

⬇ SIDE EFFECTS ⬇

SERIOUS
Wheezing, breathing difficulty, chest pain, swelling, tightness in throat or chest, dizziness, rash, itching. Such symptoms may indicate a serious allergic reaction, although this is extremely rare.

COMMON
The are no known common side effects associated with the use of folic acid.

LESS COMMON
Mild allergic reactions.

FOSINOPRIL SODIUM

Available in: Tablets
Available OTC? No   **As Generic?** Yes
Drug Class: Angiotensin-converting enzyme (ACE) inhibitor

▼ USAGE INFORMATION

WHY IT'S PRESCRIBED
To control high blood pressure; to treat congestive heart failure; to treat patients with left ventricular dysfunction (damage to the pumping chamber of the heart); and to minimize further kidney damage in diabetics with mild kidney disease.

HOW IT WORKS
Angiotensin-converting enzyme (ACE) inhibitors block an enzyme that produces angiotensin, a naturally occurring substance that causes blood vessels to constrict and stimulates production of the adrenal hormone, aldosterone, which promotes sodium retention in the body. As a result, ACE inhibitor medications relax blood vessels (causing them to widen) and reduce sodium retention, which in turn lowers blood pressure and so decreases the workload of the heart.

▼ DOSAGE GUIDELINES

RANGE AND FREQUENCY
Initial dose: 10 mg once a day. Maintenance dose: 20 to 80 mg a day, in 1 or 2 doses.

ONSET OF EFFECT
Within 1 hour.

DURATION OF ACTION
24 hours.

DIETARY ADVICE
Take fosinopril on an empty stomach, about 1 hour before mealtime. Follow your doctor's dietary advice to improve control over high blood pressure and heart disease. Avoid high-potassium foods (such as bananas and citrus fruits and juices) unless you are also taking specific medications, such as diuretics, that lower potassium levels.

STORAGE
Store in a sealed container away from heat and light. Keep away from moisture and extremes in temperature.

MISSED DOSE
Take it as soon as you remember. If it is near the time for the next dose, skip the missed dose and resume your regular dosage schedule. Do not double the next dose.

STOPPING THE DRUG
Do not stop taking this drug abruptly, as this may cause potentially serious health problems. Dosage should be reduced gradually, according to your doctor's instructions.

PROLONGED USE
Therapy with this medication may require months or years. Prolonged use may increase the risk of adverse effects.

▼ PRECAUTIONS

Over 60: Adverse reactions may be more likely and more severe.

Driving and Hazardous Work: Avoid such activities until you determine how this medication affects you.

Alcohol: Consume alcohol only in moderation since it may increase the effect of the drug and cause an excessive drop in blood pressure. Consult your doctor for advice.

Pregnancy: Do not use fosinopril if you are pregnant or trying to become pregnant. Use of this drug during the last 6 months of pregnancy may cause severe defects, even death, in the fetus.

Breast Feeding: Fosinopril passes into breast milk and may be harmful to the infant; avoid using the drug while you are nursing.

Infants and Children: Fosinopril is generally not recommended for children.

OVERDOSE
Symptoms: No specific ones have been reported.

What to Do: While overdose is unlikely, call your doctor, emergency medical services (EMS), or the nearest poison control center immediately if you suspect that someone has taken a much larger dose than prescribed.

▼ INTERACTIONS

DRUG INTERACTIONS
Consult your doctor if you are taking diuretics (especially potassium-sparing diuretics), potassium supplements or drugs containing potassium (check ingredient labels), lithium, anticoagulants (such as warfarin), indomethacin or other anti-inflammatory drugs, antacids, allopurinol, or any over-the-counter medications (especially cold remedies and diet pills).

FOOD INTERACTIONS
Avoid low-salt milk and salt substitutes. Many brands have high amounts of potassium. Avoid high-potassium foods like bananas and citrus fruits and juices.

DISEASE INTERACTIONS
Consult your doctor if you have lupus or if you have had a prior allergic reaction to ACE inhibitors. This medicine should be used with caution by patients with severe kidney disease or renal artery stenosis (narrowing of one or both of the arteries that supply blood to the kidneys).

≡ SIDE EFFECTS ≡

SERIOUS
Fever and chills, sore throat and hoarseness, sudden difficulty breathing or swallowing, swelling of the face, mouth, or extremities, impaired kidney function (ankle swelling, decreased urination), confusion, yellow discoloration of the eyes or skin (indicating liver disorder), intense itching, chest pain or palpitations, abdominal pain. Serious side effects are very rare; contact your doctor immediately.

COMMON
Dry, persistent cough.

LESS COMMON
Dizziness or fainting, skin rash, numbness or tingling in the hands, feet, or lips, unusual fatigue or muscle weakness, nausea, drowsiness, loss of taste, headache.

FUROSEMIDE

Available in: Tablets, oral solution, injection
Available OTC? No   **As Generic?** Yes
Drug Class: Loop diuretic

▼ USAGE INFORMATION

WHY IT'S PRESCRIBED
To reduce the fluid (salt and water) accumulation that can lead to edema (swelling) and breathlessness in patients who have heart disease, cirrhosis of the liver, and kidney disease. Furosemide is also sometimes used to help control high blood pressure levels.

HOW IT WORKS
Loop diuretics work on a specific portion of the kidney (the loop of Henle) to increase the excretion of water and sodium in urine.

▼ DOSAGE GUIDELINES

RANGE AND FREQUENCY
20 to 600 mg a day. Tablets and solution: dosage is given in 1, 2, or 3 divided doses daily. Injection (given in a hospital setting only): dosage given in divided doses every 2 to 3 hours or as a continuous infusion.

ONSET OF EFFECT
20 to 60 minutes.

DURATION OF ACTION
Tablets and solution: 6 to 8 hours. Injection: 2 hours.

DIETARY ADVICE
Take with food to reduce stomach irritation.

STORAGE
Keep in refrigerator, in a light-resistant container. Do not allow liquid forms to freeze.

MISSED DOSE
Take it as soon as you remember. If it is near the time for the next dose, skip the missed dose and resume your regular dosage schedule. Do not double the next dose.

STOPPING THE DRUG
The decision to stop taking the drug should be made by your doctor.

PROLONGED USE
There are no apparent problems. Regular examinations by your doctor are advised.

▼ PRECAUTIONS

Over 60: No special problems are expected.

Driving and Hazardous Work: No special precautions are required.

Alcohol: No special precautions are required.

Pregnancy: Diuretics are not useful for relieving the normal fluid retention that occurs with pregnancy. In patients who do need diuretic therapy, furosemide is generally preferred, but should be taken only after careful consultation with your primary care doctor or OB/GYN specialist.

Breast Feeding: Furosemide passes into breast milk; avoid or discontinue use while breast feeding.

Infants and Children: Use furosemide only under careful supervision by a pediatrician.

Special Concerns: To prevent sleep disruption, avoid taking furosemide in the evening. You may also have to take a potassium supplement or consume foods or fluids high in potassium while you are using this drug. Diabetic patients should monitor their blood sugar levels carefully.

OVERDOSE
Symptoms: Weakness, lethargy, mental confusion, muscle cramps.

What to Do: Call your doctor, emergency medical services (EMS), or the nearest poison control center immediately.

▼ INTERACTIONS

DRUG INTERACTIONS
Consult your doctor about any other drugs you are taking, especially antibiotics, other blood pressure drugs, any ACE inhibitor, any pain reliever, lithium, cortisone-related drugs, digitalis-related drugs, or any nonsteroidal anti-inflammatory drug.

FOOD INTERACTIONS
None reported.

DISEASE INTERACTIONS
Caution is advised when taking this medication. Consult your doctor if you have diabetes, gout, or a hearing problem, or have had a recent heart attack.

≡ SIDE EFFECTS ≡

SERIOUS
Skin rash, hives, intense itching, swelling of the mouth and throat, breathing difficulty, mood or mental changes, nausea and vomiting, unusual fatigue, black or tarry stools. Call your doctor immediately.

COMMON
Muscle cramps or pain. Potassium depletion may lead to heart palpitations and weakness. Fluid depletion may lead to dizziness, especially upon arising from a sitting or lying position, as well as thirst, dry mouth, and constipation.

LESS COMMON
Buzzing or ringing in ears, loss of hearing (particularly after intravenous treatment), diarrhea, loss of appetite, gout, increased blood sugar (a problem for diabetic patients).

GABAPENTIN

BRAND NAME

Neurontin

Available in: Capsules, tablets
Available OTC? No   **As Generic?** No
Drug Class: Anticonvulsant

▼ USAGE INFORMATION

WHY IT'S PRESCRIBED
To control certain kinds of seizures in the treatment of epilepsy. Gabapentin is often prescribed in combination with another anticonvulsant medication.

HOW IT WORKS
The drug's mechanism of action is not well understood. It is believed that gabapentin inhibits activity in certain parts of the brain and suppresses the abnormal firing of neurons that causes seizures.

▼ DOSAGE GUIDELINES

RANGE AND FREQUENCY
Adults and teenagers: 900 to 3,600 mg a day, in 3 or 4 divided doses. Some patients require higher doses. The dose is started low and then gradually increased by your doctor to achieve maximum therapeutic benefit with a minimum of side effects. Children ages 3 to 12: To start, 10 to 15 mg per 2.2 lbs (1 kg), in 3 divided doses. The dose is started low and then gradually increased by your doctor to achieve maximum therapeutic benefit with a minimum of side effects.

ONSET OF EFFECT
Several hours.

DURATION OF ACTION
Maximum effectiveness lasts 5 to 8 hours or longer; effectiveness then gradually decreases over time.

DIETARY ADVICE
No special restrictions.

STORAGE
Store in a tightly sealed container away from moisture, heat, and direct light. Refrigerate the oral solution, but do not allow the medication to freeze.

≡ SIDE EFFECTS ≡

SERIOUS
Fever, sore throat, swollen glands, red or purple point-like rash on the skin or mucous membranes, blistering or peeling skin lesions, mouth sores, easy bruising, paleness, weakness, confusion, lethargy, or seizures may be a sign of a potentially fatal blood disorder (aplastic anemia) or other complication. Call your physician immediately.

COMMON
Fatigue, dizziness, sedation, clumsiness or unsteadiness, unusual eye movements, blurred or altered vision, nausea, vomiting, tremor.

LESS COMMON
Diarrhea, muscle aches or weakness, dry mouth, headache, sleep disturbances, irritability, slurred speech. There are numerous additional side effects associated with the use of this drug; consult your doctor if you are concerned about any adverse or unusual reactions.

MISSED DOSE
Take it as soon as you remember. If your next dose is scheduled within the next 2 hours, take the missed dose, and take the next dose 1 to 2 hours later. Resume your regular dosage schedule. Do not double the next dose unless advised to do so by your doctor. Do not wait more than 12 hours between doses.

STOPPING THE DRUG
The decision to stop taking the drug should be made by your doctor. Never stop this drug abruptly because this may cause seizures. The dose is typically tapered over a period of weeks.

PROLONGED USE
Therapy with gabapentin may be required for months or years. Some side effects that are prominent during the first few weeks of therapy may subsequently diminish.

▼ PRECAUTIONS

Over 60: Older persons may require lower doses to minimize side effects.

Driving and Hazardous Work: Avoid such activities until you determine how the medication affects you.

Alcohol: May contribute to excessive drowsiness.

Pregnancy: Adequate human studies have not been done, but the use of other anticonvulsants is associated with an increased risk of birth defects. However, seizures during pregnancy can also increase the risks to the unborn child. Discuss with your doctor the potential risks and benefits of using gabapentin during pregnancy. Folate supplementation is recommended beginning 1 to 2 months before conception and throughout pregnancy.

Breast Feeding: Gabapentin may pass into breast milk, although at low levels. Consult your doctor for advice.

Infants and Children: There are few published studies about the use of gabapentin in children age 12 and younger, but effectiveness should be similar to that seen in older patients. Safety and effectiveness have not been established for children under the age of 3.

Special Concerns: Your doctor may want you to wear a medical bracelet or carry an identification card saying that you are taking this drug.

OVERDOSE
Symptoms: Few cases of overdose have been reported. Symptoms include double vision, slurred speech, drowsiness, lethargy, and diarrhea.

What to Do: Call your doctor, emergency medical services (EMS), or the nearest poison control center immediately.

▼ INTERACTIONS

DRUG INTERACTIONS
No significant interactions.

FOOD INTERACTIONS
No known food interactions.

DISEASE INTERACTIONS
Gabapentin dosage may need to be lower in patients with kidney disease.

GEMFIBROZIL

Available in: Tablets
Available OTC? No **As Generic?** Yes
Drug Class: Antilipidemic (triglyceride-lowering agent)

▼ USAGE INFORMATION

WHY IT'S PRESCRIBED
To treat high levels of blood triglyceride. Usually prescribed after other treatments, including diet, weight loss, exercise, and control of diabetes (when present), fail to lower triglyceride levels adequately.

HOW IT WORKS
Gemfibrozil speeds the removal of triglycerides from the lipoprotein known as very-low-density lipoprotein (VLDL), which is converted to low-density lipoprotein (LDL). In some people total and LDL cholesterol levels may rise while triglycerides fall.

▼ DOSAGE GUIDELINES

RANGE AND FREQUENCY
Adults: 600 milligrams, 2 times per day. Usually taken 30 to 60 minutes before morning and evening meals.

ONSET OF EFFECT
Begins in about 1 week and is noticeable in about 4 weeks.

DURATION OF ACTION
Blood triglyceride levels increase within a few weeks of stopping gemfibrozil.

DIETARY ADVICE
Follow your doctor's dietary advice to improve control over high blood pressure and help prevent heart disease. The American Heart Association publishes a "Healthy Heart" diet; discuss this with your doctor. Limit intake of alcohol, which can raise triglyceride levels.

STORAGE
Store in a tightly sealed container away from heat and direct light.

MISSED DOSE
Take your missed dose as soon as you remember that you skipped it, unless the time for your next scheduled dose is within the next 2 hours. If so, do not take the missed dose. Take your next scheduled dose at the proper time, and resume your regular dosage schedule. Do not double the next dose.

STOPPING THE DRUG
Do not stop taking gemfibrozil on your own; the level of triglycerides in your blood will increase.

PROLONGED USE
Gemfibrozil is often taken for long periods of time. If your blood triglycerides do not diminish, your physician may stop the medication.

▼ PRECAUTIONS

Over 60: Adverse reactions may be more likely and more severe in older patients.

Driving and Hazardous Work: The use of gemfibrozil should not impair your ability to perform such tasks safely.

Alcohol: Alcohol intake should be limited because it can raise triglyceride levels.

Pregnancy: Do not take gemfibrozil while pregnant unless your doctor indicates that the risks of stopping the drug are too great. Triglycerides increase substantially during pregnancy and extremely high triglycerides can trigger an attack of acute pancreatitis.

Breast Feeding: Avoid or discontinue usage while nursing.

Infants and Children: Rarely used in infants and children.

Special Concerns: The most important treatment for high levels of blood triglycerides is a proper diet, weight loss, regular moderate exercise, the avoidance of certain medications, and the control of diabetes. Because gemfibrozil has potential side effects, it is important that you maintain a healthy diet and cooperate with other treatment strategies your physician may suggest. Gemfibrozil may increase the chances of gallbladder, liver, and pancreas problems; your physician will order periodic blood tests.

OVERDOSE
Symptoms: No specific ones have been reported.

What to Do: Emergency instructions not applicable.

▼ INTERACTIONS

DRUG INTERACTIONS
Certain drugs may interact adversely with gemfibrozil, particularly anticoagulants (blood thinners, such as warfarin), niacin, and any of the group of cholesterol-lowering drugs referred to as "-statins." It may be necessary to reduce the dose of warfarin to prevent bleeding. The combination of gemfibrozil with either niacin or a statin drug can cause severe myositis (muscle inflammation), which can release a protein that damages the kidneys. Consult your doctor.

FOOD INTERACTIONS
No known food interactions.

DISEASE INTERACTIONS
Be sure to inform your doctor if you have any of the following problems: gallstones, stomach or intestinal ulcer, muscle disease, kidney or liver disease. The dose of gemfibrozil must be reduced in those with significant kidney damage.

≡ SIDE EFFECTS ≡

SERIOUS
Muscle aches and tenderness; crampy abdominal pain, especially in the area under the ribs on the right side, with nausea and vomiting (this is an uncommon, serious side effect that may indicate gallbladder disease); decreased urine output.

COMMON
Diarrhea, nausea, gas.

LESS COMMON
Decreased sexual ability; headache; weight gain; feelings similar to the flu, with muscle aches or cramps, weakness, and unusual tiredness; inflammation of mouth and lips; heartburn.

GLIMEPIRIDE

Available in: Tablets
Available OTC? No **As Generic?** Yes
Drug Class: Antidiabetic agent/sulfonylurea

▼ USAGE INFORMATION

WHY IT'S PRESCRIBED
To treat diabetes (high blood sugar) in patients who require little or no injectable insulin. It is used in conjunction with a special diet and exercise. Some patients may fail to respond initially or gradually lose their responsiveness to glimepiride. The antidiabetic agent metformin may be used with glimepiride to achieve the desired results.

HOW IT WORKS
Glimepiride stimulates the release of insulin from the pancreas and makes the tissues of your body more responsive to insulin.

▼ DOSAGE GUIDELINES

RANGE AND FREQUENCY
Adults: 1 to 4 mg once daily, 30 minutes before breakfast. Children: Not recommended.

ONSET OF EFFECT
2 to 3 hours.

DURATION OF ACTION
12 to 24 hours.

DIETARY ADVICE
Maintain any special diets that your doctor recommends. Restrict excessive intake of sugar-containing snacks. Read food labels carefully.

STORAGE
Keep away from direct light, moisture, and extremes in temperature.

MISSED DOSE
Take it as soon as you remember. If it is near the time for the next dose, skip the missed dose and resume your regular dosage schedule. Do not double the next dose.

STOPPING THE DRUG
The decision to stop taking glimepiride should be made by your doctor.

PROLONGED USE
Therapy with glimepiride may require months or years. Its prolonged use may be associated with an increased risk of side effects.

▼ PRECAUTIONS

Over 60: Adverse reactions from this drug may be more likely and more severe.

Driving and Hazardous Work: Do not drive or engage in hazardous work until you determine how the medicine affects you.

Alcohol: Use only in a moderate, responsible fashion. Consult your doctor.

Pregnancy: It should not be used during pregnancy.

Breast Feeding: It should not be used by nursing mothers.

Infants and Children: Not recommended for children.

Special Concerns: Understand the symptoms of low blood sugar. Always have easy access to sources of simple sugar—juice, candy bars, energy bars, hard candy, honey, sugar cubes, sugar dissolved in water—in the event you experience symptoms of hypoglycemia (low blood sugar). Inform your physician promptly about changes in the way you are feeling, changes in your lifestyle and level of activity, medications that you may have been prescribed by other specialists, medications that you have stopped taking, unusually high or low results for any at-home tests you use to check your urine or blood, episodes of low blood sugar, and pregnancy. Wear a special medical ID bracelet. Do not miss meals. Use caution when exercising.

OVERDOSE
Symptoms: Symptoms are similar to serious side effects.

What to Do: Call emergency medical services (EMS), your doctor, or the nearest poison control center immediately.

▼ INTERACTIONS

DRUG INTERACTIONS
Consult your doctor for specific advice if you are taking steroids and nonsteroidal anti-inflammatory drugs (such as ibuprofen, aspirin, or aspirin-containing drugs), anticoagulants, certain antibiotics, especially for fungal infections, diuretics, lithium, beta-blockers, ulcer medications, ciprofloxacin, cyclosporine, guanethidine, MAO inhibitors, quinidine, quinine, chloramphenicol, estrogen, isoniazid, thyroid hormones, theophylline, pentamidine phenothiazines, or phenytoin.

FOOD INTERACTIONS
No known food interactions.

DISEASE INTERACTIONS
Consult your doctor if you have diarrhea, persistent vomiting, malabsorption disease, liver, thyroid, kidney, or adrenal gland disease, fever, or infection.

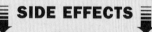

▦ SIDE EFFECTS ▦

SERIOUS
Serious side effects are related to hypoglycemia, or low blood sugar, whose symptoms include perspiration or a cold sweat, restlessness, rapid pulse, anxious feeling, nausea, feelings of dizziness, weakness, or lightheadedness, poor coordination, slurred speech, confusion, sleepiness, seizures or convulsions, weakness of an arm, leg, or an entire side of the body, fainting. Seek emergency assistance. Administer sugar-containing substances only if the patient is conscious and alert. Other serious but less common side effects include low white blood cell count and elevation of liver-associated enzymes; these problems can be detected by your doctor.

COMMON
Dizziness, weakness, nausea, headache.

LESS COMMON
Skin reactions, such as itching, peeling, rashes, and hives; blurred vision; edema (swelling due to fluid retention) of face or extremities; severe tiredness; abdominal pain.

GLIPIZIDE

Available in: Tablets, extended-release tablets
Available OTC? No   **As Generic?** Yes
Drug Class: Antidiabetic agent/sulfonylurea

▼ USAGE INFORMATION

WHY IT'S PRESCRIBED
To treat diabetes (high blood sugar) in patients who require little or no injectable insulin. It is used in conjunction with a special diet and exercise. Some patients may fail to respond initially or gradually lose their responsiveness to glipizide. Other antidiabetic agents may be used in conjunction with glipizide to achieve the desired results.

HOW IT WORKS
Glipizide stimulates the release of insulin from special cells in the pancreas and therefore helps to lower blood glucose levels.

▼ DOSAGE GUIDELINES

RANGE AND FREQUENCY
Usual starting dose: 5 mg a day, taken 30 minutes before breakfast. Dosage should be adjusted by 2.5 to 5 mg per day based on blood sugar response. If your dosage is greater than 15 mg a day, it should be divided. In the elderly or patients with liver disease, the initial dose should be 2.5 mg a day. Extended-release tablets: 5 to 10 mg, once daily, usually with breakfast.

ONSET OF EFFECT
Within 30 minutes.

DURATION OF ACTION
12 to 24 hours.

DIETARY ADVICE
Maintain special diet recommended by your doctor, nutritionist, or the American Diabetes Association. Restrict excessive intake of sugar-laden snacks. Read labels carefully when buying food.

STORAGE
Store away from direct light, moisture, and extremes in temperature.

MISSED DOSE
Take it as soon as you remember. If it is near the time for the next dose, skip the missed dose and resume your regular dosage schedule. Do not double the next dose.

STOPPING THE DRUG
The decision to stop taking it should be made by your doctor.

PROLONGED USE
Therapy may require months or years. Prolonged use may be associated with an increased risk of side effects.

▼ PRECAUTIONS

Over 60: Adverse reactions from this drug may be more likely and more severe.

Driving and Hazardous Work: Do not drive or engage in hazardous work until you determine how the medication affects you.

Alcohol: Drink in moderation.

Pregnancy: Insulin is the treatment of choice for pregnant women with diabetes.

Breast Feeding: This drug passes into breast milk, although it is uncertain whether the drug is harmful to nursing infants.

Infants and Children: Not recommended for children.

Special Concerns: Keep simple sugars (juice, candy bars, hard candy) on hand in the event of hypoglycemia. Inform your doctor promptly of changes in how you feel, unusually high or low results for any at-home tests, episodes of low blood sugar, or pregnancy. Wear a medical ID bracelet. Do not miss meals. Use caution when exercising.

OVERDOSE
Symptoms: Symptoms similar to serious side effects.

What to Do: Call emergency medical services (EMS), your doctor, or the nearest poison control center immediately.

▼ INTERACTIONS

DRUG INTERACTIONS
Consult your doctor for specific advice if you are taking anticoagulants, antibiotics (especially sulfa-containing antibiotics or those used to treat fungal infections), steroids, diuretics, seizure medications, beta-blockers (which may include eye drops for glaucoma) or other blood pressure medications, lithium, ulcer drugs, guanethidine, MAO inhibitors, quinidine, quinine, salicylates, chloramphenicol, estrogens, isoniazid, thyroid hormones, theophylline, or pentamidine.

FOOD INTERACTIONS
Food delays the absorption of immediate-release tablets.

DISEASE INTERACTIONS
Consult your doctor if you have diarrhea, persistent vomiting, malabsorption disease, liver, thyroid, kidney, or adrenal gland disease, fever, infection, or impending or recent surgery.

≡ SIDE EFFECTS ≡

▼ SERIOUS ▼
Serious side effects are related to hypoglycemia, or low blood sugar, whose symptoms include perspiration or a cold sweat, restlessness, rapid pulse, anxious feeling, nausea, feelings of dizziness, weakness, or lightheadedness, poor coordination, slurred speech, confusion, drowsiness, seizures, weakness of an arm, leg, or an entire side of the body, and fainting. Seek emergency assistance. Administer sugar-containing substances only if the patient is conscious and alert. Other serious but less common side effects include low white blood cell count and elevation of liver-associated enzymes; these can be detected by your doctor.

COMMON
Dizziness, constipation, nausea, heartburn, unusual or changed taste of food, or unusual taste in the mouth.

LESS COMMON
Peeling, red, bruised, or itching skin, pale skin, edema (swelling) of face or extremities, reduced ability to exercise, headache, fever.

GLYBURIDE

BRAND NAMES

DiaBeta, Glynase
Prestab, Micronase

Available in: Tablets
Available OTC? No   **As Generic?** Yes
Drug Class: Antidiabetic agent/sulfonylurea

▼ USAGE INFORMATION

WHY IT'S PRESCRIBED
To help control adult-onset (non-insulin-dependent, or type 2) diabetes. Glyburide is sometimes used in conjunction with metformin (another oral antidiabetic).

HOW IT WORKS
Glyburide stimulates the release of insulin by the pancreas and decreases sugar production in the liver.

▼ DOSAGE GUIDELINES

RANGE AND FREQUENCY
Starting dose is 2.5 to 5 mg daily, 30 minutes before breakfast. It can be increased by your doctor in increments of 2.5 mg to a maximum of 20 mg per day, or decreased if needed. Elderly patients or those with kidney or liver dysfunction should receive an initial dose of 1.25 mg per day. If the daily maintenance dose is increased to 10 mg or more, the total dose should be divided equally between breakfast and dinner.

ONSET OF EFFECT
1 hour.

DURATION OF ACTION
24 hours.

DIETARY ADVICE
It is usually taken 30 minutes before breakfast.

STORAGE
Store in a tightly sealed container away from heat and direct light.

MISSED DOSE
Take it as soon as you remember. If it is near the time for the next dose, skip the missed dose and resume your regular dosage schedule. Do not double the next dose.

STOPPING THE DRUG
The decision to stop taking the drug should be made by your doctor. You may need to take glyburide for the rest of your life.

PROLONGED USE
Periodic blood tests should be done to determine how prolonged use affects blood sugar levels.

▼ PRECAUTIONS

Over 60: Treatment should start with lower doses, which should be increased slowly as determined by periodic tests. Adverse reactions may be more likely and more severe in older patients.

Driving and Hazardous Work: Do not drive or engage in hazardous work until you determine how the medication affects you.

Alcohol: Avoid alcohol.

Pregnancy: Having uncontrolled blood sugar levels during pregnancy is associated with an increased risk of birth defects, so many experts recommend a switch to insulin during pregnancy.

Breast Feeding: Glyburide may pass into breast milk; caution is advised. Consult your doctor for advice.

Infants and Children: Glyburide does not work for juvenile-onset, insulin-dependent diabetes.

Special Concerns: Carry medical identification that says you have diabetes. If you are under stress due to an infection, fever, an injury, or surgery, you may need insulin therapy in addition to or instead of glyburide.

OVERDOSE
Symptoms: Symptoms are similar to serious side effects.

What to Do: An overdose of glyburide is unlikely to be life-threatening. However, if someone takes a much larger dose than prescribed, call your doctor, emergency medical services (EMS), or the nearest poison control center.

▼ INTERACTIONS

DRUG INTERACTIONS
Consult your doctor for specific advice if you are taking anabolic steroids, aspirin or other salicylates, cimetidine, gemfibrozil, fenfluramine, MAO inhibitors, phenylbutazone, ranitidine, sulfa drugs, beta-blockers, bumetanide, diazoxide, ethacrynic acid, furosemide, phenytoin, rifampin, thiazide diuretics, thyroid hormone, antacids, antifungal agents, enalapril, steroids, or warfarin.

FOOD INTERACTIONS
Glyburide is just part of the treatment for diabetes; be sure to follow the diet recommended by your doctor.

DISEASE INTERACTIONS
Use of this medication may cause complications in patients with liver or kidney disease, since these organs work together to remove the drug from the body.

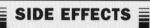

SIDE EFFECTS

SERIOUS
Serious side effects are related to hypoglycemia, or low blood sugar, whose symptoms include perspiration or a cold sweat, restlessness, rapid pulse, anxious feeling, nausea, feelings of dizziness, weakness, or lightheadedness, poor coordination, slurred speech, confusion, sleepiness, seizures, weakness of an arm, leg, or an entire side of the body, and fainting. Seek emergency assistance. Administer sugar-containing substances only if the patient is conscious and alert. Other serious but less common side effects include bone marrow suppression, hemolytic anemia, and elevation of liver-associated enzymes; these problems can be detected by your doctor.

COMMON
Bloating, heartburn, nausea, indigestion.

LESS COMMON
Blurred vision, changes in taste, itching, hives, joint or muscle pain.

HALOPERIDOL

BRAND NAMES

Haldol, Haldol Decanoate

Available in: Tablets, liquid, injection
Available OTC? No   **As Generic?** Yes
Drug Class: Neuroleptic; antipsychotic

▼ USAGE INFORMATION

WHY IT'S PRESCRIBED
To treat moderate to severe psychiatric conditions including schizophrenia, manic states, and drug-induced psychosis. It is also used to treat extreme behavior problems in children (including infantile autism), to ease the symptoms of Tourette's syndrome, and to reduce nausea and vomiting associated with chemotherapy for cancer.

HOW IT WORKS
Haloperidol blocks receptors of dopamine (a chemical that aids in the transmission of nerve impulses) in the central nervous system. Presumably, this produces a tranquilizing or antipsychotic effect.

▼ DOSAGE GUIDELINES

RANGE AND FREQUENCY
For psychotic disorders—
Adults: Initial dose is 0.5 to 5 mg, 2 or 3 times a day; maximum dose is 100 mg a day. Children ages 3 to 12: 0.05 to 0.15 mg for every 2.2 lbs (1 kg) of body weight.
For Tourette's syndrome—
Adults: 0.5 to 5 mg, 2 or 3 times a day. Children ages 3 to 12: 0.075 mg for every 2.2 lbs daily.

ONSET OF EFFECT
Sedation may occur within minutes, but onset of antipsychotic effect may take hours or may not occur until days or weeks after the beginning of therapy.

DURATION OF ACTION
12 to 24 hours, but effects may persist for several days.

DIETARY ADVICE
Take haloperidol with food or a full glass of milk or water. To prevent stomach irritation, the oral solution can be diluted in beverages such as orange, apple, or tomato juice, or cola.

STORAGE
Store in a tightly sealed container away from heat and direct light.

MISSED DOSE
Take it as soon as you remember. Do not double the next dose. Space any remaining doses for that day at regular intervals. Return to your regular schedule the next day.

STOPPING THE DRUG
The decision to stop taking the drug should be made in consultation with your doctor. Gradual reduction of doses may be required if you have taken it for a long period.

PROLONGED USE
Prolonged use may lead to tardive dyskinesia (involuntary movements of the jaw, lips, tongue, and, in rare cases, the arms, legs, hands, or body). Consult your doctor about the need for periodic evaluation and lab tests.

▼ PRECAUTIONS

Over 60: Adverse reactions are more likely and more severe in older patients.

Driving and Hazardous Work: Exercise caution until you determine how the medication affects you.

Alcohol: Avoid alcohol.

Pregnancy: Before taking haloperidol, be sure to tell your doctor if you are, or plan to become, pregnant.

Breast Feeding: Haloperidol passes into breast milk and may be harmful to the child; do not use it while nursing.

Infants and Children: Not recommended for children under age 3 or those weighing less than 33 pounds.

Special Concerns: Avoid prolonged exposure to high temperatures or hot climates. Drink plenty of fluids and stay cool in the summertime. Avoid overexposure to sunlight until you determine if the drug heightens your skin's sensitivity to ultraviolet light.

OVERDOSE
Symptoms: Shallow, slow breathing, weak or rapid pulse, muscle weakness or tremor, dizziness, confusion, seizures, deep sleep, coma.

What to Do: Call your doctor, emergency medical services (EMS), or the nearest poison control center immediately.

▼ INTERACTIONS

DRUG INTERACTIONS
Consult your doctor for specific advice if you are taking anticholinergics, anticonvulsants, antidepressants, antihistamines, antihypertensives, bupropion, central nervous system depressants such as barbiturates, clozapine, dronabinol, ethinamate, fluoxetine, guanethidine, guanfacine, lithium, methyldopa, carbamazepine, rifampin, or trihexyphenidyl.

FOOD INTERACTIONS
No known food interactions.

DISEASE INTERACTIONS
Consult your doctor if you have Parkinson's disease or any movement disorder, glaucoma, epilepsy, or liver or kidney disease.

≡ SIDE EFFECTS ≡

SERIOUS
Rapid heartbeat, profuse sweating, seizures, difficulty breathing, neck stiffness, swelling of the tongue, difficulty swallowing. Also a rare condition can develop called neuroleptic malignant syndrome, characterized by stiffness or spasms of the muscles, high fever, and confusion or disorientation. Call your doctor immediately.

COMMON
Nausea, reduced sweating, dry mouth, blurred vision, drowsiness, shaking of hands, stiffness, stooped posture.

LESS COMMON
Difficult urination, menstrual irregularities, breast pain or swelling, unexpected weight gain, uncontrolled movements of the tongue, fever, chills, sore throat, unusual bruising or bleeding, heart palpitations, skin rash, itching, increased sensitivity of the skin to sunlight.

HYDROCHLOROTHIAZIDE/TRIAMTERENE

Available in: Capsules, tablets
Available OTC? No   **As Generic?** Yes
Drug Class: Thiazide diuretic

▼ USAGE INFORMATION

WHY IT'S PRESCRIBED
To treat high blood pressure (hypertension); to treat conditions that cause edema (swelling of body tissues resulting from excess salt and water retention).

HOW IT WORKS
This drug combines a thiazide diuretic (hydrochlorothiazide) and a potassium-sparing diuretic (triamterene). Diuretics increase the excretion of salt and water in the urine. By reducing the overall fluid volume in the body, these drugs reduce blood volume and so reduce pressure within the blood vessels.

▼ DOSAGE GUIDELINES

RANGE AND FREQUENCY
Adults: 1 or 2 capsules or tablets once a day. Children: The dose must be determined by your doctor.

ONSET OF EFFECT
Within 2 hours.

DURATION OF ACTION
6 to 12 hours.

DIETARY ADVICE
This medication should be taken in the morning after eating breakfast.

STORAGE
Store in a tightly sealed container away from heat and direct light.

MISSED DOSE
Take this medication as soon as you remember. If it is near the time for the next dose, skip the missed dose and resume your regular dosage schedule. Do not double the next dose.

STOPPING THE DRUG
The decision to stop taking this prescription medication should be made by your doctor.

PROLONGED USE
See your doctor regularly for physical examinations and appropriate laboratory tests if you must take this medicine for an extended period.

▼ PRECAUTIONS

Over 60: Adverse reactions may be more likely and more severe in this age group.

Driving and Hazardous Work: No special precautions are necessary.

Alcohol: No special precautions are necessary.

Pregnancy: This drug should not be taken during pregnancy unless recommended by your doctor. Other diuretics are generally preferred.

Breast Feeding: This drug passes into breast milk; avoid or discontinue use while breast feeding.

Infants and Children: No unusual side effects are expected in children. The dose must be determined by a pediatrician.

Special Concerns: To prevent hydrochlorothiazide from interfering with sleep, take it in the morning. If you are taking it for high blood pressure, follow the diet and weight control measures that are recommended by your doctor. Avoid exposure to sunlight, use a sunblock, or wear protective clothing.

OVERDOSE
Symptoms: Dehydration, muscle weakness, cramps, heart arrhythmias.

What to Do: Call your doctor, emergency medical services (EMS), or the nearest poison control center immediately.

▼ INTERACTIONS

DRUG INTERACTIONS
Consult your doctor for specific advice if you are taking ACE inhibitors, cyclosporine, medications or dietary supplements that contain potassium, cholestyramine, colestipol, digitalis drugs, lithium, or any over-the-counter medication.

FOOD INTERACTIONS
The triamterene in this combination diuretic drug reduces excess loss of potassium in the body. For this reason, patients are usually advised not to consume large servings of potassium-rich foods. These include bananas, citrus fruits and juices, melons, prunes, (and most fruits in general), avocados, potatoes, nuts, baked beans, brussels sprouts, and skim milk.

DISEASE INTERACTIONS
Caution is advised when taking this medicine. Consult your doctor if you have diabetes, gout, kidney stones, lupus erythematosus, heart disease, pancreatitis, blood vessel disease, menstrual problems, liver disease, or kidney disease.

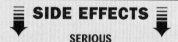

≡ SIDE EFFECTS ≡

SERIOUS
Skin rash, hives, intense itching, swelling of the mouth and throat, breathing difficulty, heart rhythm irregularities or palpitations, lightheadedness or dizziness, unusual bleeding or bruising. Call your doctor immediately.

COMMON
Fluid depletion may lead to dizziness, especially upon arising from a sitting or lying position, as well as thirst, dry mouth, and constipation.

LESS COMMON
Decreased sexual ability, increased sensitivity to sunlight, loss of appetite, gout, increased blood sugar (a problem for diabetic patients).

HYDROCHLOROTHIAZIDE (HCTZ)

Available in: Tablets, oral suspension
Available OTC? No **As Generic?** Yes
Drug Class: Thiazide diuretic

▼ USAGE INFORMATION

WHY IT'S PRESCRIBED
To treat high blood pressure (hypertension); to treat conditions that cause edema (swelling of body tissues resulting from excess salt and water retention).

HOW IT WORKS
Diuretics increase the excretion of salt and water in the urine. By reducing the overall fluid volume in the body, these drugs reduce pressure within the blood vessels.

▼ DOSAGE GUIDELINES

RANGE AND FREQUENCY
Adults—To reduce excess body water: 25 to 100 mg, 1 or 2 times a day. Your doctor may change the frequency to every other day or 3 to 5 days a week. For high blood pressure: 25 to 100 mg a day. Children, to reduce body water—Ages 2 to 12: 37.5 to 100 mg a day in 2 doses. Ages 6 months to 2 years:

12.5 to 37.5 mg a day in 2 doses. Infants under 6 months: Up to 3.3 mg per 2.2 lbs (1 kg) of body weight in 2 doses.

ONSET OF EFFECT
Within 2 hours.

DURATION OF ACTION
6 to 12 hours.

DIETARY ADVICE
It can be be taken with food to avoid stomach upset.

STORAGE
Store in a tightly sealed container away from heat and direct light. Keep the liquid form from freezing.

MISSED DOSE
Take it as soon as you remember. If it is near the time for the next dose, skip the missed dose and resume your regular dosage schedule. Do not double the next dose.

STOPPING THE DRUG
The decision to stop taking the drug should be made by your doctor.

PROLONGED USE
See your doctor regularly for examinations and tests if you must take this medicine for an extended period.

▼ PRECAUTIONS

Over 60: Adverse reactions may be more likely and more severe in older patients.

Driving and Hazardous Work: No special precautions are necessary.

Alcohol: No special precautions are necessary.

Pregnancy: Hydrochlorothiazide has caused birth defects in animals. Human studies have not been done. This medicine should not be taken during pregnancy unless recommended by your doctor; other diuretics are generally preferred for pregnant women.

Breast Feeding: Hydrochlorothiazide passes into breast milk; avoid or discontinue use during the first month of nursing.

Infants and Children: No unusual side effects are expected in children. The dose must be determined by a pediatrician.

Special Concerns: Hydrochlorothiazide is usually prescribed once a day. To prevent it from interfering with sleep, take it in the morning. If you are taking this drug for high blood pressure, follow the diet and weight control measures recommended by your doctor. Avoid exposure to sunlight,

use a sunblock, or wear protective clothing. This medicine may cause your body to lose potassium. Follow your doctor's instructions about eating potassium-rich foods or taking a potassium supplement.

OVERDOSE
Symptoms: Fainting, lethargy, dizziness, drowsiness, confusion, gastrointestinal irritation.

What to Do: Call your doctor, emergency medical services (EMS), or the nearest poison control center immediately.

▼ INTERACTIONS

DRUG INTERACTIONS
Consult your doctor for specific advice if you are taking anticoagulants, cholestyramine, colestipol, drugs for diabetes, nonsteroidal anti-inflammatory drugs, digitalis drugs, or lithium.

FOOD INTERACTIONS
No known food interactions.

DISEASE INTERACTIONS
Caution is advised when taking hydrochlorothiazide. Consult your doctor if you have any of the following: diabetes, gout, lupus erythematosus, pancreatitis, heart disease, blood vessel disease, liver disease, or kidney disease.

⬇ SIDE EFFECTS ⬇

SERIOUS
Skin rash, hives, intense itching, swelling of the mouth and throat, breathing difficulty, heart rhythm irregularities, lightheadedness, unusual bleeding or bruising. Call your doctor immediately.

COMMON
Muscle cramps or pain. Potassium depletion may lead to heart palpitations and weakness. Fluid depletion may lead to dizziness, especially upon arising from a sitting or lying position, as well as thirst, dry mouth, and constipation.

LESS COMMON
Decreased sexual ability, increased sensitivity to sunlight, loss of appetite, gout, increased blood sugar (a problem for diabetic patients), pancreatitis (rare).

HYDROCODONE BITARTRATE/ACETAMINOPHEN

Available in: Capsules, oral solution, tablets
Available OTC? No   **As Generic?** Yes
Drug Class: Opioid (narcotic) analgesic

Allay, Anexsia,
Anolor DH, Bancap-HC,
Co-Gesic, Dolacet,
Dolagesic, Duocet,
HY-PHEN, Hyco-Pap,
Hycomed, Hydrogesic,
Lorcet, Lortab, Margesic-
H, Oncet, Pancet 5/500,
Panlor, Polygesic,
Stagesic, T-Gesic, Ugesic,
Vanacet, Vendone,
Vicodin, Zydone

▼ USAGE INFORMATION

WHY IT'S PRESCRIBED
To relieve moderate to severe pain, when nonprescription pain relievers prove inadequate. When taken in combination with acetaminophen, hydrocodone may provide better pain relief at lower doses than either medication does when used alone at higher doses.

HOW IT WORKS
Hydrocodone, a narcotic, is believed to relieve pain by acting on specific areas both in the spinal cord and in the brain that process pain signals from nerves throughout the body. Acetaminophen appears to interfere with the action of prostaglandins, hormone-like chemical substances in the body that cause inflammation and make nerves more sensitive to pain impulses.

▼ DOSAGE GUIDELINES

RANGE AND FREQUENCY
Adults—Capsules: 1 every 4 to 6 hours. Oral solution: 1 to 3 teaspoons every 4 to 6 hours. Tablets: 1 or 2 that contain 2.5 mg of hydrocodone, or 1 that contains 5, 7.5, or 10 mg of hydrocodone, every 4 to 6 hours.

ONSET OF EFFECT
30 to 60 minutes.

DURATION OF ACTION
4 to 6 hours.

DIETARY ADVICE
This drug can be taken without regard to diet.

STORAGE
Store in a sealed container away from heat and light.

MISSED DOSE
If you are taking this medicine on a fixed schedule, take it as soon as you remember. If it is near the time for the next dose, skip the missed dose and resume your regular dosage schedule. Do not double the next dose.

STOPPING THE DRUG
The decision to stop taking the drug should be made by your doctor.

PROLONGED USE
See your doctor regularly for tests and examinations. Prolonged use can cause mental or physical dependence.

▼ PRECAUTIONS

Over 60: Adverse reactions may be more likely and more severe in older patients.

Driving and Hazardous Work: Do not drive or engage in hazardous work until you determine how the medicine affects you.

Alcohol: Avoid alcohol.

Pregnancy: Overuse during pregnancy can cause drug dependence in the fetus.

Breast Feeding: It is not known whether this drug passes into breast milk; caution is advised. Consult your doctor for specific advice.

Infants and Children: Adverse reactions may be more likely and more severe in children.

Special Concerns: If you feel the medication is not working properly after a few weeks of use, do not increase the dose on your own. See your doctor for advice.

OVERDOSE
Symptoms: Severe dizziness or drowsiness; cold, clammy skin; slow breathing or shortness of breath; seizures; severe confusion; stomach cramps or pain; diarrhea; sweating; constricted pupils; nausea or vomiting; irregular heartbeat; severe weakness.

What to Do: Call your doctor, emergency medical services (EMS), or the nearest poison control center immediately.

▼ INTERACTIONS

DRUG INTERACTIONS
Consult your doctor for specific advice if you are taking any prescription or over-the-counter medications, especially drugs with acetaminophen or central nervous system depressants such as barbiturates, seizure medicine, muscle relaxants, anesthetics, tranquilizers, or sedatives.

FOOD INTERACTIONS
No known food interactions.

DISEASE INTERACTIONS
Consult your doctor if you have a head injury or brain disease, hypothyroidism, an enlarged prostate, seizures, kidney or liver disease, gall bladder problems, a blood disorder, or a history of alcohol or drug abuse.

≡ SIDE EFFECTS ≡

SERIOUS
Bloody, dark, or cloudy urine; severe pain in lower back or side; pale or black, tarry stools; yellow-tinged eyes or skin; hallucinations; frequent urge to urinate; painful or difficult urination; sudden decrease in amount of urine; increased sweating; unusual bleeding or bruising; irregular heartbeat; skin rash, hives, or itching; unusual excitement; irregular breathing or wheezing; ringing or buzzing in ears; pinpoint red spots on skin; sore throat and fever; confusion; trembling or uncontrolled muscle movements; flushing or swelling of face. Call your doctor immediately.

COMMON
Dizziness, lightheadedness, nausea or vomiting, drowsiness, constipation, itching.

LESS COMMON
Stomach pain, allergic reaction, false sense of well-being, depression, loss of appetite, blurring or change in vision, feeling of illness, headache, nervousness, insomnia.

IBUPROFEN

Available in: Tablets, oral solution, chewable tablets
Available OTC? Yes **As Generic?** Yes
Drug Class: Nonsteroidal anti-inflammatory drug (NSAID)

▼ USAGE INFORMATION

WHY IT'S PRESCRIBED
To treat mild to moderate pain and inflammation caused by tendinitis, arthritis, bursitis, gout, soft tissue injuries, migraine and other vascular headaches, menstrual cramps, and other conditions. It is also used to reduce fever.

HOW IT WORKS
NSAIDs work by interfering with the formation of prostaglandins, substances that cause inflammation and make nerves more sensitive to pain impulses. NSAIDs also have other modes of action that are less well understood.

▼ DOSAGE GUIDELINES

RANGE AND FREQUENCY
Adults—For mild to moderate pain, arthritis, and menstrual pain: 200 to 400 mg every 4 to 6 hours. For fever: 200 to 400 mg every 4 to 6 hours, but not more than 1,200 mg a day. Children ages 6 months to 12 years—For fevers below 102.5°F, 5 mg for every 2.2 lbs (1 kg) of body weight every 6 to 8 hours. For higher fevers, 10 mg per 2.2 lbs every 6 to 8 hours, but not more than 40 mg per 2.2 lbs a day.

ONSET OF EFFECT
For pain and fever, 30 minutes. For arthritis, up to 3 weeks before relief.

DURATION OF ACTION
4 hours or more.

DIETARY ADVICE
Take ibuprofen with food.

STORAGE
Store in a tightly sealed container away from moisture, heat, and direct light.

MISSED DOSE
Take it as soon as you remember. However, if it is near the time for the next dose, skip the missed dose and resume your regular dosage schedule. Do not double the next dose.

STOPPING THE DRUG
If you're taking this drug by prescription, do not stop without consulting the doctor.

PROLONGED USE
Prolonged use can cause gastrointestinal problems, which may include ulceration and bleeding, kidney dysfunction, and liver inflammation. See your doctor regularly for laboratory tests and physical examinations.

▼ PRECAUTIONS

Over 60: Because of the potentially greater consequences of gastrointestinal side effects, the dose of NSAIDs for older patients, especially those over age 70, is often cut in half.

Driving and Hazardous Work: Do not drive or engage in hazardous work until you determine how the medicine affects you.

Alcohol: Avoid alcohol, as it may increase the risk of stomach irritation.

Pregnancy: Avoid or discontinue this drug if you are pregnant or are planning to become pregnant.

Breast Feeding: Ibuprofen passes into breast milk; avoid using it while nursing.

Infants and Children: May be used in exceptional circumstances; consult your doctor.

Special Concerns: Because NSAIDs can interfere with blood coagulation, this drug should be stopped at least 3 days prior to any surgery.

OVERDOSE
Symptoms: Severe nausea, vomiting, headache, confusion, seizures.

What to Do: Call your doctor, emergency medical services (EMS), or the nearest poison control center immediately.

▼ INTERACTIONS

DRUG INTERACTIONS
Do not take this drug with aspirin or any other NSAIDs without your doctor's approval. In addition, consult your doctor if you are taking antihypertensives, steroids, anticoagulants, antibiotics, itraconazole or ketoconazole, plicamycin, penicillamine, valproic acid, phenytoin, cyclosporine, digitalis drugs, lithium, methotrexate, probenecid, triamterene, or zidovudine.

FOOD INTERACTIONS
No known food interactions.

DISEASE INTERACTIONS
Consult your doctor if you have any of the following: bleeding problems, gastrointestinal inflammation or ulcers, diabetes mellitus, systemic lupus erythematosus (SLE), anemia, asthma, epilepsy, Parkinson's disease, kidney stones, or a history of heart disease or alcohol abuse. Use of ibuprofen may cause complications in patients with liver or kidney disease, since these organs work together to remove the medication from the body.

≡ SIDE EFFECTS ≡

SERIOUS
Shortness of breath or wheezing, with or without swelling of legs or other signs of heart failure; chest pain; peptic ulcer disease with vomiting of blood; black, tarry stools; decreasing kidney function. Call your doctor immediately.

COMMON
Nausea, vomiting, heartburn, diarrhea, constipation, headache, dizziness, sleepiness.

LESS COMMON
Ulcers or sores in mouth, depression, rashes or blistering of skin, ringing sound in the ears, unusual tingling or numbness of the hands or feet, seizures, blurred vision. Also: elevated potassium levels, decreased blood counts; such problems can be detected by your doctor.

INDINAVIR

BRAND NAME

Crixivan

Available in: Capsules
Available OTC? No   **As Generic?** No
Drug Class: Antiviral/protease inhibitor

▼ USAGE INFORMATION

WHY IT'S PRESCRIBED
To treat advanced HIV (human immunodeficiency virus) infection and AIDS (acquired immunodeficiency syndrome), usually in combination with other drugs. While not a cure for HIV infection, this drug may suppress the replication of the virus and delay the progression of the disease.

HOW IT WORKS
Indinavir blocks the activity of a viral protease, an enzyme that is needed by HIV to reproduce. Blocking the protease causes HIV to make copies that cannot infect new cells.

▼ DOSAGE GUIDELINES

RANGE AND FREQUENCY
800 mg every 8 hours, alone or in combination with other antiviral agents. Higher or lower doses are sometimes prescribed when indinavir is being combined with medications such as nevirapine and delavirdine, which alter indinavir blood levels.

ONSET OF EFFECT
Unknown. With most anti-retroviral drugs, an early response can be seen within the first few days of therapy, but the maximum effect may take 12 to 16 weeks.

DURATION OF ACTION
Unknown. Effects of the drug may be prolonged if indinavir is used in combination with other effective drugs and the virus is maximally suppressed.

DIETARY ADVICE
Indinavir should be taken with plenty of water or other liquid, preferably at least 1 hour before or 2 hours after a meal. It may also be taken with a light, nonfat snack. Drink at least 48 ounces of water per day.

STORAGE
Store in a tightly sealed container away from moisture, heat, and direct light.

MISSED DOSE
Take it as soon as you remember. However, if it is near the time for the next dose, skip the missed dose and resume your regular dosage schedule. Do not double the next dose.

STOPPING THE DRUG
The decision to stop taking the drug should be made by your doctor.

PROLONGED USE
See your doctor regularly for tests and examinations.

▼ PRECAUTIONS

Over 60: No special precautions are necessary.

Driving and Hazardous Work: Do not drive or engage in hazardous work until you determine how the medicine affects you.

Alcohol: Avoid alcohol if liver function is impaired.

Pregnancy: Indinavir has been shown to cause birth defects in animals. Human studies have not been done. Nevertheless, indinavir is increasingly used in combination with other antiretroviral drugs to treat pregnant HIV-infected women.

Breast Feeding: Women infected with HIV should not breast-feed, so they can avoid transmitting the virus to an uninfected child.

Infants and Children: Safety and effectiveness of indinavir for children under the age of 16 have not been established.

Special Concerns: Indinavir should not be taken concurrently with the herb St. John's wort; it can increase blood levels of the drug in the body, which may lead to possible resistance to indinavir. It is important to drink at least 48 ounces of water or other liquids every 24 hours to help prevent kidney stones. Indinavir therapy may be interrupted for patients who develop kidney stones. Tell any doctors or dentists treating you that you are taking this medication.

OVERDOSE
Symptoms: Pain in the lower back, blood in the urine, nausea, vomiting, diarrhea.

What to Do: An overdose is unlikely to be life-threatening. However, if someone takes a much larger dose than prescribed, call your doctor, emergency medical services (EMS), or the nearest poison control center immediately.

▼ INTERACTIONS

DRUG INTERACTIONS
Consult your doctor for specific advice if you are taking any other prescription or over-the-counter drug, especially astemizole, cisapride, didanosine, delavirdine, efavirenz, itraconazole, ketoconazole, midazolam, triazolam, didanosine, rifabutin, rifampin, phenobarbital, phenytoin, carbamazepine, cholesterol-lowering drugs, or dexamethasone.

FOOD INTERACTIONS
Food, especially fatty foods, will decrease absorption of the drug.

DISEASE INTERACTIONS
Use of indinavir may cause complications in patients with liver disease.

≣ SIDE EFFECTS ≣

SERIOUS
Blood in urine and sharp back pain caused by kidney stones. High blood sugar (diabetes) has occurred in patients taking drugs of this class, although a cause-and-effect relationship has not been established. Call your doctor if you develop increased thirst or excessive urination.

COMMON
Weakness, abdominal pains, diarrhea, nausea, vomiting, headache, insomnia, changes in taste, dry skin, chapped lips.

LESS COMMON
Dizziness, drowsiness, depression, memory changes, abdominal bloating, muscle wasting.

INSULIN GLARGINE (RDNA ORIGIN)

Available in: Injection
Available OTC? No   **As Generic?** No
Drug Class: Antidiabetic agent

▼ USAGE INFORMATION

WHY IT'S PRESCRIBED
For long-term treatment of diabetes mellitus. All patients with type 1 diabetes require lifelong insulin treatment. Patients with type 2 diabetes may require insulin if they are unable to control their blood glucose (sugar) levels with diet and oral medications. Insulin glargine is a slightly modified form of human insulin that maintains a relatively constant glucose-lowering effect over a 24-hour period and thus permits dosing once a day.

HOW IT WORKS
Insulin, a hormone secreted by the beta cells of the pancreas, plays an essential role in controlling the metabolism and storage of carbohydrates, fat, and protein. Insulin is secreted in response to a rise in blood sugar (glucose). Insulin lowers blood glucose by increasing its uptake by body cells, especially muscle, and by reducing the release of glucose from the liver between meals.

▼ DOSAGE GUIDELINES

RANGE AND FREQUENCY
Injected under the skin (of the stomach, thigh, or upper arm) once a day at bedtime. Doses are determined by your doctor. The solution should be clear and colorless, without any visible particles. Insulin glargine must not be diluted or mixed with any other insulin or solution.

ONSET OF EFFECT
About 1 to 2 hours.

DURATION OF ACTION
At least 24 hours.

≡ SIDE EFFECTS ≡

SERIOUS
Symptoms of hypoglycemia can be caused by the release of adrenaline or by an inadequate supply of glucose to the brain. With severe hypoglycemia, lack of sufficient glucose to the brain may cause slurred speech, impaired concentration, confusion, seizures, coma, irreversible brain damage, and death. Mild hypoglycemia may cause restless sleep, nightmares, or a cold sweat that awakens patients at night.

COMMON
Symptoms resulting from release of adrenaline are common manifestations of mild to moderate hypoglycemia. They include cold sweats, anxiety, shakiness, hunger, rapid heartbeat, headache, and nervousness. Weight gain is common when taking insulin.

LESS COMMON
Allergic reactions, lipoatrophy (depressions in the skin due to loss of fat tissue), and lipohypertrophy (excessive accumulation of fat tissue).

DIETARY ADVICE
All patients with diabetes should follow the general dietary recommendations of the American Diabetes Association. While intake of simple sugars is not forbidden, consuming large amounts of sugary foods at one time may trigger a rapid rise in blood glucose that can increase urination and thirst. In addition, patients who take insulin must remain consistent from day to day in the timing and caloric content of their meals. Depending on the timing, dose, and types of insulin prescribed, snacks may be recommended in the late afternoon, before bedtime, or prior to unusual physical activity. Diabetic patients must always have available a juice, food, or tablets that can rapidly raise blood glucose levels to counter an episode of hypoglycemia.

STORAGE
Refrigerate insulin but do not allow it to freeze. If refrigeration is not possible, the 10 milliliter (mL) vial or 3 mL cartridge in use can be kept unrefrigerated for up to 28 days away from direct heat and light, as long as the temperature is not greater than 86°F. Unrefrigerated 10 mL vials and 3 mL cartridges must be used within the 28-day period or they must be discarded. If refrigeration is not possible, the 5 mL vial in use can be kept unrefrigerated for up to 14 days away from direct heat and light, as long as the temperature is not greater than 86°F. Unrefrigerated 5 mL vials must be used within the 14-day period or they must be discarded. If refrigerated, the 5 mL vial in use can be kept for up to 28 days. Once the 3 mL cartridge is placed into an OptiPen One, it should not be put in the refrigerator.

MISSED DOSE
Timing of insulin doses is extremely important. The best approach is to measure blood glucose and add a dose of regular insulin if glucose levels are too high. Otherwise, wait for the next scheduled dose.

STOPPING THE DRUG
Do not stop taking insulin injections unless ordered to do so by your doctor. Patients with diabetes are often given general instructions for modifying their insulin doses based on home blood glucose measurements.

PROLONGED USE
After many years with diabetes, some patients become insensitive to the symptoms of hypoglycemia and are at risk for serious brain complications of prolonged, unrecognized hypoglycemia.

▼ PRECAUTIONS

Over 60: No special warnings. Some older people may, however, have vision problems that may make it difficult to draw up the correct dose of insulin.

Driving and Hazardous Work: Patients taking insulin must be very careful to avoid hypoglycemia when driving or engaging in hazardous work.

Alcohol: Moderate alcohol intake, especially when taken with large meals, does not

(continued)

adversely affect control of diabetes or alter the dose of insulin. However, large amounts of alcohol increase the risk of hypoglycemia.

Pregnancy: Strict metabolic control—using insulin injections in most women—must be maintained during pregnancy to reduce the risk of birth defects, fetal complications, or death at the time of delivery. In women who had diabetes before the onset of pregnancy, the dose of insulin is often smaller during the first third (trimester) of pregnancy and then higher during the final two trimesters. When women first develop diabetes during pregnancy (gestational diabetes), insulin requirements drop rapidly after delivery and most do not need to continue with insulin treatment.

Breast Feeding: Insulin requirements tend to be lower during breast feeding.

Home glucose monitoring is important to avoid hypoglycemia. Insulin glargine may pass into breast milk; consult your doctor for advice.

Infants and Children: Treatment with insulin in young patients age 6 and older is the same as that in older people with diabetes. The safety and effectiveness of insulin glargine in children under the age of 6 have not been established.

Special Concerns: Inadequate amounts of insulin in type 1 diabetes may lead to the serious complication of diabetic ketoacidosis, characterized by loss of appetite, excessive thirst and urination, nausea, vomiting, deep breathing, fruity breath odor, drowsiness, confusion, and loss of consciousness. Insulin glargine is not the insulin of choice for treating diabetic ketoacidosis. An intravenous short-acting insulin is the preferred treatment.

OVERDOSE

Symptoms: Insulin overdose results in hypoglycemia (see Side Effects for symptoms).

What to Do: For mild to moderate hypoglycemia, ingest drinks or food containing sugar. For more severe hypoglycemia, administer injections of glucagon or call emergency medical services (EMS) immediately.

▼ INTERACTIONS

DRUG INTERACTIONS
A large number of drugs can promote either elevated blood glucose levels or hypoglycemia. Be sure that your doctor knows about all of the medications you take and is informed before you start taking any new drugs, either by prescription or over the counter. Corticosteroids in particular are likely to raise blood glucose levels and insulin requirements. Beta-

blockers (commonly prescribed for hypertension) may cause either high blood glucose levels or hypoglycemia; in addition, because these medications may dampen the symptoms of hypoglycemia that are caused by adrenaline release, mild degrees of hypoglycemia may progress unnoticed to more serious hypoglycemia affecting the brain.

FOOD INTERACTIONS
Insulin requirements are increased by the ingestion of large amounts of calories, especially simple sugars and other carbohydrates.

DISEASE INTERACTIONS
Insulin requirements are increased by infections, psychological stress, or an uncontrolled overactive thyroid, and often at a time of surgery. Requirements may diminish with kidney disease or an underactive adrenal or pituitary gland.

INSULIN LISPRO (RDNA ORIGIN)

Available in: Injection
Available OTC? No   **As Generic?** No
Drug Class: Antidiabetic agent

▼ USAGE INFORMATION

WHY IT'S PRESCRIBED
For long-term treatment of diabetes mellitus. All patients with type 1 diabetes require lifelong insulin treatment. Patients with type 2 diabetes may require insulin if they are unable to control their blood glucose (sugar) levels with diet and oral medications.

HOW IT WORKS
Insulin, a hormone secreted by the beta cells of the pancreas, plays an essential role in controlling the metabolism and storage of carbohydrates, fat, and protein. Insulin is secreted in response to a rise in blood sugar (glucose). Insulin lowers blood glucose by increasing its uptake by body cells, especially muscle, and by reducing the release of glucose from the liver between meals.

▼ DOSAGE GUIDELINES

RANGE AND FREQUENCY
It may be taken 1 to 4 times daily, before meals and possibly at bedtime. Doses and frequency are determined by your doctor. Rapid-acting (lispro rDNA origin) insulin should be administered 15 minutes before a meal.

ONSET OF EFFECT
Within 30 to 45 minutes; the peak effect occurs within 1 hour.

DURATION OF ACTION
From 3 to 4 hours.

DIETARY ADVICE
All patients with diabetes should follow the general dietary recommendations of the American Diabetes Association. Though intake of simple sugars is not forbidden, consuming a large amount of sugary foods at one time may trigger a rapid rise in blood glucose that can increase urination and thirst. In addition, patients who take insulin must remain consistent from day to day in the timing and caloric content of their meals. Depending on the timing, dose, and types of insulin prescribed, snacks may be recommended for the late afternoon, before bedtime, or prior to unusual physical activity. Diabetic patients must always have available a juice, food, or tablets that can raise blood glucose levels rapidly to counter an episode of hypoglycemia.

STORAGE
Refrigerate insulin but do not allow it to freeze. Insulin does not have to be kept refrigerated when you're traveling for short periods, but exposure to high temperatures must be avoided.

MISSED DOSE
Timing of insulin doses is extremely important. The best approach is to measure blood glucose and add a dose of regular insulin if your glucose levels are too high. Otherwise, wait for the next scheduled dose.

STOPPING THE DRUG
Do not stop taking insulin injections unless ordered to do so by your doctor. Patients with diabetes are often given general instructions for modifying their insulin doses based on their home blood glucose measurements.

PROLONGED USE
After many years with diabetes, some patients become insensitive to the symptoms of hypoglycemia and are at risk for serious brain complications from prolonged, unrecognized hypoglycemia.

▼ PRECAUTIONS

Over 60: No special warnings. Some older people may, however, have vision problems that may make it difficult to draw up the correct dose of insulin.

Driving and Hazardous Work: Patients taking insulin must be very careful to avoid hypoglycemia when driving or engaging in hazardous work.

Alcohol: Moderate alcohol intake, especially when taken with large meals, does not adversely affect control of diabetes or alter the dose of insulin. However, large amounts of alcohol increase the risk of hypoglycemia.

Pregnancy: Strict metabolic control—using insulin injections in most women—must be maintained during pregnancy to reduce the risk of birth defects, fetal complications, or death at the time of delivery. In women who had diabetes before the onset of pregnancy, the dose of insulin is often smaller during the first third (trimester) of pregnancy and then higher during the final two trimesters. When women first develop diabetes during pregnancy (gestational diabetes), insulin requirements drop rapidly after delivery and most do not need to continue with insulin treatment.

Breast Feeding: Insulin requirements tend to be

▤ SIDE EFFECTS ▤

SERIOUS
Symptoms of hypoglycemia can be caused by the release of adrenaline or by an inadequate supply of glucose to the brain. With severe hypoglycemia, lack of sufficient glucose to the brain may cause slurred speech, impaired concentration, confusion, seizures, coma, irreversible brain damage, and death. Mild hypoglycemia may cause restless sleep, nightmares, or a cold sweat that awakens patients at night.

COMMON
Symptoms resulting from release of adrenaline are common manifestations of mild to moderate hypoglycemia. They include cold sweats, anxiety, shakiness, hunger, rapid heartbeat, headache, and nervousness. Weight gain is common when taking insulin.

LESS COMMON
Allergic reactions, lipoatrophy (depressions in the skin due to loss of fat tissue), and lipohypertrophy (excessive accumulation of fat tissue).

lower during breast feeding. Home glucose monitoring is important to avoid hypoglycemia. Insulin is not present in breast milk.

Infants and Children: Treatment with insulin in young patients is the same as that in older people with diabetes.

Special Concerns: Inadequate amounts of insulin in type 1 diabetes may lead to the serious complication of diabetic ketoacidosis, characterized by loss of appetite, excessive thirst and urination, nausea, vomiting, deep breathing, fruity breath odor, drowsiness, confusion, and loss of consciousness.

OVERDOSE

Symptoms: Insulin overdose results in hypoglycemia (see Side Effects for symptoms).

What to Do: For mild to moderate hypoglycemia, ingest drinks or food containing sugar. For more severe hypoglycemia, administer injections of glucagon or call emergency medical services (EMS) immediately.

▼ INTERACTIONS

DRUG INTERACTIONS

A large number of drugs can promote either elevated blood glucose levels or hypoglycemia. Be sure your doctor knows about all of the medications you take and is informed before you start taking any new drugs, either by prescription or over the counter. Corticosteroids in particular are likely to raise blood glucose levels and insulin requirements. Beta-blockers (commonly prescribed for hypertension) may cause either high blood glucose levels or hypoglycemia; in addition, because these medications may dampen the symptoms of hypoglycemia that are caused by adrenaline release, mild degrees of hypoglycemia may progress unnoticed over time to more serious hypoglycemia affecting the brain.

FOOD INTERACTIONS

Insulin requirements are increased when larger amounts of calories are ingested, especially simple sugars and carbohydrates.

DISEASE INTERACTIONS

Insulin requirements are increased by infections, psychological stress, or an uncontrolled overactive thyroid, and often at a time of surgery. Requirements may diminish with kidney disease or an underactive adrenal or pituitary gland.

INTERFERON BETA-1B (RIFN-B)

Betaseron

Available in: Powder for injection
Available OTC? No   **As Generic?** No
Drug Class: Immunomodulator

▼ USAGE INFORMATION

WHY IT'S PRESCRIBED
To treat relapsing-remitting multiple sclerosis (the most common form of MS, in which periods of active disease alternate with periods of remission or reduced severity of symptoms).

HOW IT WORKS
It acts in the same way as the body's natural interferons, which are proteins released by the immune system to fight viruses, cancer cells, and other types of disease. The exact way in which this drug fights MS is unknown, but it appears to interfere with the immune system's attack on healthy tissue.

▼ DOSAGE GUIDELINES

RANGE AND FREQUENCY
8 million units (0.25 mg) by injection every other day.

ONSET OF EFFECT
Unknown.

DURATION OF ACTION
Unknown.

DIETARY ADVICE
Drink plenty of fluids to reduce the risk of excessively low blood pressure.

STORAGE
Keep the liquid form refrigerated but do not allow it to freeze.

MISSED DOSE
If you miss a dose, do not take the missed dose and do not double the next dose. Notify your doctor.

STOPPING THE DRUG
The decision to stop taking the drug should be made by your doctor.

PROLONGED USE
See your doctor regularly for tests and examinations if you must take this drug for a prolonged period.

▼ PRECAUTIONS

Over 60: Adverse reactions may be more likely and more severe in older patients.

Driving and Hazardous Work: Do not drive or engage in hazardous work until you determine how the medicine affects you.

Alcohol: Avoid alcohol.

Pregnancy: Adequate studies have not been done. Consult your doctor for advice.

Breast Feeding: Interferon beta-1b may pass into breast milk; caution is advised. Consult your doctor for advice.

Infants and Children: No special studies have been done on the effects of beta interferon in children.

Special Concerns: Interferon beta-1b should be used with caution in patients with a history of depression, since it has been linked to an increase in suicidal impulses. Try to avoid people with infections, because this drug can lower white blood cell levels temporarily and increase susceptibility to disease. Be careful when using a toothbrush, dental floss, or toothpick. Your doctor or dentist may recommend other ways to clean your teeth. Check with your doctor before having any dental work done. Be careful not to cut yourself when using sharp objects such as a razor. Avoid contact sports or other situations where bruising could occur. Do not touch your eyes or the inside of your mouth unless you have just washed your hands.

OVERDOSE
Symptoms: No specific ones have been reported.

What to Do: Call your doctor or emergency medical services (EMS) immediately if you suspect an overdose.

▼ INTERACTIONS

DRUG INTERACTIONS
Consult your doctor for specific advice if you are taking any prescription or over-the-counter medication.

FOOD INTERACTIONS
None are known.

DISEASE INTERACTIONS
Caution is advised when taking interferon beta-1b. Consult your doctor if you have a history of bleeding or clotting disorders, chicken pox, shingles, psychological or neurological disorders, diabetes, autoimmune disorders, heart disease, kidney disease, liver disease, lung disease, or thyroid disease.

≡ SIDE EFFECTS ≡

SERIOUS
Seizures, swelling and fluid retention, pelvic pain, pounding in the chest, breast pain, frequent urination, sweating, anxiety, confusion, joint pain, breathing difficulty, depression, suicidal thoughts or impulses. Call your doctor right away.

COMMON
Pain, inflammation, or allergic reaction at injection site (most common side effect); flu-like symptoms, including headache, fever, muscle aches, general weakness, and fatigue (these symptoms tend to diminish as the body adjusts to therapy); insomnia; increased susceptibility to infection; nausea and vomiting; diarrhea; abdominal pain; temporary hair loss.

LESS COMMON
Dizziness, dry mouth, dry or itching skin, increased sweating, joint pain, vision or hearing problems. Tissue death at the site of injection has occurred in a few patients.

IPRATROPIUM BROMIDE

Available in: Inhalation aerosol, inhalation solution
Available OTC? No **As Generic?** Yes
Drug Class: Respiratory inhalant

▼ USAGE INFORMATION

WHY IT'S PRESCRIBED
To control the symptoms of lung diseases, such as asthma, chronic bronchitis, and emphysema.

HOW IT WORKS
It inhibits the cough reflex by blocking the activity of acetylcholine, a chemical that, in the lungs, causes the smooth muscles surrounding the airways to constrict. Therefore, when inhaled, ipratropium bromide causes the airways to widen (bronchodilation).

▼ DOSAGE GUIDELINES

RANGE AND FREQUENCY
The drug may be used as needed to relieve respiratory symptoms. For chronic obstructive lung disease such as bronchitis or emphysema– Inhalation aerosol: Adults and children 6 and over: 2 to 4 inhalations 3 or 4 times a day at regularly spaced intervals. Some patients may need 6 to 8 inhalations a day. Inhalation solution, adults and children 12 and over: 250 to 500 micrograms in a nebulizer 3 or 4 times a day, every 6 to 8 hours.

ONSET OF EFFECT
5 to 15 minutes.

DURATION OF ACTION
3 to 4 hours.

DIETARY ADVICE
Sugarless hard candy or gum can be taken to relieve dry mouth.

STORAGE
Store in a tightly sealed container away from heat and direct light. Open bottles of the solution should be refrigerated, but do not allow the solution to freeze.

MISSED DOSE
Take it as soon as you remember. If it is near the time for the next dose, skip the missed dose and resume your regular dosage schedule. Do not double the next dose.

STOPPING THE DRUG
It may not be necessary to continue using the medication for as long as originally prescribed; consult your doctor.

PROLONGED USE
You should see your doctor regularly if you must take this drug for a prolonged period.

▼ PRECAUTIONS

Over 60: Ipratropium is not expected to cause different problems in older patients than in younger persons.

Driving and Hazardous Work: Do not drive or engage in hazardous work until you determine how the medicine affects you.

Alcohol: No special precautions are necessary.

Pregnancy: Ipratropium has not caused birth defects in animals. Human studies have not been done. Before you take ipratropium, tell your doctor if you are pregnant or plan to become pregnant.

Breast Feeding: It is not known whether ipratropium passes into breast milk; caution is advised. Consult your doctor for specific advice.

Infants and Children: Ipratropium has been tested in children and has not been shown to cause different effects than in adults.

Special Concerns: To test the inhaler, insert the canister into the mouthpiece, take the cap off the mouthpiece, shake the inhaler 3 or 4 times, and spray once into the air. To use the inhaler, hold it upright, with the mouthpiece end down, shake it 3 or 4 times, then breathe out. Spray into open mouth or with mouth closed over inhaler, as recommended by your doctor. Clean the inhaler, mouthpiece, and spacer at least twice a week. To take the inhalation solution, use a power-operated nebulizer with a face mask or mouthpiece. Get instructions for using the nebulizer from your doctor.

OVERDOSE
Symptoms: No specific ones have been reported.

What to Do: An overdose of ipratropium is unlikely to be life-threatening. However, if someone takes a much larger dose than prescribed, call your doctor, emergency medical services (EMS), or the nearest poison control center.

▼ INTERACTIONS

DRUG INTERACTIONS
Before you use ipratropium, tell your doctor if you are using any other prescription or over-the-counter drug.

FOOD INTERACTIONS
No known food interactions.

DISEASE INTERACTIONS
Consult your doctor if you have glaucoma or difficulty urinating.

≡ SIDE EFFECTS ≡

SERIOUS
Persistent constipation; lower abdominal pain or bloating; wheezing or difficulty breathing; tightness in chest; severe eye pain; skin rash or hives; swelling of face, lips, or eyelids. Call your doctor immediately.

COMMON
Dry mouth, cough, unpleasant taste.

LESS COMMON
Blurred vision, other changes in vision, burning eyes, difficult urination, dizziness, headache, nausea, pounding heartbeat, nervousness, sweating, trembling.

IRBESARTAN

Available in: Tablets
Available OTC? No   **As Generic?** No
Drug Class: Antihypertensive/angiotensin II antagonist

▼ USAGE INFORMATION

WHY IT'S PRESCRIBED
To control high blood pressure. This drug appears to have the same benefits as the class of antihypertensive drugs known as ACE inhibitors, without producing the common side effect (experienced by as many as 30% of patients) of a dry cough. The drug may be used by itself or in conjunction with other antihypertensive medications.

HOW IT WORKS
Irbesartan blocks the effects of angiotensin II, a naturally occurring substance that causes blood vessels to narrow. Irbesartan causes the blood vessels to dilate, thereby lowering blood pressure and decreasing the workload of the heart.

▼ DOSAGE GUIDELINES

RANGE AND FREQUENCY
To start, 150 mg once a day. It may be increased by your doctor to a maximum dose of 300 mg per day.

ONSET OF EFFECT
Within 2 to 4 hours.

DURATION OF ACTION
More than 24 hours.

DIETARY ADVICE
No special restrictions, unless your doctor has advised a low-sodium diet or other dietary modifications to help control your blood pressure.

STORAGE
Store in a tightly sealed container away from moisture, heat, and direct light.

MISSED DOSE
If you miss a dose on one day, do not double the dose the next day. Resume your regular dosage schedule.

STOPPING THE DRUG
Take it as prescribed for the full treatment period. The decision to stop taking the drug should be made in consultation with your physician.

PROLONGED USE
Lifelong therapy may be necessary. However, if you do change certain health habits (for example, losing weight or increasing exercise), a reduced dose may be possible under a doctor's supervision.

▼ PRECAUTIONS

Over 60: Adverse reactions may be more likely and more severe in older patients.

Driving and Hazardous Work: Do not drive or engage in hazardous work until you determine how the medicine affects you.

Alcohol: No special precautions are necessary.

Pregnancy: Irbesartan should not be used by pregnant women. Discontinue taking the drug as soon as possible when pregnancy is detected and discuss treatment alternatives with your doctor.

Breast Feeding: Irbesartan may pass into breast milk; caution is advised. Consult your doctor for advice.

Infants and Children: The safety and effectiveness of use in children have not been established.

Special Concerns: Irbesartan may cause excessively low blood pressure with dizziness or lightheadedness, which is most noticeable when you change position. This may lead to fainting, falls, and injury. Sit or lie down immediately if you feel dizzy or lightheaded. This side effect may be worsened by alcohol, hot weather, dehydration, salt depletion from diuretic use, fever, prolonged standing, prolonged sitting, or exercise.

OVERDOSE

Symptoms: No cases of overdose have been reported. If you take a much larger dose than your doctor prescribes, however, you may experience extremely low blood pressure or heartbeat irregularities.

What to Do: If you take a much larger dose than prescribed, contact your doctor.

▼ INTERACTIONS

DRUG INTERACTIONS
No drug interactions have yet been observed with irbesartan. Consult your doctor for specific advice if you are taking any other medication, including other drugs for high blood pressure. Irbesartan can be taken together with diuretics or other medications for high blood pressure, if your doctor approves.

FOOD INTERACTIONS
No known food interactions.

DISEASE INTERACTIONS
Patients with liver or kidney disease are advised to exercise caution when they are taking irbesartan.

⇛ SIDE EFFECTS ⇚

SERIOUS
No serious side effects are associated with the use of irbesartan. (In clinical trials, the incidence of adverse effects was not significantly greater with the medication than with a placebo.)

COMMON
No common side effects are associated with the use of irbesartan.

LESS COMMON
Diarrhea, indigestion, heartburn, fatigue, muscle pain, edema, sexual dysfunction, low blood pressure.

ISOSORBIDE MONONITRATE

Available in: Tablets, extended-release tablets
Available OTC? No   **As Generic?** Yes
Drug Class: Nitrate

▼ USAGE INFORMATION

WHY IT'S PRESCRIBED
To prevent or relieve attacks of angina (chest pain associated with heart disease).

HOW IT WORKS
Isosorbide relaxes the smooth muscle of the blood vessels and increases the supply of blood and oxygen to the heart. It also reduces the heart's workload and demand for oxygen.

▼ DOSAGE GUIDELINES

RANGE AND FREQUENCY
To prevent angina attacks—Tablets: 20 mg, 2 times a day, with doses 7 hours apart. Extended-release tablets: 30 to 240 mg once a day.

ONSET OF EFFECT
60 minutes.

DURATION OF ACTION
Unknown.

DIETARY ADVICE
Take tablets on an empty stomach, at least 30 minutes before or 1 to 2 hours after a meal.

STORAGE
Store in a tightly sealed container away from heat and direct light.

MISSED DOSE
Take it as soon as you remember. If it is near the time for the next dose, skip the missed dose and resume your regular dosage schedule as prescribed. Do not double the next dose.

STOPPING THE DRUG
The decision to stop taking the drug should be made by your doctor.

PROLONGED USE
You should see your doctor regularly if you take this medicine for an extended period.

▼ PRECAUTIONS

Over 60: Adverse reactions may be more likely and more severe in older patients.

Driving and Hazardous Work: Avoid such activities until you determine how the medicine affects you.

Alcohol: Avoid alcohol.

Pregnancy: Animal tests have shown that the drug has adverse effects on the fetus. Human tests have not been done. Before taking isosorbide, tell your doctor if you are pregnant or if you plan to become pregnant.

Breast Feeding: Isosorbide mononitrate may pass into breast milk; caution is advised. Consult your doctor for specific advice.

Infants and Children: No studies on the use of this medicine in children have been done. Use and dose should be determined by your doctor.

Special Concerns: Do not stop taking this medicine suddenly because it can cause a spasm of the blood vessels in the heart. Consult your doctor about reducing the dose gradually. Use extra care in hot weather or during exercise, or when you must stand for long periods. This medicine may cause headaches at the beginning of therapy. Headaches can be treated with aspirin or acetaminophen and usually stop after your body becomes accustomed to the medication. The dose may be reduced temporarily because of headaches. The effectiveness of the drug may decrease over time; notify your doctor if this occurs.

OVERDOSE
Symptoms: Bluish fingernails, lips or palms; extreme dizziness or fainting; unusual weakness, fever, weak and fast heartbeat, seizures.

What to Do: Call your doctor, emergency medical services (EMS), or the nearest poison control center immediately.

▼ INTERACTIONS

DRUG INTERACTIONS
Do not take isosorbide mononitrate within 24 hours of taking sildenafil citrate. Sildenafil can enhance the action of nitrates (such as isosorbide), causing potentially dangerous decreases in blood pressure. Consult your doctor for specific advice if you are taking other heart medicines or antihypertensive drugs.

FOOD INTERACTIONS
No known food interactions.

DISEASE INTERACTIONS
Consult your doctor if you have any of the following: anemia, glaucoma, a recent head injury or stroke, an overactive thyroid, or a recent heart attack. Use of isosorbide mononitrate may cause complications in patients with severe liver or kidney disease, since these organs work together to remove the medication from the body.

▦ SIDE EFFECTS ▦

SERIOUS
Blurred vision, dry mouth, severe or prolonged headache. Call your doctor immediately.

COMMON
Dizziness or lightheadedness, especially when rising suddenly to a standing position, flushing of the face and neck, rapid pulse or heartbeat, nausea or vomiting, restlessness.

LESS COMMON
Skin rash.

LANSOPRAZOLE

Available in: Delayed-release capsules
Available OTC? No   **As Generic?** No
Drug Class: Antacid/proton pump inhibitor

▼ USAGE INFORMATION

WHY IT'S PRESCRIBED
To treat stomach and duodenal ulcers, gastroesophageal reflux disease (chronic heartburn caused by the backwash of stomach acid into the esophagus), and conditions that cause increased stomach acid secretion. To treat and prevent stomach ulcers associated with nonsteroidal anti-inflammatory drugs (NSAIDs). Lansoprazole is also prescribed in conjunction with the antibiotics amoxicillin and clarithromycin to eradicate the bacterium H. pylori and thus prevent the recurrence of duodenal ulcers caused by this bacterium.

HOW IT WORKS
Lansoprazole blocks the action of a specific enzyme in the cells that line the stomach, decreasing the production of stomach acid. Reduction of stomach acid creates a more favorable environment for the eradication of H. pylori and promotes ulcer healing.

▼ DOSAGE GUIDELINES

RANGE AND FREQUENCY
Prevacid–To treat duodenal ulcers: Initial dose is 15 mg once a day; it may later be increased. To treat gastro-esophageal reflux disease: 15 mg once a day for up to 8 weeks. To treat NSAID-associated stomach ulcers: 30 mg once a day for 8 weeks. To reduce the risk of NSAID-associated stomach ulcer: 15 mg once a day for up to 12 weeks. To treat other conditions: Initial dose is 60 mg once a day; it may be increased. Treatment usually runs 4 to 8 weeks. A second course of treatment may be necessary. Prevpac–To prevent duodenal ulcers: 30 mg lansoprazole, 1 gram amoxicillin, and 500 mg clarithromycin every 12 hours for 14 days.

ONSET OF EFFECT
1 to 3 hours.

DURATION OF ACTION
More than 24 hours.

DIETARY ADVICE
The drug is best taken 30 minutes or more before a meal, preferably in the morning before breakfast.

STORAGE
Store in a tightly sealed container away from moisture, heat, and direct light.

MISSED DOSE
Take it as soon as you remember. However, if it is near the time for the next dose, skip the missed dose and resume your regular dosage schedule. Do not double the next dose.

STOPPING THE DRUG
Take as prescribed for the full treatment period, even if your symptoms improve before the scheduled end of therapy.

PROLONGED USE
See your doctor regularly for tests and examinations if you must take this drug for a prolonged period. Lansoprazole should not be used indefinitely as maintenance therapy for esophagitis or a duodenal ulcer; other treatments are recommended.

▼ PRECAUTIONS

Over 60: No special problems are expected.

Driving and Hazardous Work: Do not drive or engage in hazardous activities until you determine how lansoprazole affects you. Taking it may be a disqualification for piloting aircraft.

Alcohol: Avoid alcohol for the duration of therapy.

Pregnancy: Adequate human studies have not been done. Before taking lansoprazole, tell your doctor if you are pregnant or if you plan to become pregnant.

Breast Feeding: Lansoprazole may pass into breast milk; caution is advised. Consult your doctor for advice.

Infants and Children: Use and dose for anyone under 18 should be determined by your doctor or pediatrician.

Special Concerns: Tell any doctor or dentist whom you see for treatment that you are taking lansoprazole. Do not chew the capsules. If you have trouble swallowing them, you may open them and sprinkle the contents on one tablespoon of applesauce, cottage cheese, yogurt, or similar food. If your doctor so directs, you may take an antacid along with lansoprazole.

OVERDOSE
Symptoms: No cases of overdose have been reported.

What to Do: An overdose is unlikely to be life-threatening. However, if someone takes a much larger dose than prescribed, call your doctor, emergency medical services (EMS), or the nearest poison control center immediately.

▼ INTERACTIONS

DRUG INTERACTIONS
Consult your doctor for specific advice if you are taking ampicillin, sucralfate, iron salts or supplements, cyclosporine, diazepam, disulfiram, ketoconazole, phenytoin, or theophylline.

FOOD INTERACTIONS
No significant food interactions have been reported.

DISEASE INTERACTIONS
Caution is advised when taking lansoprazole. Consult your doctor if you have liver disease, since it may increase the risk of side effects.

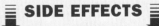
≡ SIDE EFFECTS ≡

SERIOUS
No serious side effects have been reported.

COMMON
Diarrhea, itching or rash, headache, dizziness.

LESS COMMON
Abdominal or stomach pain, nausea, increase or decrease in appetite, anxiety, flu-like symptoms, constipation, coughing, mental depression, muscle pain.

LATANOPROST

Available in: Ophthalmic solution
Available OTC? No   **As Generic?** No
Drug Class: Antiglaucoma agent

▼ USAGE INFORMATION

WHY IT'S PRESCRIBED
To treat glaucoma.

HOW IT WORKS
Glaucoma, a sight-threatening disorder, occurs when the aqueous humor (fluid inside the eye) cannot drain properly, causing increased pressure within the eyeball (intraocular pressure). Increased eye pressure can damage the optic nerve and lead to a gradually progressive loss of vision. Latanoprost promotes outflow of aqueous humor, thereby reducing intraocular pressure.

▼ DOSAGE GUIDELINES

RANGE AND FREQUENCY
1 drop of latanoprost in each eye once daily in the evening.

ONSET OF EFFECT
3 to 4 hours.

DURATION OF ACTION
24 hours or more.

DIETARY ADVICE
This medication can be used without regard to diet.

STORAGE
Store in a tightly sealed container away from moisture, heat, and direct light. Do not allow the medicine to freeze.

MISSED DOSE
Apply it as soon as you remember. If it is near the time for the next dose, skip the missed dose and resume your regular dosage schedule. Do not double the next dose.

STOPPING THE DRUG
The decision to stop using the drug should be made by your doctor.

PROLONGED USE
See your doctor regularly for tests and examinations if you must take this drug for an extended period.

▼ PRECAUTIONS

Over 60:
No special problems are expected.

Driving and Hazardous Work:
Do not drive or engage in hazardous work until you determine how the medicine affects your vision.

Alcohol:
No special precautions are necessary.

Pregnancy:
Latanoprost has not caused birth defects in animals. Human studies have not been done. Before you take latanoprost, tell your doctor if you are pregnant or plan to become pregnant.

Breast Feeding:
Latanoprost may pass into breast milk; caution is advised. Consult your doctor for advice.

Infants and Children:
The safety and effectiveness of latanoprost in infants and children have not been established.

Special Concerns:
To use the eye drops, first wash your hands. Tilt your head back. Gently apply pressure to the inside corner of the eyelid and with the index finger of the same hand, pull downward on the lower eyelid to make a space. Drop the medicine into this space and close your eye. Apply pressure for 1 or 2 minutes while keeping the eye closed without blinking. Then wash your hands again. Make sure the tip of the dropper does not touch your eye, finger, or any other surface. Latanoprost may make your eyes more sensitive to sunlight. If this occurs, wear sunglasses or avoid exposure to bright light as necessary. Latanoprost may change eye color, increasing the brown pigment in the iris over a period of months or years. The color change may be permanent. Latanoprost contains ingredients that may damage contact lenses. Contact lenses should be removed 15 minutes before applying the medication and reinserted 15 minutes or more afterward.

OVERDOSE
Symptoms: No specific ones have been reported.

What to Do: An overdose of latanoprost is unlikely to be life-threatening. If a large volume enters the eyes, flush with water. If someone ingests the medication accidentally, immediately call your doctor, emergency medical services (EMS), or the nearest poison control center.

▼ INTERACTIONS

DRUG INTERACTIONS
Other drugs may interact with latanoprost. Consult your doctor for specific advice if you are taking any other prescription or over-the-counter medication. If you are using other ophthalmic medications to reduce fluid pressure in the eye, administer them at least 5 minutes apart.

FOOD INTERACTIONS
No known food interactions.

DISEASE INTERACTIONS
Use of latanoprost may cause complications in patients with liver or kidney disease, since these organs work together to remove the drug from the body.

≡ SIDE EFFECTS ≡

SERIOUS
Chest pain, difficulty breathing. Call your doctor right away.

COMMON
Blurred vision, burning and stinging of the eye, sensation of something in the eye, increased brown pigmentation of the iris, eye redness.

LESS COMMON
Dry eye, excessive tearing, eye pain, lid crusting, swollen eyelid, eyelid pain or discomfort, sensitivity to light, upper respiratory tract infection, double vision, pain in the chest and back.

LEVODOPA

BRAND NAMES

Dopar, Larodopa

Available in: Tablets, capsules
Available OTC? No **As Generic?** Yes
Drug Class: Antiparkinsonism drug

▼ USAGE INFORMATION

WHY IT'S PRESCRIBED
To treat Parkinson's disease and Parkinson-like syndromes. Such syndromes can occur following injury to or infection of the central nervous system, damage to the blood vessels in the brain (for example, after a stroke), or exposure to certain toxins.

HOW IT WORKS
Levodopa replenishes the supply of dopamine in the brain. Dopamine is a chemical in the central nervous system that plays an essential role in the initiation and smooth control of voluntary muscle movement.

▼ DOSAGE GUIDELINES

RANGE AND FREQUENCY
Adults: To start, 0.5 g per day in 2 or more divided doses. The dose is increased gradually (by 0.5 to 0.75 g per day) over the course of 4 to 7 days, until the desired therapeutic response is achieved. The onset of adverse side effects may preclude the use of higher doses. The maximum beneficial dose is usually 5 to 6 g per day. Children: Smaller doses are used; consult your pediatrician for specific information.

ONSET OF EFFECT
Within 1 to 2 hours.

DURATION OF ACTION
From 4 to 5 hours.

DIETARY ADVICE
Eating food shortly after taking this medication may minimize the chance of stomach upset. Eating food before taking the medicine or at the same time may blunt levodopa's effects.

STORAGE
Store in a tightly sealed container away from moisture, heat, and direct light.

MISSED DOSE
Take it as soon as you remember. However, if it is near the time for the next dose, skip the missed dose and resume your regular dosage schedule. Do not double the next dose.

STOPPING THE DRUG
Consult your doctor for the best approach to stopping this drug. The dose should be decreased very gradually. Abruptly stopping the drug can cause an acute (sudden-onset) adverse reaction.

PROLONGED USE
Prolonged use of levodopa can result in a less predictable therapeutic response and bothersome involuntary muscle movements.

▼ PRECAUTIONS

Over 60: Adverse reactions to levodopa may be more likely and more severe in older patients. The dose should be increased very gradually in this age group.

Driving and Hazardous Work: Do not drive or engage in hazardous work until the full dose has been attained and you determine how the drug affects you.

Alcohol: Do not consume alcohol. Alcohol can cause pronounced confusion or delirium in patients taking this medication.

Pregnancy: Adequate human studies have not been done, and the effects of levodopa during pregnancy have not been determined. Pregnant women should therefore avoid taking levodopa.

Breast Feeding: Levodopa passes into breast milk; this medication should not be used by nursing mothers.

Infants and Children: Levodopa should be used with caution by infants and children. The dose should be smaller than that for adults and should be determined by your pediatrician.

Special Concerns: Patients taking levodopa should not eat a high-protein diet, because it can reduce the medication's effectiveness.

OVERDOSE
Symptoms: The symptoms of levodopa overdose are unknown.

What to Do: If you have any reason to suspect an overdose, call your doctor, emergency medical services (EMS), or the nearest poison control center.

▼ INTERACTIONS

DRUG INTERACTIONS
Consult your doctor for specific advice if you are taking any of the following drugs: MAO inhibitor antidepressants (such as phenelzine sulfate or tranylcypromine sulfate) or antihypertensives.

FOOD INTERACTIONS
A high-protein diet can reduce the effectiveness of levodopa. Persons taking levodopa should therefore decrease their protein intake if it is high.

DISEASE INTERACTIONS
Caution is advised when taking levodopa. Consult your doctor if you have any of the following: heart disease or heart rhythm abnormalities, bronchial asthma, glaucoma, malignant melanoma, or changes in mental state.

≡ SIDE EFFECTS ≡

▼ SERIOUS ▼
Irregular heartbeat, heart rhythm abnormalities, low blood pressure, fainting or near fainting, hallucinations.

COMMON
Nausea, confusion.

LESS COMMON
Breathing difficulty.

LEVOFLOXACIN

Available in: Tablets, injection
Available OTC? No **As Generic?** No
Drug Class: Fluoroquinolone antibiotic

▼ USAGE INFORMATION

WHY IT'S PRESCRIBED
To treat pneumonia, chronic bronchitis, and other infections caused by bacteria.

HOW IT WORKS
Levofloxacin inhibits the activity of a bacterial enzyme (gyrase) that is necessary for proper DNA formation and replication. This fights infection by preventing bacteria cells from reproducing.

▼ DOSAGE GUIDELINES

RANGE AND FREQUENCY
Adults: 250 to 500 mg once a day for 7 to 14 days. After an initial dose of 250 to 500 mg, patients with kidney problems receive 250 mg every day for 7 to 14 days.

ONSET OF EFFECT
Varies depending on the infection being treated.

DURATION OF ACTION
Unknown.

DIETARY ADVICE
Drink plenty of fluids.

STORAGE
Store in a tightly sealed container away from heat and direct light. Do not allow the injection form to freeze.

MISSED DOSE
Take it as soon as you remember. If it is near the time for the next dose, skip the missed dose and resume your regular dosage schedule. Do not double the next dose.

STOPPING THE DRUG
It is very important to take this drug as prescribed for the full treatment period, even if you begin to feel better before the scheduled end of therapy (unless you experience intolerable side effects, including increased sensitivity to sunlight).

PROLONGED USE
See your doctor regularly for tests and examinations if you must take this medicine for an extended period.

▼ PRECAUTIONS

Over 60: No special problems are expected.

Driving and Hazardous Work: Do not drive or engage in hazardous work until you determine how the medicine affects you.

Alcohol: It is advisable to abstain from alcohol when fighting an infection.

Pregnancy: In some animal tests, levofloxacin has caused birth defects. Adequate studies in humans have not been done. The drug should be used during pregnancy only if potential benefits clearly justify the risks. Before you take levofloxacin, tell your doctor if you are pregnant or plan to become pregnant.

Breast Feeding: Levofloxacin passes into breast milk and may cause serious side effects in the nursing infant; use of the drug is discouraged when nursing.

Infants and Children: Levofloxacin is not recommended for use by persons under the age of 18, as it has been shown to interfere with bone development.

Special Concerns: If levofloxacin causes sensitivity to sunlight, stop taking the drug and try to avoid exposure to sunlight for the next 5 days; also wear protective clothing and use a sunblock. Levofloxacin should not be taken by patients whose work makes it impossible to avoid exposure to sunlight. It is important to drink plenty of fluids while taking this drug.

OVERDOSE
Symptoms: No specific ones have been reported.

What to Do: If you have any reason to suspect an overdose, call your doctor, the emergency medical services (EMS), or the nearest poison control center.

▼ INTERACTIONS

DRUG INTERACTIONS
Consult your doctor for specific advice if you are taking aminophylline, antacids, didanosine, iron supplements, sucralfate, or zinc salts. Also tell your doctor if you are taking any other prescription or over-the-counter drug.

FOOD INTERACTIONS
No known food interactions.

DISEASE INTERACTIONS
Caution is advised when taking levofloxacin. Consult your doctor if you have any other medical condition. Use of the drug can cause complications in patients with kidney disease, since this organ works to remove the medication from the body.

⬇ SIDE EFFECTS ⬇

SERIOUS
Serious reactions to levofloxacin are rare and include seizures, mental confusion, hallucinations, agitation, nightmares, depression, shortness of breath, unusual swelling in the face or extremities, and loss of consciousness. Also skin burning, redness, blisters, rash, or itching after exposure to sunlight; increased risk of tendinitis or tendon rupture. Call your doctor immediately.

COMMON
Increased sensitivity to sunlight (and increased risk of sunburn) for days following therapy.

LESS COMMON
Diarrhea, nausea and vomiting, stomach pain and upset, gas, headache, dizziness, restlessness, insomnia, changes in taste perception, drowsiness, itching, dry mouth, unusual body aches or pains.

LEVONORGESTREL IMPLANTS

Available in: Implanted capsule
Available OTC? No   **As Generic?** No
Drug Class: Progestin (hormone)

▼ USAGE INFORMATION

WHY IT'S PRESCRIBED
As a birth control method.

HOW IT WORKS
The implant slowly releases levonorgestrel, a synthetic hormone, into the bloodstream. It prevents a woman's egg from developing fully and causes changes in the uterine lining that make it difficult for sperm to reach the egg. It may prevent ovulation in some patients.

▼ DOSAGE GUIDELINES

RANGE AND FREQUENCY
6 capsules are implanted under the skin of the upper arm. The capsules are placed in a fanlike position, 15 degrees apart. They are removed after 5 years.

ONSET OF EFFECT
Within 24 hours if implanted within 7 days of the menstrual period.

DURATION OF ACTION
Up to 5 years.

DIETARY ADVICE
No special restrictions.

STORAGE
Not applicable.

MISSED DOSE
Not applicable; the drug is delivered continuously from the implant under the skin.

STOPPING THE DRUG
The decision to stop using the implant can be made whenever you choose, but the implants should be removed by your doctor.

PROLONGED USE
See your doctor at least once a year for periodic examinations and lab tests.

▼ PRECAUTIONS

Over 60: Not normally prescribed for postmenopausal women.

Driving and Hazardous Work: No special precautions are necessary.

Alcohol: No special precautions are necessary.

Pregnancy: Extensive studies have shown that no special risks to mother or child are associated with pregnancies occurring prior to or shortly after implantation of levonorgestrel capsules. Nevertheless, it is advisable to have the implants removed if pregnancy does occur.

Breast Feeding: Levonorgestrel passes into breast milk but has not been shown to cause problems. It can be used by nursing mothers who desire contraception.

Infants and Children: Levonorgestrel implants have not been shown to cause problems in teenagers. However, birth control methods that protect against sexually transmitted diseases (for example, condoms) are preferred for those in this age group.

Special Concerns: Do not have this implant inserted until you are sure you are not pregnant. Call your doctor immediately if one of the capsules falls out before the skin heals over the implant. No contraceptive method is perfect: If you suspect a pregnancy, you should call your doctor immediately. If you have any laboratory test, tell the health professional that you are using these contraceptives. Cigarette smoking or alcohol abuse can increase the risk of osteoporosis and blood clot formation. Implants should be removed if you develop active thrombophlebitis (pain caused by a blot clot lodged in a blood vessel), thromboembolic disease, or jaundice (yellowish tinge to the eyes or skin), or if you will be immobilized for a significant period of time because of illness or some other factor. If you have a sudden unexplained vision problem, including changes in tolerance for contact lenses, you should be evaluated by an ophthalmologist.

OVERDOSE
Symptoms: Not applicable.

What to Do: Emergency instructions not applicable.

▼ INTERACTIONS

DRUG INTERACTIONS
Consult your doctor for specific advice if you are taking aminoglutethimide, carbamazepine, phenytoin, rifabutin, or rifampin.

FOOD INTERACTIONS
No known food interactions.

DISEASE INTERACTIONS
Caution is advised when using this contraceptive. Consult your doctor if you have any of the following: asthma, epilepsy, heart or circulation problems, kidney disease, liver disease, migraine headaches, breast disease, bleeding disorders, central nervous system disorders (including depression), diabetes, or high blood cholesterol.

≣ SIDE EFFECTS ≣

SERIOUS
Changes in or cessation of menstrual bleeding, unexpected or increased flow of breast milk, mental depression, skin rash, loss of or change in speech, impaired coordination or vision, severe and sudden shortness of breath. Call your doctor immediately.

COMMON
Stomach pain, swelling of face, ankles, or feet, mild headache, mood changes, unusual fatigue, weight gain, pain or irritation at site of implant.

LESS COMMON
Acne, breast pain or tenderness, hot flashes, insomnia, loss of sexual desire, loss or gain of scalp hair or body hair, brown spots on skin.

LEVOTHYROXINE SODIUM

Available in: Tablets, injection
Available OTC? No **As Generic?** Yes
Drug Class: Hypothyroid agent

▼ USAGE INFORMATION

WHY IT'S PRESCRIBED
To treat patients with an underactive thyroid gland, goiter (enlarged thyroid gland), and benign (noncancerous) and malignant (cancerous) thyroid nodules.

HOW IT WORKS
Levothyroxine acts in the body as a substitute for natural thyroid hormone.

▼ DOSAGE GUIDELINES

RANGE AND FREQUENCY
Tablets—Adults and teenagers: 0.0016 mg per 2.2 lbs (1 kg) a day. Children less than 6 months old: 0.025 to 0.05 mg once a day. Children 6 to 12 months old: 0.05 to 0.075 mg once a day. Children ages 1 to 5: 0.075 to 0.1 mg once a day. Children ages 6 to 12: 0.1 to 0.15 mg a day. Injection—Adults and teenagers: 0.05 to 0.1 mg into a vein or muscle once a day. Children less than 6 months old: 0.019 to 0.038 mg once a day. Children 6 to 12 months old: 0.038 to 0.056 mg once a day. Children ages 1 to 5: 0.056 to 0.075 mg once a day. Children ages 6 to 10: 0.075 to 0.113 mg once a day. Children ages 10 to 12: 0.113 to 0.15 mg once a day.

ONSET OF EFFECT
24 hours.

DURATION OF ACTION
1 to 3 weeks.

DIETARY ADVICE
Take it before breakfast on an empty stomach.

STORAGE
Store in a tightly sealed container away from moisture, heat, and direct light.

MISSED DOSE
If you miss your dose on one day, you may double the dose on the next day. If you miss two or more doses in a row, call your doctor.

STOPPING THE DRUG
The decision to stop taking the drug should be made in consultation with your doctor.

PROLONGED USE
If you must take this drug, it is very likely that lifelong therapy will be necessary. See your doctor regularly for routine tests and examinations to evaluate your condition.

▼ PRECAUTIONS

Over 60: Modification of the dosage may be required.

Driving and Hazardous Work: Avoid such activities until you determine how the medicine affects you.

Alcohol: Avoid alcohol.

Pregnancy: Using the recommended dose of levothyroxine has not been shown to cause birth defects. The dose may need to be changed during pregnancy. Consult your doctor for specific advice.

Breast Feeding: Using the recommended dose of levothyroxine has not been shown to cause problems while nursing. Consult your doctor for specific advice.

Infants and Children: No special problems are expected.

Special Concerns: You should wear a medical bracelet or carry an identification card indicating that you are taking this medication.

OVERDOSE
Symptoms: Rapid heartbeat, chest pain, shortness of breath.

What to Do: Call your doctor, emergency medical services (EMS), or the nearest poison control center immediately.

▼ INTERACTIONS

DRUG INTERACTIONS
Consult your doctor for advice if you are taking anticoagulants, cholestyramine, colestipol, amphetamines, appetite suppressants, asthma medication, or cold, sinus, or allergy medications.

FOOD INTERACTIONS
No known food interactions.

DISEASE INTERACTIONS
Caution is advised when taking levothyroxine. Consult your doctor if you have any of the following: diabetes mellitus, diabetes insipidus, myxedema, an overactive thyroid gland, atherosclerosis (so-called hardening of the arteries), heart disease, high blood pressure, an underactive adrenal gland, or an underactive pituitary gland.

⬇ SIDE EFFECTS ⬇

SERIOUS
In rare instances levothyroxine may cause severe headaches, skin rash, hives, rapid or irregular heartbeat, chest pain, or shortness of breath. These symptoms may signal an overdose or an allergic reaction. Seek emergency medical assistance immediately.

COMMON
No common side effects are associated with the use of levothyroxine.

LESS COMMON
Leg cramps, diarrhea, changes in menstrual cycle, changes in appetite, sweating, sensitivity to heat, shaking of the hands, fever, headache, insomnia, irritability, weight loss, vomiting, nervousness. These symptoms may indicate your dose needs adjustment by your doctor.

LISINOPRIL

Available in: Tablets
Available OTC? No   **As Generic?** No
Drug Class: Angiotensin-converting enzyme (ACE) inhibitor

▼ USAGE INFORMATION

WHY IT'S PRESCRIBED
To control high blood pressure (hypertension). Also used to treat congestive heart failure (CHF) and left ventricular dysfunction (damage to the primary pumping chamber of the heart), and to minimize further kidney damage in diabetic patients with mild kidney disease.

HOW IT WORKS
Angiotensin-converting enzyme (ACE) inhibitors block an enzyme that produces angiotensin, a naturally occurring substance that causes blood vessels to constrict and also stimulates production of the adrenal hormone, aldosterone, which promotes sodium retention in the body. As a result, ACE inhibitor medications relax blood vessels (causing them to widen) and reduce sodium retention, which in turn lowers blood pressure and so decreases the workload of the heart.

▼ DOSAGE GUIDELINES

RANGE AND FREQUENCY
For high blood pressure: 5 to 40 mg once a day. For congestive heart failure: 2.5 to 20 mg once a day.

ONSET OF EFFECT
Within 1 hour.

DURATION OF ACTION
24 hours.

DIETARY ADVICE
Take lisinopril on an empty stomach, about 1 hour before mealtime. Follow your doctor's dietary advice (including low-salt or low-cholesterol restrictions) to improve control over high blood pressure and heart disease. Avoid high-potassium foods like bananas and citrus fruits and juices, unless you are also taking medications, such as diuretics, that lower potassium levels.

STORAGE
Store in a tightly sealed container away from heat and direct light.

MISSED DOSE
Take it as soon as you remember. If it is near the time for the next dose, skip the missed dose and resume your regular dosage schedule. Do not double the next dose.

STOPPING THE DRUG
Do not stop taking this drug abruptly, as this may cause potentially serious health problems. Dosage should be reduced gradually, according to your doctor's instructions.

PROLONGED USE
Lifelong therapy with lisinopril may be necessary. See your doctor regularly for examinations and tests if you must take this medicine for an extended period.

▼ PRECAUTIONS

Over 60: No unusual problems are expected in older patients.

Driving and Hazardous Work: Do not drive or engage in hazardous work until you determine how the medicine affects you.

Alcohol: Consume alcohol only in moderation since it may increase the effect of the drug and cause an excessive drop in blood pressure. Consult your doctor for advice.

Pregnancy: Use of lisinopril during the last 6 months of pregnancy may cause severe defects, even death, in the fetus. The drug should be discontinued if you are pregnant or plan to become pregnant.

Breast Feeding: Lisinopril may pass into breast milk; caution is advised. Consult your doctor for advice.

Infants and Children: Children may be especially sensitive to the effects of lisinopril. Benefits must be weighed against potential risks; consult your pediatrician for advice.

OVERDOSE
Symptoms: Dizziness, confusion, faintness.

What to Do: Call your doctor, emergency medical services (EMS), or the nearest poison control center immediately.

▼ INTERACTIONS

DRUG INTERACTIONS
Consult your doctor if you are taking diuretics (especially potassium-sparing diuretics), potassium supplements or drugs containing potassium (check ingredient labels), lithium, anticoagulants (such as warfarin), indomethacin or other anti-inflammatory drugs, or any over-the-counter medications (especially diet pills and cold remedies).

FOOD INTERACTIONS
Avoid low-salt milk and salt substitutes. Many of these products contain potassium.

DISEASE INTERACTIONS
Consult your doctor if you have systemic lupus erythematosus (SLE) or if you have had a prior allergic reaction to ACE inhibitor drugs. Lisinopril should be used with caution by patients with severe kidney disease or renal artery stenosis (narrowing of one or both of the arteries that supply blood to the kidneys).

≡ SIDE EFFECTS ≡

SERIOUS
Fever and chills, sore throat and hoarseness, sudden difficulty breathing or swallowing, swelling of the face, mouth, or extremities, impaired kidney function (ankle swelling, decreased urination), confusion, yellow discoloration of the eyes or skin (indicating liver disorder), intense itching, chest pain or palpitations, abdominal pain. Serious side effects are very rare; contact your doctor immediately.

COMMON
Dry, persistent cough.

LESS COMMON
Dizziness or fainting, skin rash, numbness or tingling in the hands, feet, or lips, unusual fatigue or muscle weakness, nausea, drowsiness, loss of taste, headache.

LISINOPRIL/HYDROCHLOROTHIAZIDE

BRAND NAMES

Prinzide, Zestoretic

Available in: Tablets
Available OTC? No **As Generic?** No
Drug Class: Angiotensin-converting enzyme (ACE) inhibitor/diuretic

▼ USAGE INFORMATION

WHY IT'S PRESCRIBED
To treat high blood pressure (hypertension).

HOW IT WORKS
Angiotensin-converting enzyme (ACE) inhibitors such as lisinopril block an enzyme that produces angiotensin, a naturally occurring substance that causes blood vessels to constrict and stimulates production of the adrenal hormone, aldosterone, which promotes sodium retention in the body. As a result, ACE inhibitors relax blood vessels (causing them to widen) and also reduce sodium retention, which lowers blood pressure and so decreases the workload of the heart. Hydrochlorothiazide (HCTZ), a diuretic, increases sodium and water in the urine output. By reducing the overall fluid volume in the body, diuretics reduce blood volume and so lower blood pressure.

▼ DOSAGE GUIDELINES

RANGE AND FREQUENCY
This combination medication comes in three strengths: lisinopril/hydrochlorothiazide 10/12.5, 20/12.5, and 20/25. The dose ranges from 10 to 40 mg of lisinopril and 12.5 to 50 mg of hydrochlorothiazide per day. 1 or 2 tablets are taken once a day in the morning after breakfast.

ONSET OF EFFECT
Within 1 hour.

DURATION OF ACTION
Unknown.

DIETARY ADVICE
Follow your doctor's dietary advice (such as low-salt or low-fat restrictions) to improve control over high blood pressure and heart disease.

STORAGE
Store in a tightly sealed container away from moisture, heat, and direct light.

MISSED DOSE
Take it as soon as you remember. If it is near the time for the next dose, skip the missed dose and resume your regular dosage schedule. Do not double the next dose.

STOPPING THE DRUG
Discontinuing this drug abruptly may cause potentially serious problems. The dosage should be reduced gradually, according to your doctor's instructions.

PROLONGED USE
Lifelong therapy may be required; see your doctor regularly for evaluation.

▼ PRECAUTIONS

Over 60: Adverse reactions may be more likely and more severe in older patients.

Driving and Hazardous Work: Do not drive or engage in hazardous work until you determine how the medicine affects you.

Alcohol: Consume alcohol only in moderation since it may increase the effect of the drug and cause an excessive drop in blood pressure. Consult your doctor for advice.

Pregnancy: Before taking this medication, tell your doctor if you are pregnant or plan to become pregnant. Use of this medicine during the last 6 months of pregnancy may cause severe defects, even death, in the fetus.

Breast Feeding: Lisinopril may pass into breast milk; caution is advised. Consult your doctor for advice.

Infants and Children: Children may be especially sensitive to the effects of lisinopril. Consult your pediatrician about the relative risks and benefits.

OVERDOSE
Symptoms: Overdose has not been reported; symptoms might include dizziness, faintness, or confusion.

What to Do: While overdose is unlikely, call your doctor, emergency medical services (EMS), or the nearest poison control center immediately if you suspect that someone has taken a much larger dose than prescribed.

▼ INTERACTIONS

DRUG INTERACTIONS
Consult your doctor for specific advice if you are taking cholestyramine, colestipol, digitalis drugs, lithium, potassium-containing drugs or supplements, or any over-the-counter drug (especially cold remedies and diet pills).

FOOD INTERACTIONS
Avoid low-salt milk and salt substitutes. Many of these products contain potassium.

DISEASE INTERACTIONS
Consult your doctor if you have systemic lupus erythematosus or if you have had a prior allergic reaction to ACE inhibitors. This medication should be used with caution by patients with severe kidney disease or renal artery stenosis (narrowing of one or both of the arteries that supply blood to the kidneys).

≡ SIDE EFFECTS ≡

SERIOUS
Fever and chills, sore throat and hoarseness, sudden difficulty breathing or swallowing, swelling of the face, mouth, or extremities, impaired kidney function (ankle swelling, decreased urination), confusion, yellow discoloration of the eyes or skin (indicating liver disorder), intense itching, chest pain or heartbeat irregularities, abdominal pain. Serious side effects are very rare; contact your doctor immediately.

COMMON
Dry, persistent cough.

LESS COMMON
Dizziness or fainting, skin rash, numbness or tingling in the hands, feet, or lips, change in color of the hands from white to blue to red (Raynaud's phenomenon) in cold weather, unusual fatigue or muscle weakness, loss of taste, nausea, drowsiness, headache, unusual dreams.

LORATADINE

Available in: Tablets, syrup
Available OTC? No   **As Generic?** No
Drug Class: Antihistamine

▼ USAGE INFORMATION

WHY IT'S PRESCRIBED
To prevent or relieve symptoms of hay fever and other allergies, such as watery or itchy eyes, sneezing, runny nose, or itchy skin. The drug loratadine is also used sometimes to treat chronic (or persistent) hives.

HOW IT WORKS
Loratadine blocks the effects of histamine, a naturally occurring substance that causes swelling, itching, sneezing, watery eyes, hives, and other symptoms of allergic reaction.

▼ DOSAGE GUIDELINES

RANGE AND FREQUENCY
Tablets and syrup—Adults and children age 10 and older: 10 mg once a day. Children ages 2 to 9: 5 mg once a day. Do not increase the dose in an attempt to achieve quicker relief of symptoms.

ONSET OF EFFECT
Within 1 hour.

DURATION OF ACTION
24 hours or more.

DIETARY ADVICE
Loratadine can be taken without regard to diet, but taking this medicine with food may be beneficial because it can increase absorption of the drug from the gastrointestinal tract by up to 40%.

STORAGE
Store in a tightly sealed container at room temperature, away from heat, moisture, and direct light.

MISSED DOSE
Take it as soon as you remember. However, if it is near the time for the next dose, skip the missed dose and resume your regular dosage schedule. Do not double the next dose.

STOPPING THE DRUG
The decision to stop taking the drug should be made in consultation with your doctor.

PROLONGED USE
Loratadine can be taken safely for extended periods. Long-term use is not linked to decreased effectiveness of the drug (a problem with certain allergy medications and other drugs).

▼ PRECAUTIONS

Over 60: Adverse reactions may be more likely and more severe in older patients.

Driving and Hazardous Work: The use of loratadine, at recommended doses, should not impair your ability to perform such tasks safely.

Alcohol: No special precautions are necessary.

Pregnancy: Before you take loratadine, tell your doctor if you are pregnant or plan to become pregnant.

Breast Feeding: Loratadine passes into breast milk; avoid or discontinue use while breast feeding.

Infants and Children: Adverse reactions may be more likely and more severe in children.

Special Concerns: Stop taking loratadine 4 to 7 days before you have an allergy skin test.

OVERDOSE
Symptoms: Rapid heartbeat, headache, drowsiness.

What to Do: An overdose of loratadine is unlikely to be life-threatening. However, if someone takes a much larger dose than prescribed, call your doctor, emergency medical services (EMS), or the nearest poison control center.

▼ INTERACTIONS

DRUG INTERACTIONS
Be sure to consult your doctor for advice if you are taking clarithromycin, erythromycin, troleandomycin, itraconazole, or ketoconazole.

FOOD INTERACTIONS
There are no known interactions between loratadine and specific foods.

DISEASE INTERACTIONS
There are no known disease interactions.

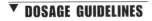

≣ SIDE EFFECTS ≣

SERIOUS
No serious side effects are associated with the use of loratadine.

COMMON
No common side effects are associated with the use of loratadine.

LESS COMMON
In rare cases adverse reactions have been reported in persons taking loratadine, but none of these reactions is clearly linked to use of the drug.

LORATADINE/PSEUDOEPHEDRINE

BRAND NAMES

Claritin-D

Available in: Extended-release tablets
Available OTC? No   **As Generic?** No
Drug Class: Antihistamine/decongestant

▼ USAGE INFORMATION

WHY IT'S PRESCRIBED
To relieve the symptoms of seasonal allergic rhinitis (hay fever), which include runny nose, nasal congestion, and sneezing.

HOW IT WORKS
Loratadine blocks the effects of histamine, a naturally occurring substance that causes swelling, itching, sneezing, nasal discharge and congestion, and other symptoms of an allergic reaction. Pseudoephedrine narrows and constricts blood vessels to reduce blood flow to swollen nasal passages, which reduces nasal secretions, shrinks swollen nasal mucous membranes, and improves airflow through the nasal passages.

▼ DOSAGE GUIDELINES

RANGE AND FREQUENCY
The 12-hour formulation may be taken twice a day (every 12 hours). The 24-hour formulation should only be taken once a day. Tablets should be taken with a full glass of water.

ONSET OF EFFECT
Within 1 to 3 hours.

DURATION OF ACTION
12 to 24 hours or more.

DIETARY ADVICE
This drug can be taken without regard to meals. Take it with a full glass of water.

STORAGE
Store in a tightly sealed container away from moisture, heat, and direct light.

MISSED DOSE
Not applicable. This drug is taken as needed.

STOPPING THE DRUG
Not applicable. This drug is taken as needed.

PROLONGED USE
This drug is prescribed for short-term (seasonal) use only.

▼ PRECAUTIONS

Over 60: Adequate studies have not been done. However, older patients are more susceptible to the effects of the pseudoephedrine component.

Driving and Hazardous Work: The use of this drug should not impair your ability to perform such tasks safely. However, exercise caution if the drug makes you drowsy.

Alcohol: No special warnings.

Pregnancy: Adequate human studies have not been done. Discuss with your doctor the relative risks and benefits of using this drug while pregnant.

Breast Feeding: Both drugs pass into breast milk. Discuss with your doctor the relative risks and benefits of using this drug while nursing.

Infants and Children: Not recommended for use by children under age 12.

Special Concerns: Do not break or chew the tablet. Patients with a history of esophageal narrowing or swallowing difficulty should not take this drug.

OVERDOSE
Symptoms: Drowsiness, heartbeat irregularities, headache, giddiness, nausea, vomiting, sweating, increased thirst, chest pain, urination difficulties, muscle weakness and tenseness, anxiety, restlessness, insomnia, hallucinations, delusions, seizures, difficulty breathing.

What to Do: Call your doctor, emergency medical services (EMS), or the nearest poison control center immediately.

▼ INTERACTIONS

DRUG INTERACTIONS
This drug and MAO inhibitors should not be used within 14 days of each other. Consult your doctor for specific advice if you are taking beta-blockers, digitalis drugs, or over-the-counter antihistamines or decongestants.

FOOD INTERACTIONS
No known food interactions.

DISEASE INTERACTIONS
You should not take this drug if you have narrow-angle glaucoma, urinary retention, severe hypertension, or severe coronary artery disease. Caution is advised when taking this drug if you have any of the following: high blood pressure, heart disease, diabetes mellitus, increased eye pressure, hyperthyroidism, or enlarged prostate. Use of this drug may cause complications in patients with liver or kidney disease, since these organs work together to remove the medication from the body.

≡ SIDE EFFECTS ≡

SERIOUS
No serious side effects are associated with the use of loratadine/pseudoephedrine.

COMMON
Insomnia, dry mouth, drowsiness.

LESS COMMON
Nervousness, dizziness, indigestion.

LORAZEPAM

BRAND NAME

Ativan

Available in: Oral solution, tablets, injection
Available OTC? No   **As Generic?** Yes
Drug Class: Benzodiazepine tranquilizer; antianxiety agent

▼ USAGE INFORMATION

WHY IT'S PRESCRIBED
To treat anxiety and insomnia. Administered in a hospital setting, the injection form of lorazepam is used to treat a type of seizure disorder (status epilepticus) and is given before surgery to sedate patients prior to the administration of anesthesia.

HOW IT WORKS
Lorazepam produces mild sedation by depressing activity in the central nervous system. In particular, the drug appears to enhance the effect of gamma-aminobutyric acid (GABA), a natural chemical that inhibits the firing of neurons and dampens the transmission of nerve signals, decreasing nervous excitation.

▼ DOSAGE GUIDELINES

RANGE AND FREQUENCY
For anxiety—Adults and teenagers: 1 to 2 mg every 8 or 12 hours, up to 6 mg a day. Older adults: 0.5 mg, 2 times a day to start; the dose may be increased. For insomnia—Adults and teenagers: 1 to 2 mg taken at bedtime. Note: In all cases, use and dosage for children under 12 years of age must be determined by your doctor.

ONSET OF EFFECT
30 minutes to 2 hours for oral forms.

DURATION OF ACTION
12 to 24 hours.

DIETARY ADVICE
Can be taken with food to prevent gastrointestinal upset.

STORAGE
Store in a tightly sealed container away from moisture, heat, and direct light.

MISSED DOSE
Take it as soon as you remember. However, if it is near the time for the next dose, skip the missed dose and resume your regular dosage schedule. Do not double the next dose. For insomnia, do not take it unless your schedule allows a full night's sleep.

STOPPING THE DRUG
Never stop taking the drug abruptly, as this can cause withdrawal symptoms. Dosage should be reduced gradually as directed by your doctor.

PROLONGED USE
Lorazepam may slowly lose its effectiveness with prolonged use. See your doctor for periodic evaluation if you must take this drug for an extended length of time.

▼ PRECAUTIONS

Over 60: Adverse reactions may be more likely and more severe in older patients. A lower dose may be warranted.

Driving and Hazardous Work: Lorazepam can impair mental alertness and physical coordination. Adjust your activities accordingly.

Alcohol: Avoid drinking alcoholic beverages.

Pregnancy: Use of lorazepam during pregnancy should be avoided if possible. Tell your doctor if you are pregnant or plan to become pregnant.

Breast Feeding: Lorazepam passes into breast milk; do not take this medication while you are nursing.

Infants and Children: Lorazepam should be used by children only under close medical supervision.

Special Concerns: Lorazepam use can lead to psychological or physical dependence. Short-term therapy (8 weeks or less) is typical; do not take the drug for a longer period unless so advised by your doctor. Never take more than the prescribed daily dose.

OVERDOSE
Symptoms: Extreme drowsiness, confusion, slurred speech, slow reflexes, poor coordination, staggering gait, tremor, slowed breathing, loss of consciousness.

What to Do: Call your doctor, emergency medical services (EMS), or the nearest poison control center immediately.

▼ INTERACTIONS

DRUG INTERACTIONS
Consult your doctor for specific advice if you are taking any drugs that depress the central nervous system (such as antihistamines, antidepressants or other psychiatric medications, barbiturates, sedatives, cough medicines, decongestants, and painkillers). Be sure your doctor knows about any over-the-counter drug you may take.

FOOD INTERACTIONS
None reported.

DISEASE INTERACTIONS
Consult your doctor if you have a history of alcohol or drug abuse, stroke or other brain disease, any chronic lung disease, hyperactivity, depression or other mental illness, myasthenia gravis, sleep apnea, epilepsy, porphyria, kidney disease, or liver disease.

≡ SIDE EFFECTS ≡

SERIOUS
Difficulty concentrating, outbursts of anger, other behavior problems, depression, hallucinations, low blood pressure (causing faintness or confusion), memory impairment, muscle weakness, skin rash or itching, sore throat, fever and chills, sores or ulcers in throat or mouth, unusual bruising or bleeding, extreme fatigue, yellowish tinge to eyes or skin. Call your doctor immediately.

COMMON
Drowsiness, loss of coordination, unsteady gait, dizziness, lightheadedness, slurred speech.

LESS COMMON
Change in sexual desire or ability, constipation, false sense of well-being, nausea and vomiting, urinary problems, unusual fatigue.

LOSARTAN POTASSIUM

Available in: Tablets
Available OTC? No   **As Generic?** No
Drug Class: Antihypertensive/angiotensin II antagonist

▼ USAGE INFORMATION

WHY IT'S PRESCRIBED
To control high blood pressure (hypertension). This drug appears to have the same benefits as the class of antihypertensive drugs known as ACE inhibitors, but without producing the common side effect (experienced by as many as 30% of patients) of a dry cough. Losartan may be used alone or in conjunction with other antihypertensive medications.

HOW IT WORKS
Losartan blocks the effects of angiotensin II, a naturally occurring substance that causes blood vessels to narrow. This medication causes the blood vessels to dilate, thereby lowering blood pressure and decreasing the workload of the heart.

▼ DOSAGE GUIDELINES

RANGE AND FREQUENCY
Adults: To start, 25 to 50 mg once a day. The usual maintenance dose is 25 to 100 mg, taken once a day or divided into 2 doses. Children: Losartan is not recommended for children.

ONSET OF EFFECT
Within 1 hour.

DURATION OF ACTION
24 hours.

DIETARY ADVICE
Follow a healthy diet (low-salt, low-fat, low-cholesterol) as advised by your doctor to help control blood pressure and prevent heart disease.

STORAGE
Store in a tightly sealed container away from moisture, heat, and direct light.

MISSED DOSE
Take it as soon as you remember. If it is near the time for the next dose, skip the missed dose and resume your regular dosage schedule. Do not double the next dose.

STOPPING THE DRUG
Take it as prescribed for the full treatment period. The decision to stop taking the drug should be made in consultation with your physician.

PROLONGED USE
Lifelong therapy may be necessary. However, if you do change certain health habits (for example, increasing exercise or losing weight), it may be possible, under your doctor's supervision, to reduce the dose.

▼ PRECAUTIONS

Over 60: Adverse reactions may be more likely and more severe in older patients.

Driving and Hazardous Work: Do not drive or engage in hazardous work until you determine how the medicine affects you.

Alcohol: Drink only in careful moderation. (See Special Concerns.)

Pregnancy: In certain ways losartan is similar to a class of drugs that have caused damage to the unborn child when taken in the second or third trimester of pregnancy. Because safer, more effective medications can lower blood pressure during pregnancy, and because adequate studies on the use of losartan during pregnancy have not been done, women who are pregnant or who are planning to become pregnant should not take this drug.

Breast Feeding: Losartan passes into breast milk; avoid use while nursing.

Infants and Children: The safety and effectiveness of this drug have not been established for children.

Special Concerns: Losartan may cause dizziness or lightheadedness, which is most noticeable when you change position. This may lead to fainting, falls, and injury. Sit or lie down immediately if you feel dizzy or lightheaded. This side effect may be worsened by alcohol, hot weather, dehydration, fever, prolonged standing, prolonged sitting, or exercise.

OVERDOSE
Symptoms: Fainting, dizziness, weak pulse that might be very slow or very fast, nausea and vomiting, chest pain.

What to Do: Call your doctor, emergency medical services (EMS), or the nearest poison control center immediately.

▼ INTERACTIONS

DRUG INTERACTIONS
Consult your doctor for specific advice if you are taking diuretics, potassium-containing medicines or supplements, salt substitutes, low-salt milk, NSAIDs, allopurinol, over-the-counter medications for colds, coughs, hay fever, asthma, sinus problems, or appetite control, or other prescription medications.

FOOD INTERACTIONS
No known food interactions.

DISEASE INTERACTIONS
Use of losartan may cause complications in patients with liver or kidney disease, since these organs work together to remove the medication from the body.

≡ SIDE EFFECTS ≡

SERIOUS
Sudden difficulty breathing or swallowing, hoarseness, swelling of the face, mouth, hands, or throat, dizziness, cough, fever or sore throat. Call your doctor immediately.

COMMON
Headache.

LESS COMMON
Back pain, fatigue, diarrhea, nasal congestion.

LOVASTATIN

Available in: Tablets
Available OTC? No   **As Generic?** No
Drug Class: Antilipidemic (cholesterol-lowering agent)

▼ USAGE INFORMATION

WHY IT'S PRESCRIBED
To treat high cholesterol. Usually prescribed after first lines of treatment—diet, weight loss, and exercise—fail to reduce total and low-density lipoprotein (LDL) cholesterol to acceptable levels. Lovastatin has also been approved for the primary prevention of coronary artery disease (CAD) in persons with no symptoms of CAD, but who have average to modestly elevated levels of total and LDL cholesterol and below average HDL.

HOW IT WORKS
Lovastatin blocks the action of an enzyme required for the manufacture of cholesterol, thereby interfering with its formation. By lowering the amount of cholesterol in the liver cells, lovastatin increases the formation of receptors for LDL, and thereby reduces blood levels of total and LDL cholesterol. In addition to lowering LDL cholesterol levels, lovastatin also modestly reduces triglyceride levels and raises HDL (the so-called "good") cholesterol.

▼ DOSAGE GUIDELINES

RANGE AND FREQUENCY
20 to 80 mg per day, taken with meals. The 20 mg dose is taken with the evening meal; doses greater than 20 mg per day are taken in the morning and evening.

ONSET OF EFFECT
2 to 4 weeks.

DURATION OF ACTION
The effect persists for the duration of therapy.

DIETARY ADVICE
Cholesterol-lowering drugs are only one part of a total program that should include regular exercise and a healthy diet. The American Heart Association publishes a "Healthy Heart" diet, which is widely recommended.

STORAGE
Store in a tightly sealed container away from moisture, heat, and direct light.

MISSED DOSE
Take your missed dose as soon as you remember. Take your next scheduled dose at the proper time, and resume your regular dosage schedule. Do not take a double dose.

STOPPING THE DRUG
The decision to stop taking the drug should be made in consultation with your doctor. Once the medication is discontinued, blood cholesterol is likely to return to original elevated levels.

PROLONGED USE
Side effects are more likely with prolonged use. As you continue with lovastatin, your doctor will periodically order blood tests to evaluate liver function.

▼ PRECAUTIONS

Over 60: No special problems are expected in older patients.

Driving and Hazardous Work: The use of lovastatin should not impair your ability to perform such tasks safely.

Alcohol: No special precautions are necessary.

Pregnancy: Lovastatin should not be used during pregnancy nor by women who are trying to become pregnant.

Breast Feeding: This drug is not recommended for women who are nursing.

Infants and Children: The drug can be effective, but safety is not known; rarely used in children. Consult your pediatrician.

Special Concerns: Important elements of treatment for high cholesterol include proper diet, weight loss, regular moderate exercise, and the avoidance of certain medications that may increase cholesterol levels. Because lovastatin has potential side effects, it is important that you maintain a recommended healthy diet and cooperate with other treatments your physician may suggest.

OVERDOSE
Symptoms: An overdose of lovastatin is unlikely.

What to Do: Emergency instructions not applicable.

▼ INTERACTIONS

DRUG INTERACTIONS
Consult your doctor if you are taking cyclosporine, gemfibrozil, niacin, antibiotics (especially erythromycin), or medications for fungal infections. All of these drugs may increase the risk of myositis (muscle inflammation) when taken with lovastatin and may lead to kidney failure.

FOOD INTERACTIONS
None reported.

DISEASE INTERACTIONS
Consult your doctor if you have any of the following problems: liver, kidney, or muscle disease, or a medical history involving organ transplant or recent surgery.

≡ SIDE EFFECTS ≡

SERIOUS
Fever, unusual or unexplained muscle aches and tenderness. Call your doctor right away.

COMMON
Side effects occur in only 1% to 2% of patients. These include constipation or diarrhea, dizziness or lightheadedness, bloating or gas, heartburn, nausea, skin rash, stomach pain, rise in liver enzymes.

LESS COMMON
Sleeping difficulty.

LYME DISEASE VACCINE (RECOMBINANT OSPA)

Available in: Injection
Available OTC? No   **As Generic?** No
Drug Class: Vaccine

▼ USAGE INFORMATION

WHY IT'S PRESCRIBED
To protect against, but not treat, Lyme disease in people ages 15 to 70. The vaccine is recommended for people who live or work in grassy or wooded areas that are infested with ticks infected with Borrelia burgdorferi (the bacteria that causes Lyme disease); the vaccine is also for people planning to travel to tick-infested areas.

HOW IT WORKS
This Lyme disease vaccine stimulates the body's immune system to produce antibodies against a protein on the outer surface of the tick. When infected ticks bite vaccinated humans, the vaccine-induced antibodies then enter the tick and attack the B. burgdorferi inside the gut of the tick, thereby preventing transmission of the disease.

▼ DOSAGE GUIDELINES

RANGE AND FREQUENCY
All doses need to be administered by a health care professional. Adults and teenagers: 1 dose injected into a muscle in the upper arm. Booster doses are given at 1 month and 12 months

after the first dose. All three doses are required to confer optimal protection.

ONSET OF EFFECT
Unknown.

DURATION OF ACTION
Unknown.

DIETARY ADVICE
No special restrictions.

STORAGE
Not applicable; the dose is administered only at a health care facility.

MISSED DOSE
If you miss a scheduled vaccination, contact your doctor. According to the Centers for Disease Control and Prevention (CDC), if you miss the one-month booster, you may take it as soon as possible within the first year. All 3 injections should be completed within 1 year.

STOPPING THE DRUG
The full schedule of injections should be followed unless a medical problem intervenes. A full course of injections must be completed to ensure adequate immunization.

PROLONGED USE
Periodic booster shots may be recommended.

▼ PRECAUTIONS

Over 60: Lyme disease vaccine is not expected to cause different or more severe side effects in older patients than in younger persons.

Driving and Hazardous Work: The vaccine should not impair your ability to perform such tasks safely.

Alcohol: No special precautions are necessary.

Pregnancy: Adequate human studies have not been done. Before taking Lyme disease vaccine, tell your physician if you are pregnant or planning to become pregnant.

Breast Feeding: Lyme disease vaccine may pass into breast milk; caution is advised. Consult your doctor for more specific advice.

Infants and Children: Not recommended for use by children under the age of 15. No special problems are expected in persons over the age of 15.

Special Concerns: Previous infection with B. burgdorferi does not mean that you are immune to future infections of Lyme disease. As with any vaccine, Lyme disease vaccine may not protect all individuals. In clinical studies, the vaccine was effective in approximately 78% of cases in which the individuals received all three doses. In addition to being vaccinated, people can decrease their chances of acquiring tick-borne infections by wearing pants and long-sleeved shirts, tucking pants into socks,

spraying tick repellent on clothing, checking for ticks in a tick-infested area, and removing attached ticks.

OVERDOSE
Symptoms: Not applicable.

What to Do: No cases of overdose have been reported.

▼ INTERACTIONS

DRUG INTERACTIONS
No drug interactions have been reported. However, as with other intramuscular injections, Lyme disease vaccine should not be given to people taking anticoagulant drugs such as warfarin unless the potential benefit outweighs the risks.

FOOD INTERACTIONS
No known food interactions.

DISEASE INTERACTIONS
No known disease interactions. However, as with other intramuscular injections, Lyme disease vaccine should not be administered to people with blood clotting disorders. The safety of the vaccine has not been tested in people who have joint or neurological complications from Lyme disease, in those who have disorders associated with chronic joint swelling, or in those who have a pacemaker.

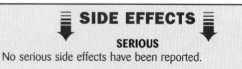

≡ SIDE EFFECTS ≡

SERIOUS
No serious side effects have been reported.

COMMON
Soreness or redness at the site of injection.

LESS COMMON
Muscle pain, chills, fever, flu-like symptoms.

MEDROXYPROGESTERONE ACETATE

Available in: Tablets, injection
Available OTC? No   **As Generic?** Yes
Drug Class: Progestin (hormone)

▼ USAGE INFORMATION

WHY IT'S PRESCRIBED
To treat amenorrhea (cessation of menstrual periods) and abnormal uterine bleeding. This drug also may be used as a contraceptive.

HOW IT WORKS
Medroxyprogesterone inhibits the secretion of pituitary hormones that in turn then regulate menstrual and reproductive cycles. The drug also alters activity of uterine cells, resulting in, among other changes, a thickening of the cervical mucus. Such changes make it less likely that a partner's sperm will reach and fertilize an egg.

▼ DOSAGE GUIDELINES

RANGE AND FREQUENCY
For amenorrhea: Tablets, 5 to 10 mg a day for 5 to 10 days. For abnormal uterine bleeding: Tablets, 5 to 10 mg a day for 5 to 10 days beginning on the 16th or 21st day of the menstrual cycle. For contraception: 1 depo (Depo-Provera) injection (150 mg) every 3 months. For use in treating menopause: Tablets, 10 mg a day for 10 to 14 days, together with estrogen in each 25-day cycle.

ONSET OF EFFECT
Varies with mode of delivery. Protection against pregnancy can begin immediately if injection is given within 5 days of the menstrual period.

DURATION OF ACTION
Tablets: 24 hours or more.
Injection: More than 3 months.

DIETARY ADVICE
Take it with meals to prevent gastrointestinal upset.

STORAGE
Store in a tightly sealed container away from heat and direct light.

MISSED DOSE
Take a missed dose of the tablet as soon as you remember. If it is near the time for the next dose, skip the missed dose and resume your regular dosage schedule. Do not double the next dose.

STOPPING THE DRUG
The decision to stop taking the drug should be made by your doctor.

PROLONGED USE
Consult your doctor about the need for periodic examinations and laboratory tests if you use this drug for an extended period.

▼ PRECAUTIONS

Over 60: No special problems are expected in older patients.

Driving and Hazardous Work: Do not drive or engage in hazardous work until you determine how the medicine affects you.

Alcohol: No special problems are expected.

Pregnancy: Before you use medroxyprogesterone, tell your doctor if you are pregnant or if you plan to become pregnant. This drug must not be used during pregnancy.

Breast Feeding: Medroxyprogesterone passes into breast milk; avoid or discontinue use while nursing.

Infants and Children: This medication is not recommended for young patients.

Special Concerns: Remember that no contraceptive method is foolproof; 1% of women using the medroxyprogesterone injections have become pregnant.

OVERDOSE
Symptoms: No specific ones have been reported.

What to Do: An overdose of medroxyprogesterone is unlikely to be life-threatening. However, if someone takes a much larger dose than prescribed, call your doctor, emergency medical services (EMS), or the nearest poison control center immediately.

▼ INTERACTIONS

DRUG INTERACTIONS
Consult your doctor for specific advice if you are taking aminoglutethimide, carbamazepine, phenytoin, rifabutin, or rifampin.

FOOD INTERACTIONS
No known food interactions.

DISEASE INTERACTIONS
Do not take medroxyprogesterone if you have: known or suspected breast malignancies or tumors, acute liver disease or liver tumors, or active thrombophlebitis or thromboembolic disease. Consult your doctor if you have any of the following: asthma, epilepsy, migraine headaches, heart or circulation problems, bleeding problems, a history of thrombophlebitis or thromboembolic disease, diabetes mellitus, high blood cholesterol, kidney disease, risk factors for osteoporosis, or central nervous system disorders such as depression.

≡ SIDE EFFECTS ≡

SERIOUS
Abnormal menstrual bleeding; unexpected or increased flow of breast milk; mental depression; skin rash; loss of or change in speech, coordination, or vision; severe and sudden shortness of breath. Call your doctor immediately.

COMMON
Stomach pain, swelling of face, ankles, or feet, mild headache, mood changes, unusual fatigue, weight gain.

LESS COMMON
Acne, breast pain or tenderness, hot flashes, insomnia, loss of sexual desire, loss or gain of scalp hair or body hair, brown spots on skin.

MEFLOQUINE HYDROCHLORIDE

Available in: Tablets
Available OTC? No   **As Generic?** No
Drug Class: Anti-infective/antimalarial

▼ USAGE INFORMATION

WHY IT'S PRESCRIBED
To treat mild to moderate acute malaria caused by strains of plasmodia (the parasite that causes malaria) that are susceptible to mefloquine–specifically, Plasmodium falciparum and P. vivax. Also used to prevent malaria caused by these strains.

HOW IT WORKS
Mefloquine is poisonous to the malarial parasite.

▼ DOSAGE GUIDELINES

RANGE AND FREQUENCY
Adults–To treat: 5 tablets (1,250 mg each) taken as a single dose. Patients with acute P. vivax malaria, treated with mefloquine, are at high risk of relapse. To avoid relapse after the initial treatment, patients should be treated with another antimalarial such as primaquine. To prevent: 250 mg once a week. Begin taking mefloquine one week prior to departure and continue taking the drug for 4 weeks upon return. Children 6 months of age and older–To treat, 20 to 25 mg per 2.2 lbs (1 kg) of body weight. Split the total dose into 2 doses 6 to 8 hours apart in order to reduce the risk and severity of side effects. To prevent: Your pediatrician will determine the appropriate dose.

ONSET OF EFFECT
Unknown.

DURATION OF ACTION
Up to 3 weeks.

DIETARY ADVICE
Do not take on an empty stomach. Take with at least 8 oz of water.

STORAGE
Store in a tightly sealed container away from moisture, heat, and direct light.

MISSED DOSE
If taking 1 or more doses a day, take it as soon as you remember. If it is near the time for the next dose, skip the missed dose and resume your regular dosage schedule. Do not double the next dose. If taking 1 weekly dose, take it as soon as possible, then resume regular schedule.

STOPPING THE DRUG
Take it as prescribed for the full treatment period.

PROLONGED USE
Periodic liver function tests and eye exams are recommended.

▼ PRECAUTIONS

Over 60: Adverse reactions may be more likely and more severe among this age group.

Driving and Hazardous Work: Avoid such activities until you determine how the medicine affects you. Dizziness and coordination difficulties may occur after the drug is discontinued.

Alcohol: No special warnings.

Pregnancy: The use of mefloquine is discouraged during pregnancy because of the risks it poses to the unborn child. Women of child-bearing age should practice contraception during preventive therapy.

Breast Feeding: Mefloquine passes into breast milk; extreme caution is advised. Consult your physician for specific advice.

Infants and Children: Safety and effectiveness have not been established for children under the age of 6 months. Early vomiting has been associated with mefloquine use in children and with treatment failure. If a second dose is not tolerated, alternative antimalarial measures should be considered.

Special Concerns: If you take mefloquine once a week, take it on the same day every week. Malaria is spread by mosquitoes. Take appropriate precautions, such as using mosquito netting, to guard against being bitten by malaria-carrying mosquitoes.

OVERDOSE
Symptoms: Side effects may be more pronounced. (See Side Effects.)

What to Do: If you have reason to suspect overdose, call your doctor, emergency medical services (EMS), or the nearest poison control center immediately.

▼ INTERACTIONS

DRUG INTERACTIONS
Consult a doctor for advice if you are taking a beta-blocker, quinidine, quinine, chloroquine, antiarrhythmic drugs, calcium channel blockers, halofantrine, antihistamines, histamine (H1) blockers, tricyclic antidepressants, phenothiazines, or anticonvulsants. Also, tell your physician if you are taking any other prescription or over-the-counter drug.

FOOD INTERACTIONS
No known food interactions.

DISEASE INTERACTIONS
Consult your doctor for specific advice if you have a seizure or psychiatric disorder, impaired liver function, any eye condition, or heart disease.

≡ SIDE EFFECTS ≡

▼ SERIOUS ▼
Slowed heartbeat, seizures. Severe anxiety, depression, restlessness, or confusion during preventive therapy may be signs of more serious psychiatric problems. Call your doctor immediately.

COMMON
Treatment-related: dizziness, muscle pain, nausea, fever, headache, vomiting, chills, diarrhea, skin rash, abdominal pain, fatigue, loss of appetite, ringing in the ears. Prevention-related: vomiting, nausea.

LESS COMMON
Treatment-related: hair loss, emotional problems, itching, fatigue. Prevention-related: dizziness, lightheadedness.

METFORMIN

Available in: Tablets, extended-release tablets
Available OTC? No   **As Generic?** No
Drug Class: Antidiabetic agent/biguanide

▼ USAGE INFORMATION

WHY IT'S PRESCRIBED
Used to lower abnormally high blood glucose (sugar) levels in patients with non-insulin-dependent (type 2) diabetes whose blood sugar levels cannot be adequately controlled by diet or exercise alone. The drug may be used alone or in conjunction with sulfonylurea drugs or insulin.

HOW IT WORKS
Metformin decreases the liver's production of glucose, inhibits the breakdown of fatty acids used to produce glucose, and increases the removal of glucose from muscle, the liver, and other body tissues where it is stored.

▼ DOSAGE GUIDELINES

RANGE AND FREQUENCY
Available in 500 mg, 850 mg, or 1,000 mg tablets; the extended-release tablets are available in 500-mg strength only and should not be used by patients under the age of 17. Initial dose: 500 mg a day, taken with dinner. If tolerated, a second dose can be added, taken with breakfast. The dose may be slowly increased (1 tablet every 1 or 2 weeks) to a maximum of 2,500 mg a day. Alternatively, 850 mg daily, increased by 850 mg every other week to a maximum of 2,550 mg per day.

ONSET OF EFFECT
Within 2 hours.

DURATION OF ACTION
From 12 to 15 hours.

DIETARY ADVICE
Take with meals to reduce risk of stomach upset.

STORAGE
Store in a sealed container at room temperature away from heat and direct light.

▼ SIDE EFFECTS

SERIOUS
In rare cases, metformin may lead to lactic acidosis, an abnormal and potentially life-threatening buildup of lactic acid in the blood. Symptoms include rapid, shallow breathing, unusual sleepiness or weakness, muscle pain, and abdominal distress. Metformin also occasionally causes abnormally low blood glucose levels (hypoglycemia); symptoms include blurred vision, cold sweats, confusion, anxiousness, rapid heartbeat, shakiness, and nausea. Seek medical assistance immediately.

COMMON
Diarrhea, nausea, vomiting, abdominal bloating, gas, diminished appetite. Usually such symptoms are mild and transient. Consult your doctor if the symptoms persist or increase in severity.

LESS COMMON
Unpleasant or metallic taste in mouth.

MISSED DOSE
Take it with food as soon as you remember. However, if it is almost time for the next dose, skip the missed dose and resume your regular dosage schedule. Do not double the next dose.

STOPPING THE DRUG
Stop taking metformin only when your doctor advises.

PROLONGED USE
Because metformin helps to manage diabetes but does not cure the disease, its use will be ongoing as long as your blood glucose levels are being adequately controlled. If not, the metformin dosage may be adjusted or a different treatment prescribed.

▼ PRECAUTIONS

Over 60: Because metformin is metabolized in the kidneys, extra caution is warranted in thin, elderly patients with mild adrenal insufficiency (not often detected by the usual tests for kidney impairment).

Driving and Hazardous Work: No special precautions are necessary.

Alcohol: Excessive amounts of alcohol can increase the effect of metformin, possibly resulting in abnormally low blood glucose levels.

Pregnancy: Taking metformin is not advised during pregnancy. Consult your doctor if you become pregnant or plan to become pregnant; insulin is usually the treatment of choice for pregnant women who have diabetes.

Breast Feeding: Metformin passes into breast milk, although it has not been shown to cause harm to nursing infants.

Infants and Children: Glucophage may be used in children 10 years of age and older; Glucophage XR may be used in children 17 years of age and older.

OVERDOSE
Symptoms: Symptoms of lactic acidosis or hypoglycemia (see Serious Side Effects).

What to Do: Seek emergency medical assistance right away.

▼ INTERACTIONS

DRUG INTERACTIONS
Consult your doctor if you are taking any of the following: amiloride, calcium channel blockers, cimetidine, digoxin, furosemide, morphine, procainamide, quinidine, quinine, ranitidine, trimethoprim, triamterene, or vancomycin.

FOOD INTERACTIONS
The amount and type of food you eat affect your blood glucose levels and must be taken into account while you receive metformin therapy.

DISEASE INTERACTIONS
Do not take metformin if you have a condition requiring careful control of blood glucose levels, such as severe infection; any condition contributing to abnormally low blood oxygen levels, such as congestive heart failure; metabolic acidosis (buildup of acid in the blood); a history of alcohol abuse; or kidney or liver disease.

METHOTREXATE

Available in: Tablets, injection
Available OTC? No   **As Generic?** Yes
Drug Class: Antineoplastic agent/antimetabolite; antipsoriatic; antirheumatic

▼ USAGE INFORMATION

WHY IT'S PRESCRIBED
To treat certain kinds of cancer, psoriasis, and rheumatoid arthritis.

HOW IT WORKS
Methotrexate interferes with the activity of an enzyme needed for the maintenance and replication of cells, especially those that divide and proliferate rapidly. Such cells include many types of cancer cells, as well as those that compose the bone marrow and the cells that line the mouth, intestine, and bladder. Consequently, in addition to its cancer-fighting effects, methotrexate may also harm healthy tissues in the body, causing unpleasant or serious side effects. It is unknown how methotrexate works to ease rheumatoid arthritis, but this medication appears to modify the function of the immune system, whose activity is believed to play an important role in the progression of the disease.

▼ DOSAGE GUIDELINES

RANGE AND FREQUENCY
For psoriasis or rheumatoid arthritis—Tablets: 2.5 to 5 mg every 12 hours for 3 doses in 1 week; or 7.5 to 10 mg once a week. Injection: 10 mg, once a week. For cancer—Use and dose depends on type and stage of disease. Your doctor may alter dosage as needed. Consult pediatrician for children's dose.

ONSET OF EFFECT
Unknown.

DURATION OF ACTION
Unknown.

DIETARY ADVICE
This drug is best taken 1 to 2 hours before meals.

STORAGE
Store in a tightly sealed container away from moisture, heat, and direct light.

MISSED DOSE
If you miss a dose, do not take the missed dose and do not double the next dose. Resume your regular schedule and check with your doctor.

STOPPING THE DRUG
The decision to stop taking the drug should be made by your doctor.

PROLONGED USE
See your doctor regularly for tests and examinations.

▼ PRECAUTIONS

Over 60: Adverse reactions may be more likely and more severe in older patients.

Driving and Hazardous Work: Avoid such activities until you determine how the medicine affects you.

Alcohol: Avoid alcohol.

Pregnancy: Methotrexate can cause birth defects and other problems; avoid use during pregnancy.

Breast Feeding: Methotrexate passes into breast milk and may cause serious side effects in the nursing infant; do not use while breast feeding.

Infants and Children: Infants are more sensitive to the effects of methotrexate. No special problems are expected in older children.

Special Concerns: Methotrexate may lower your resistance to infection by reducing the number of white blood cells in the blood. Do not have any immunizations without your doctor's approval. Avoid people with infections. Use care when shaving, trimming nails, or using sharp objects. Inform your doctor immediately if you have fever, chills, unusual bleeding or bruising, diarrhea, or a cough. Methotrexate may increase skin sensitivity to sunlight. Limit sun exposure until you see how the medicine affects you. After you stop taking methotrexate, you may experience back pain, blurred vision, confusion, seizures, dizziness, fever, or unusual fatigue; consult your doctor immediately.

OVERDOSE
Symptoms: Severe damage to the liver, kidneys, stomach, intestines, bone marrow, and lungs, causing a wide array of symptoms.

What to Do: If you suspect an overdose, seek medical assistance immediately.

▼ INTERACTIONS

DRUG INTERACTIONS
A number of drugs may interact with methotrexate. Ask your doctor for specific advice if you are taking any drugs that may affect the liver such as azathioprine, retinoids, and sulfasalazine; or any other prescription or over-the-counter medication.

FOOD INTERACTIONS
No known food interactions.

DISEASE INTERACTIONS
Consult your doctor if you have any of the following: a history of alcohol abuse, chicken pox, shingles, colitis, any disease of the immune system, kidney stones, any infection, intestinal blockage, kidney disease, liver disease, mouth sores or inflammation, or stomach ulcers.

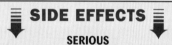

SIDE EFFECTS

SERIOUS
Black, tarry stools, bloody vomit, diarrhea, flushing or redness of skin, sores in mouth and on lips, stomach pain, blood in urine or stools, confusion, seizures, cough or hoarseness, fever or chills, pain in lower back or side, painful or difficult urination, red spots on skin, shortness of breath, swollen feet or lower legs, unusual bleeding or bruising, back pain, dark urine, drowsiness, dizziness, headache, joint pain, unusual fatigue, yellow-tinged eyes or skin. Call your doctor immediately.

COMMON
Loss of appetite, nausea and vomiting, minor mouth ulcers.

LESS COMMON
Acne, boils, pale skin, skin rash, or itching.

METHYLPHENIDATE HYDROCHLORIDE

BRAND NAMES

Methylin, Ritalin, Ritalin-SR

Available in: Tablets, extended-release tablets
Available OTC? No   **As Generic?** Yes
Drug Class: Central nervous system stimulant

▼ USAGE INFORMATION

WHY IT'S PRESCRIBED
To treat attention-deficit hyperactivity disorder (ADHD). It is also used to treat narcolepsy.

HOW IT WORKS
Methylphenidate is thought to stimulate the release of norepinephrine, a natural hormone that promotes the transmission of nerve impulses in the brain. It works by decreasing restlessness and increasing attention in adults and children who cannot concentrate for very long, are easily distracted, or are unusually impulsive.

▼ DOSAGE GUIDELINES

RANGE AND FREQUENCY
For ADHD—Tablets: Adults and teenagers: 5 to 20 mg, 2 to 3 times a day, taken with or after meals. Children ages 6 to 12: To start, 5 mg, 2 times a day. If needed, your doctor may increase the dose by 5 to 10 mg a week. Extended-release tablets: Adults, teenagers and children ages 6 to 12: 20 mg, 1 to 3 times a day, every 8 hours. For narcolepsy— Tablets: Adults and teenagers: 5 to 20 mg, 3 or 4 times a day, taken with or after meals. Extended-release tablets: Adults and teenagers: 20 mg, 2 to 3 times a day.

ONSET OF EFFECT
Tablets: Usually within 30 minutes. Extended-release tablets: Usually between 30 and 60 minutes.

DURATION OF ACTION
Tablets: 4 to 6 hours. Extended-release tablets: 6 hours or longer.

DIETARY ADVICE
For attention-deficit hyperactivity disorder, this medicine should be taken with or after meals. For narcolepsy, it should be taken 30 to 45 minutes before meals.

STORAGE
Store in a tightly sealed container away from moisture, heat, and direct light.

MISSED DOSE
Take it as soon as you remember. If it is near the time for the next dose, skip the missed dose and resume your regular dosage schedule. Do not double the next dose.

STOPPING THE DRUG
The decision to stop taking the drug should be made by your doctor.

PROLONGED USE
See your doctor regularly for tests and examinations.

▼ PRECAUTIONS

Over 60: No special problems are expected.

Driving and Hazardous Work: Do not drive or engage in hazardous work until you determine how the medicine affects you.

Alcohol: Avoid alcohol.

Pregnancy: Adequate human studies have not been completed. Before taking methylphenidate, tell your doctor if you are pregnant or plan to become pregnant.

Breast Feeding: It is not known whether methylphenidate passes into breast milk; caution is advised. Consult your doctor for advice.

Infants and Children: This drug is not recommended for use by children under the age of 6. Older children may be especially likely to experience side effects such as loss of appetite, stomach pain, and weight loss.

Special Concerns: To prevent insomnia, do not take methylphenidate too close to bedtime. Your prescription cannot be refilled, so you must get a new one from your doctor to obtain more medication.

OVERDOSE
Symptoms: Agitation, confusion, delirium, seizures, dry mouth, false sense of well-being, rapid, pounding, or irregular heartbeat, fever, sweating, severe headache, increased blood pressure, muscle twitching, trembling or tremors, vomiting.

What to Do: Call your doctor, emergency medical services (EMS), or the nearest poison control center immediately.

▼ INTERACTIONS

DRUG INTERACTIONS
Call your doctor for specific advice if you are taking caffeine, amantadine, appetite suppressants, tricyclic antidepressants, chlophedianol, pemoline, asthma medicine, amphetamines, medicine for colds or sinus problems or allergies, nabilone, pimozide, or MAO inhibitors.

FOOD INTERACTIONS
Do not drink large amounts of caffeinated beverages, such as coffee, tea, soft drinks, cocoa, or chocolate milk.

DISEASE INTERACTIONS
Consult your doctor if you have Tourette's syndrome or other tics, glaucoma, epilepsy or another seizure disorder, high blood pressure, psychosis, severe anxiety, depression, or a history of alcohol or drug abuse.

☰ SIDE EFFECTS ☰

SERIOUS
Fast heartbeat, unusual bleeding or bruising, chest pain, fever, joint pain, increased heartbeat, skin rash or hives, uncontrolled body movements, blurred vision or other vision changes, seizures, sore throat and fever, unusual fatigue, weight loss, mood or mental changes. Call your doctor immediately.

COMMON
Loss of appetite, insomnia, nervousness.

LESS COMMON
Dizziness, stomach pain, drowsiness, nausea, headache.

METHYLPRESNISOLONE

Available in: Tablets, injection, enema
Available OTC? No **As Generic?** Yes
Drug Class: Corticosteroid

▼ USAGE INFORMATION

WHY IT'S PRESCRIBED
To treat numerous conditions that involve inflammation (a response by body tissues, producing redness, warmth, swelling, and pain). Such conditions include arthritis, allergic reactions, asthma, some skin diseases, multiple sclerosis flare-ups, and other autoimmune diseases. Also prescribed to treat deficiency of natural steroid hormones.

HOW IT WORKS
This hormone mimics the effects of the body's natural corticosteroids. It depresses the synthesis, release, and activity of inflammation-producing body chemicals. It also suppresses the activity of the immune system.

▼ DOSAGE GUIDELINES

RANGE AND FREQUENCY
Tablets: 4 to 160 mg a day, depending on condition, in

1 or more doses. Injection: 10 to 160 mg a day injected into a muscle or vein, or 4 to 120 mg as needed, injected into a muscle, joint, or lesion. Enema: 40 mg, 3 to 7 times a week. Consult your pediatrician for children's dose.

ONSET OF EFFECT
Varies widely depending on form used.

DURATION OF ACTION
30 to 36 hours with tablets; 1 to 4 weeks after muscle injection; 1 to 5 weeks after other injections.

DIETARY ADVICE
Take it with food or milk to minimize stomach upset. Your doctor may recommend a low-salt, high-potassium, high-protein diet.

STORAGE
Store in a tightly sealed container away from moisture, heat, and direct light. Do not freeze the liquid form of the medication.

MISSED DOSE
If you take several doses a day and it is close to the next dose, double the next dose. If you take 1 dose a day and you do not remember until the next day, skip the missed dose and do not double the next dose.

STOPPING THE DRUG
With long-term therapy, do not stop taking the drug abruptly; the dosage should be decreased gradually.

PROLONGED USE
Long-term use may lead to cataracts, diabetes, hypertension, or osteoporosis; see your doctor for regular visits.

▼ PRECAUTIONS

Over 60: Adverse reactions may be more likely and more severe in older patients.

Driving and Hazardous Work: Avoid such activities until you determine how the medicine affects you.

Alcohol: May cause stomach problems; avoid it unless your physician approves occasional moderate drinking.

Pregnancy: Overuse during pregnancy can impair growth and development of the child.

Breast Feeding: Do not use this drug while nursing.

Infants and Children: Methylprednisolone may retard the development of bone and other tissues.

Special Concerns: This drug can lower your resistance to infection. Avoid immuniza-

tions with live vaccines. Patients undergoing long-term therapy should wear a medical-alert bracelet. Call a doctor if you develop a fever.

OVERDOSE
Symptoms: Fever, muscle or joint pain, nausea, dizziness, fainting, difficulty breathing. Prolonged overuse: Moon-face, obesity, unusual hair growth, acne, loss of sexual function, muscle wasting.

What to Do: Seek medical assistance immediately.

▼ INTERACTIONS

DRUG INTERACTIONS
Consult your doctor for specific advice if you are taking aminoglutethimide, antacids, barbiturates, carbamazepine, griseofulvin, mitotane, phenylbutazone, phenytoin, primidone, rifampin, injectable amphotericin B, oral antidiabetes agents, insulin, digitalis drugs, diuretics, or medications containing potassium or sodium.

FOOD INTERACTIONS
Avoid excess sodium.

DISEASE INTERACTIONS
Consult your doctor if you have a history of bone disease, chicken pox, measles, gastrointestinal disorders, diabetes, recent serious infection, glaucoma, heart disease, hypertension, liver or kidney disorders, high blood cholesterol, thyroid problems, myasthenia gravis, or lupus.

≡ SIDE EFFECTS ≡

SERIOUS
Vision problems, frequent urination, increased thirst, rectal bleeding, blistering skin, confusion, hallucinations, paranoia, euphoria, depression, mood swings, redness and swelling at injection site. Call your doctor immediately.

COMMON
Increased appetite, indigestion, nervousness, insomnia, greater susceptibility to infections, increased blood pressure, slowed wound healing, weight gain, easy bruising, fluid retention.

LESS COMMON
Change in skin color, dizziness, headache, increased sweating, unusual growth of body or facial hair, increased blood sugar, peptic ulcers, adrenal insufficiency, muscle weakness, cataracts, glaucoma, osteoporosis.

METOPROLOL

Available in: Tablets, extended-release tablets (Injection is for hospital use only.)
Available OTC? No   **As Generic?** Yes
Drug Class: Beta-blocker

▼ USAGE INFORMATION

WHY IT'S PRESCRIBED
To treat mild to moderate high blood pressure or angina; to prevent or control heartbeat irregularities (cardiac arrhythmias); to treat congestive heart failure.Injection is used in hospitals for emergency treatment of heart attack, followed by maintenance with oral forms.

HOW IT WORKS
Metoprolol slows the rate and force of contraction of the heart by blocking certain nerve impulses, thus reducing blood pressure. By modifying nerve impulses to the heart, the drug also helps to stabilize heart rhythm.

▼ DOSAGE GUIDELINES

RANGE AND FREQUENCY
For high blood pressure or angina—Adults: 100 to 400 mg a day in divided doses. Extended-release tablets: Up to 400 mg once a day. For treatment after a heart attack—Initial dose is 50 mg every 6 hours, followed by a maintenance dose of 100 mg or more (up to 400 mg a day), 2 times a day for as long as the physician recommends. For congestive heart failure (Toprol-XL)—The exact dose will be determined by your doctor. Average dose is 25 mg once a day for 2 weeks in people with stable heart failure (NYHA class II) and 12.5 mg once a day in those with more severe heart failure. The dose may gradually be doubled every 2 weeks, up to 200 mg a day.

ONSET OF EFFECT
Within 15 minutes.

DURATION OF ACTION
6 to 12 hours; up to 24 hours with the extended-release tablet.

DIETARY ADVICE
Take it with food. Follow a low-salt or low-cholesterol diet to improve control over high blood pressure and heart disease.

STORAGE
Store in a tightly sealed container away from heat and direct light.

MISSED DOSE
Take it as soon as you remember. However, if it is within 4 hours of your next dose (8 hours if using extended-release tablet), skip the missed dose and resume your regular dosage schedule. Do not double the next dose.

STOPPING THE DRUG
This drug should not be stopped suddenly, as this may lead to angina and possibly a heart attack in patients with advanced heart disease. Slow reduction of the dose under doctor's close supervision for 2 to 3 weeks is advised.

PROLONGED USE
Lifelong therapy may be necessary. See your doctor for regular examinations.

▼ PRECAUTIONS

Over 60: Adverse reactions may be more likely and more severe in older patients.

Driving and Hazardous Work: Use caution until you determine how the medicine affects you.

Alcohol: Drink alcoholic beverages in careful moderation, if at all. Alcohol may interact with the medication and cause a dangerous drop in blood pressure.

Pregnancy: Discuss with your doctor the relative risks and benefits of using this medication during the time you are pregnant.

Breast Feeding: Adverse effects in infants have not been documented.

Infants and Children: No special problems are expected.

OVERDOSE
Symptoms: Unusually slow or rapid heartbeat, severe dizziness or fainting, poor circulation in the hands (bluish skin), breathing difficulty, seizures.

What to Do: Call your doctor, emergency medical services (EMS), or the nearest poison control center immediately.

▼ INTERACTIONS

DRUG INTERACTIONS
Consult your doctor if you are taking amphetamines, oral antidiabetic agents, asthma medication, calcium channel blockers, clonidine; guanabenz, halothane, immunotherapy for allergies, insulin, MAO inhibitors, reserpine, other beta-blockers, or any over-the-counter medicine.

FOOD INTERACTIONS
None reported.

DISEASE INTERACTIONS
Metoprolol should be used with caution in people with diabetes, especially type 1, since the drug may mask symptoms of hypoglycemia. Consult your doctor if you have allergies or asthma, heart or blood vessel disease, hyperthyroidism, irregular (slow) heartbeat, myasthenia gravis, psoriasis, respiratory problems such as bronchitis or emphysema, kidney or liver disease, or a history of mental depression.

≡ SIDE EFFECTS ≡

SERIOUS
Shortness of breath, wheezing; irregular or slow heartbeat (50 beats per minute or less); chest pain or tightness; swelling of the ankles, feet, and lower legs; mental depression. If you experience such symptoms, stop taking metoprolol and call your doctor immediately.

COMMON
Dizziness or lightheadedness, especially when rising suddenly to a standing position; decreased sexual ability; unusual fatigue, weakness, or drowsiness; insomnia.

LESS COMMON
Anxiety, irritability, nervousness; constipation; diarrhea; dry, sore eyes; itching; nausea or vomiting; nightmares or intensely vivid dreams; numbness or tingling.

MOMETASONE FUROATE NASAL

Available in: Nasal spray
Available OTC? No   **As Generic?** No
Drug Class: Nasal corticosteroid

▼ USAGE INFORMATION

WHY IT'S PRESCRIBED
To prevent and treat the symptoms of allergic rhinitis (seasonal and perennial allergies such as hay fever).

HOW IT WORKS
Respiratory corticosteroids such as mometasone reduce or prevent inflammation of the lining of the airways, reduce the allergic response to inhaled allergens, and inhibit the secretion of mucus within the airways.

▼ DOSAGE GUIDELINES

RANGE AND FREQUENCY
Adults and teenagers: 2 sprays (50 micrograms [mcg] in each spray) in each nostril once a day, for a maximum daily dose of 200 mcg. To prevent the symptoms of allergic rhinitis from developing, it is recommended that patients with known seasonal allergies begin taking mometasone 2 to 4 weeks before the anticipated start of the pollen season.

ONSET OF EFFECT
From 11 hours to 2 days.

DURATION OF ACTION
Mometasone is effective as long as you continue to take the medication.

DIETARY ADVICE
Mometasone can be used without regard to diet.

STORAGE
Store in a tightly sealed container away from moisture, heat, and direct light.

MISSED DOSE
If you miss a dose on one day, resume your regular dosage schedule the next day. Do not double the next dose.

STOPPING THE DRUG
No special instructions.

PROLONGED USE
Consult your doctor about any need for periodic physical examinations and lab tests.

▼ PRECAUTIONS

Over 60: No special problems are expected.

Driving and Hazardous Work: Mometasone should not impair your ability to perform such tasks safely.

Alcohol: No special precautions are necessary.

Pregnancy: Nasal steroids have not been reported to cause birth defects if taken during pregnancy. Before using this drug, tell your doctor if you are pregnant or plan to become pregnant.

Breast Feeding: Mometasone may pass into breast milk; caution is advised. Consult your doctor for advice.

Infants and Children: Not recommended for use by children under age 12.

Special Concerns: Prior to your initial use of the inhaler, you must prime it by depressing the pump 10 times or until a fine mist appears. You may store the inhaler for up to 1 week without repriming. If it is unused for more than 1 week, reprime it by depressing the pump 2 times or until a fine mist appears. Avoid spraying the medication into the eyes.

OVERDOSE
Symptoms: No cases of overdose have been reported.

What to Do: An overdose with mometasone is unlikely. If someone takes a much larger dose than prescribed, call your doctor.

▼ INTERACTIONS

DRUG INTERACTIONS
Consult your doctor for advice if you are taking systemic corticosteroids, other inhaled corticosteroids, or any drugs that suppress the immune system.

FOOD INTERACTIONS
No known food interactions.

DISEASE INTERACTIONS
Consult your doctor if you have any other medical problem, particularly glaucoma, a herpes infection of the eye, a history of tuberculosis, liver disease, an underactive thyroid, or osteoporosis.

≡ SIDE EFFECTS ≡
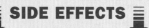

SERIOUS
No serious side effects are associated with mometasone.

COMMON
Headache, increased susceptibility to viral infection, sore throat, nosebleeds or bloody nasal secretions.

LESS COMMON
Cough, increased susceptibility to upper respiratory infection, menstrual irregularities, bone pain, sinus pain.

MONTELUKAST

Available in: Tablets, chewable tablets
Available OTC? No **As Generic?** No
Drug Class: Leukotriene receptor antagonist

▼ USAGE INFORMATION

WHY IT'S PRESCRIBED
To prevent and treat the symptoms of chronic asthma by preventing bronchospasm (contraction of the smooth muscle tissue surrounding the airways, which results in narrowing and obstruction of the air passages). Montelukast may be used in conjunction with other asthma treatments.

HOW IT WORKS
Montelukast blocks cell receptors for leukotrienes, naturally formed substances that cause inflammation and constriction of the airways. Unlike bronchodilators, which relieve the acute symptoms of an asthma attack, montelukast is prescribed to be taken regularly when no symptoms are present, to reduce the chronic inflammation of the airways that causes asthma, thus preventing asthma attacks.

▼ DOSAGE GUIDELINES

RANGE AND FREQUENCY
Adults and children age 15 and over: One 10 mg tablet per day, taken in the evening.

Children ages 6 to 14: One 5 mg chewable tablet per day, taken in the evening. Children ages 2 to 5: One 4 mg chewable tablet per day, taken in the evening.

ONSET OF EFFECT
Unknown.

DURATION OF ACTION
Unknown.

DIETARY ADVICE
Montelukast can be taken without regard to diet.

STORAGE
Store in a tightly sealed container away from moisture, heat, and direct light.

MISSED DOSE
If you miss a dose one day, do not double the dose the next day. Resume your regular dosage schedule.

STOPPING THE DRUG
The decision to stop taking the drug should be made in consultation with your doctor.

PROLONGED USE
No special problems are expected.

▤ SIDE EFFECTS ▤

SERIOUS
Skin rash (indicating potentially life-threatening allergic reaction); gastroenteritis (causing loss of appetite, nausea, vomiting, stomach upset, fever, and diarrhea). Call your doctor immediately.

COMMON
Headache.

LESS COMMON
Weakness, fatigue, fever, abdominal pain, indigestion, mouth ulcers, dizziness, nasal congestion, cough, flulike symptoms.

▼ PRECAUTIONS

Over 60: Adverse reactions may be more likely and more severe among this age group.

Driving and Hazardous Work: No special precautions are necessary.

Alcohol: No special precautions are necessary.

Pregnancy: Adequate human studies have not been done. Before taking montelukast, tell your doctor if you are pregnant or plan to become pregnant.

Breast Feeding: Montelukast may pass into breast milk; caution is advised. Consult your doctor for advice.

Infants and Children: Not recommended for use by children under age 2.

Special Concerns: Montelukast has no effect on an asthma attack that has already started. You should have a fast-acting inhaled bronchodilator on hand to treat an acute asthma attack in progress. Consult your doctor if you need to use inhaled bronchodilators more often than usual, or if you are taking more than the maximum number of inhalations in a 24-hour period. Continue to take montelukast even when you are not experiencing any symptoms, as well as during periods of worsening asthma. In rare cases, if doses of systemic corticosteroids are reduced, montelukast may cause Churg-Strauss syndrome, a tissue disorder that sometimes strikes adult asthma patients and, if left untreated, can destroy organs. Early symptoms include fever, muscle aches, and weight loss. Montelukast should not be used as the sole treatment for exercise-induced bronchospasm.

OVERDOSE
Symptoms: No cases of overdose have been reported.

What to Do: An overdose with montelukast is unlikely. If someone takes a much larger dose than prescribed, call your doctor, emergency medical services (EMS), or the nearest poison control center immediately.

▼ INTERACTIONS

DRUG INTERACTIONS
Consult your doctor for specific advice if you are already taking phenobarbital or rifampin. Before you take montelukast, tell your doctor if you are allergic to any other prescription or over-the-counter medicine.

FOOD INTERACTIONS
No known food interactions.

DISEASE INTERACTIONS
If you have phenylketonuria, you should not use the chewable tablet form of montelukast, since it contains phenylalanine. Use of the drug may cause complications in those patients with severe liver disease, since this organ works to remove the medication from the body.

MUPIROCIN

BRAND NAME

Bactroban

Available in: Ointment, cream
Available OTC? No **As Generic?** Yes
Drug Class: Antibiotic

▼ USAGE INFORMATION

WHY IT'S PRESCRIBED
Mupirocin is prescribed for topical therapy of certain bacteria-related skin infections. Mupirocin may be used alone or is occasionally used in combination with a second antibiotic (which is usually taken in an oral form).

HOW IT WORKS
Mupirocin works by preventing bacterial cells from manufacturing vital cell proteins and forming protective cell walls. This action ultimately destroys the infecting bacterial organisms.

▼ DOSAGE GUIDELINES

RANGE AND FREQUENCY
Apply to affected skin 3 times a day. The site may be covered with a gauze dressing if desired.

ONSET OF EFFECT
Mupirocin begins antibacterial activity as soon as the ointment or cream is applied. Several days may be required, however, before its full effects become noticeable.

DURATION OF ACTION
Unknown.

DIETARY ADVICE
No special restrictions.

STORAGE
Store in a tightly sealed container away from heat and direct light. Keep away from moisture and extremes in temperature.

MISSED DOSE
Apply it as soon as you remember. If it is near the time for the next application, skip the missed one and resume your regular dosage schedule. Do not increase the quantity of medication with the next application.

STOPPING THE DRUG
Apply as prescribed for the full treatment period, even if you begin to feel the affected area is better before the scheduled end of therapy.

PROLONGED USE
Therapy with this medication should not require more than 14 days in most cases. Extended use of mupirocin may increase the risk of undesirable side effects.

▼ PRECAUTIONS

Over 60: No special precautions for older patients.

Driving and Hazardous Work: The use of mupirocin should not impair your ability to perform such tasks safely.

Alcohol: No special precautions are necessary.

Pregnancy: Mupirocin has not been evaluated in pregnant women. It is likely that mupirocin is safe for use during pregnancy in certain situations. This should be determined by your doctor.

Breast Feeding: The drug is not thought to be significantly absorbed into the bloodstream. If excessive amounts of mupirocin were absorbed, however, it could pass into breast milk; consult your doctor for advice.

Infants and Children: Consult your pediatrician.

Special Concerns: Mupirocin should not be used by anyone with a history of allergic reaction to mupirocin or any of the ingredients in the ointment or cream (carefully check the label). As with any other antibiotic, mupirocin is useful only against types of bacteria that are susceptible to its effects. Therefore, it is important to tell your doctor if your condition has not improved—or if it has worsened—within 3 to 5 days of starting the drug. The particular bacteria causing your illness may be resistant to mupirocin, and a different antibiotic may be required. Avoid using this medicine near or around the eyes.

OVERDOSE
Symptoms: No cases of overdose have been reported.

What to Do: Overapplication of mupirocin is unlikely to be harmful. However, if someone swallows the medication, call your doctor, emergency medical services (EMS), or the nearest poison control center.

▼ INTERACTIONS

DRUG INTERACTIONS
No specific interactions have been reported. Consult your doctor or pharmacist if you are concerned about taking another prescription or non-prescription medication while you are using mupirocin.

FOOD INTERACTIONS
No known food interactions.

DISEASE INTERACTIONS
No disease interactions have been reported.

≡ SIDE EFFECTS ≡

SERIOUS
There are no serious side effects associated with the use of mupirocin.

COMMON
Mild stinging or burning sensation with initial application.

LESS COMMON
Persistent irritation or skin allergy with pain or discomfort (stinging or burning) at application site; itching, redness, rash, or dryness of the skin; nausea.

NABUMETONE

Available in: Tablets
Available OTC? No   **As Generic?** No
Drug Class: Nonsteroidal anti-inflammatory drug (NSAID)

▼ USAGE INFORMATION

WHY IT'S PRESCRIBED
To treat mild to moderate pain and inflammation caused by tendinitis, arthritis, bursitis, gout, soft tissue injuries, migraine and other vascular headaches, menstrual cramps, and other conditions. When patients fail to respond to one NSAID, another may be tried. The greatest effectiveness often requires trial and error of several different NSAIDs.

HOW IT WORKS
NSAIDs work by interfering with the formation of prosta- glandins, naturally occurring substances in the body that cause inflammation and make nerves more sensitive to pain impulses. NSAIDs also have other modes of action that are less well understood.

▼ DOSAGE GUIDELINES

RANGE AND FREQUENCY
Adults: 1,000 mg once a day. It may be increased to a maximum of 2,000 mg a day. For children's dose, consult your pediatrician.

ONSET OF EFFECT
From 30 minutes to several hours or longer.

DURATION OF ACTION
Variable.

DIETARY ADVICE
Take with food; maintain your usual food and fluid intake.

STORAGE
Store in a tightly sealed con- tainer away from moisture, heat, and direct light.

MISSED DOSE
Take it as soon as you remember. However, if it is near the time for the next dose, skip the missed dose and resume your regular dosage schedule. Do not double the next dose.

STOPPING THE DRUG
The decision to stop taking the drug should be made in consultation with your doctor.

PROLONGED USE
Extended use can cause gas- trointestinal problems, such as ulceration and bleeding, kidney dysfunction, and liver inflammation. Consult your doctor about the need for medical exams and lab tests.

▼ PRECAUTIONS

Over 60: Because of the potentially greater conse- quences of gastrointestinal side effects, the dose of NSAIDs for older patients, especially those over age 70, is often cut in half.

Driving and Hazardous Work: Avoid such activities until you determine how the medicine affects you.

Alcohol: Avoid alcohol when using this medication because it increases the risk of stom- ach irritation.

Pregnancy: Avoid or discon- tinue this medication if you are pregnant or if you plan to become pregnant.

Breast Feeding: Nabumetone passes into breast milk; avoid use while breast feeding.

Infants and Children: May be used in exceptional circum- stances; consult your doctor.

Special Concerns: Because NSAIDs can interfere with blood coagulation, this drug should be stopped at least 3 days prior to any surgery.

OVERDOSE
Symptoms: Severe nausea, vomiting, headache, confu- sion, seizures.

What to Do: Call your doctor, emergency medical services (EMS), or the nearest poison control center immediately.

▼ INTERACTIONS

DRUG INTERACTIONS
Do not take this drug with aspirin or any other NSAIDs without your doctor's ap- proval. In addition, consult your doctor if you are taking antihypertensives, steroids, anticoagulants, antibiotics, itraconazole or ketoconazole, plicamycin, penicillamine, valproic acid, phenytoin, cyclosporine, digitalis drugs, lithium, methotrexate, probenecid, triamterene, or zidovudine.

FOOD INTERACTIONS
No known food interactions.

DISEASE INTERACTIONS
Consult your doctor if you have any of the following: bleeding problems, ulcers or inflammation of the stomach and intestines, diabetes mellitus, systemic lupus erythematosus (SLE, lupus), anemia, asthma, epilepsy, Parkinson's disease, kidney stones, or a history of heart disease or alcohol abuse. Use of nabumetone may cause complications in patients with liver or kidney disease, since these organs work together to remove the medication from the body.

≡ SIDE EFFECTS ≡

SERIOUS
Shortness of breath or wheezing, with or without swelling of legs or other signs of heart failure; chest pain; peptic ulcer disease with vomiting of blood; black, tarry stools; decreasing kidney function. Call your doctor immediately.

COMMON
Nausea, vomiting, heartburn, diarrhea, constipation, headache, dizziness, sleepiness.

LESS COMMON
Ulcers or sores in mouth, depression, rashes or blistering of skin, ringing sound in the ears, unusual tingling or numbness of the hands or feet, seizures, blurred vision. Also elevated potassium levels, decreased blood counts; such problems can be detected by your doctor.

NAPROXEN

Available in: Tablets, oral suspension, gelcaps
Available OTC? Yes   **As Generic?** Yes
Drug Class: Nonsteroidal anti-inflammatory drug (NSAID)

▼ USAGE INFORMATION

WHY IT'S PRESCRIBED
To relieve minor pain or inflammation associated with headaches, the common cold, toothache, muscle aches, backache, arthritis, gout, tendinitis, bursitis, or menstrual cramps; also, to reduce fever. When patients fail to respond to one NSAID, several others may be tried.

HOW IT WORKS
NSAIDs work by interfering with the formation of prostaglandins, naturally occurring substances in the body that cause inflammation and make nerves more sensitive to pain impulses. NSAIDs also have other modes of action that are less well understood.

▼ DOSAGE GUIDELINES

RANGE AND FREQUENCY
Adults: 440 to 1,500 mg daily. Maximum dose is 1,500 mg a day, taken in 2 to 3 evenly divided doses.

ONSET OF EFFECT
Rapid; relieves pain within 1 hour. However, it may take up to 2 weeks to suppress inflammation.

DURATION OF ACTION
Up to 12 hours.

DIETARY ADVICE
Take with food; maintain your usual food and fluid intake.

STORAGE
Store tablets in a tightly sealed container away from heat, moisture, and direct light. Store oral suspension in refrigerator, but do not allow it to freeze.

MISSED DOSE
Take it as soon as you remember. However, if it is near the time for the next dose, skip the missed dose and resume your regular dosage schedule. Do not double the next dose.

STOPPING THE DRUG
If you are taking this drug by prescription, do not stop taking it without first consulting your doctor.

PROLONGED USE
Extended use can cause gastrointestinal problems such as ulceration and bleeding, kidney dysfunction, and liver inflammation. Consult your doctor about the need for medical examinations and lab studies.

▼ PRECAUTIONS

Over 60: Because of the potentially greater consequences of gastrointestinal side effects, the dose of NSAIDs for older patients, especially those over age 70, is often cut in half.

Driving and Hazardous Work: Do not drive or engage in hazardous work until you determine how the medication affects you.

Alcohol: Avoid drinking alcohol when taking this drug; the combination of naproxen and alcohol can be highly toxic to the liver.

Pregnancy: Avoid or discontinue this drug if you are pregnant or if you plan to become pregnant.

Breast Feeding: Naproxen passes into breast milk; avoid or discontinue use while breast feeding.

Infants and Children: Naproxen may be given to children only in exceptional circumstances; consult your pediatrician for advice.

Special Concerns: Because NSAIDs can interfere with blood coagulation, this drug should be stopped at least 3 days prior to any surgery.

OVERDOSE
Symptoms: Severe nausea, vomiting, headache, confusion, seizures.

What to Do: Call your doctor, emergency medical services (EMS), or the nearest poison control center immediately.

▼ INTERACTIONS

DRUG INTERACTIONS
Do not take this drug with aspirin or any other NSAIDs without your doctor's approval. In addition, consult your doctor if you are taking antihypertensives, steroids, anticoagulants, antibiotics, itraconazole or ketoconazole, plicamycin, penicillamine, valproic acid, phenytoin, cyclosporine, digitalis drugs, lithium, methotrexate, probenecid, triamterene, or zidovudine.

FOOD INTERACTIONS
No known food interactions.

DISEASE INTERACTIONS
Consult your doctor if you have any of the following: bleeding problems, ulcers or inflammation of the stomach and intestines, diabetes mellitus, systemic lupus erythematosus (SLE, lupus), anemia, asthma, epilepsy, Parkinson's disease, kidney stones, or a history of heart disease or alcohol abuse. The use of naproxen may cause complications in patients with liver or kidney disease, since these organs work together to remove the medication from the body.

≡ SIDE EFFECTS ≡

SERIOUS
Shortness of breath or wheezing, with or without swelling of legs or other signs of heart failure; chest pain; peptic ulcer disease with vomiting of blood; black, tarry stools; decreasing kidney function. Call your doctor immediately.

COMMON
Nausea, vomiting, heartburn, diarrhea, constipation, headache, dizziness, sleepiness.

LESS COMMON
Ulcers or sores in mouth, depression, rashes or blistering of skin, ringing sound in the ears, unusual tingling or numbness of the hands or feet, seizures, blurred vision. Also elevated potassium levels, decreased blood counts; such problems can be detected by your doctor.

NARATRIPTAN HYDROCHLORIDE

Available in: Tablets
Available OTC? No **As Generic?** No
Drug Class: Antimigraine/antiheadache drug

▼ USAGE INFORMATION

WHY IT'S PRESCRIBED
To treat severe, acute migraine headaches. Naratriptan is not intended as a migraine preventive or for use against any other kinds of pain or headache, including basilar and hemiplegic migraines. Your doctor will determine whether this medication is appropriate in your particular case.

HOW IT WORKS
The exact mechanism of action of the drug naratriptan is unknown.

▼ DOSAGE GUIDELINES

RANGE AND FREQUENCY
A single tablet of 1 or 2.5 mg taken with water is generally effective. If the migraine returns or there is only partial symptomatic relief, the dose may be repeated once after 4 hours, but no more than 5 mg should be taken in any 24-hour period. Since individuals may vary in their response to naratriptan, your experience with the drug will determine the most appropriate initial dosage for you.

ONSET OF EFFECT
Within 1 to 3 hours.

DURATION OF ACTION
Up to 24 hours.

DIETARY ADVICE
The medication can be taken with or without food.

STORAGE
Store in a tightly sealed container away from moisture, heat, and direct light.

MISSED DOSE
Not applicable, since the drug is taken only when necessary.

STOPPING THE DRUG
Consult your doctor before discontinuing naratriptan.

PROLONGED USE
No special problems are expected. However, if you are at risk for coronary artery disease (see Special Concerns), you should undergo periodic medical tests and evaluation.

▼ PRECAUTIONS

Over 60:
Naratriptan is not recommended for use in older patients.

Driving and Hazardous Work:
Some people feel drowsy or dizzy during or following a migraine attack or after taking naratriptan. Avoid driving or other tasks requiring concentration if you have such symptoms.

Alcohol:
No special warnings, although alcohol may trigger or exacerbate migraine headaches.

Pregnancy:
Adequate human studies have not been done. Discuss with your doctor the relative risks and benefits of using the drug while pregnant.

Breast Feeding:
Naratriptan may pass into breast milk; caution is advised. Consult your doctor for advice.

Infants and Children:
The safety and effectiveness of naratriptan have not been established for patients under age 18. Consult your pediatrician for advice.

Special Concerns:
Serious, but rare, heart-related problems may occur after using naratriptan. Anyone at risk for unrecognized coronary artery disease, such as postmenopausal women, men over age 40, or those with risk factors for coronary artery disease (hypertension, high blood cholesterol levels, obesity, diabetes, strong family history of heart disease, or cigarette smoking) should have the first dose of naratriptan administered in a doctor's office. Naratriptan should not be used by any individual with any symptoms of heart disease (including chest pain or tightness, or shortness of breath).

OVERDOSE

Symptoms:
Increase in blood pressure resulting in lightheadedness, tension in the neck, fatigue, and loss of coordination.

What to Do:
An overdose with naratriptan is unlikely. If someone takes a much larger dose than prescribed, call your doctor, emergency medical services (EMS), or the nearest poison control center immediately.

▼ INTERACTIONS

DRUG INTERACTIONS
Do not take naratriptan within 24 hours of taking almotriptan, sumatriptan, rizatriptan, zolmitriptan, ergotamine-containing medication, dihydroergotamine mesylate, or methysergide mesylate. Oral contraceptives may interact with naratriptan. Consult your doctor for advice.

FOOD INTERACTIONS
No known food interactions.

DISEASE INTERACTIONS
You should not take naratriptan if you have a history of angina, heart disease, stroke, uncontrolled hypertension, heartbeat irregularities, peripheral vascular disease, or severely impaired kidney or liver function.

≡ SIDE EFFECTS ≡

SERIOUS
Chest pain or tightness, sudden or severe abdominal pain, shortness of breath, wheezing, heartbeat irregularities or palpitations, skin rash, hives, swelling of the eyelids, face, or lips. Seek emergency medical assistance immediately.

COMMON
Tingling, hot flashes, flushing, weakness, drowsiness or dizziness, fatigue, general feeling of illness.

LESS COMMON
There are no less-common side effects associated with the use of naratriptan.

NEFAZODONE HYDROCHLORIDE

Available in: Tablets
Available OTC? No **As Generic?** No
Drug Class: Antidepressant

▼ USAGE INFORMATION

WHY IT'S PRESCRIBED
To treat symptoms of major depression.

HOW IT WORKS
Nefazodone affects the levels of serotonin and norepinephrine, brain chemicals that are thought to be linked to mood, emotions, and mental state.

▼ DOSAGE GUIDELINES

RANGE AND FREQUENCY
Adults: To start, 100 mg once a day. The dose may then be gradually increased by your doctor to a maximum of 600 mg a day. Older adults: To start, 50 mg 1 or 2 times a day. The dose may then be gradually increased over time by your doctor.

ONSET OF EFFECT
The full effect may take several weeks.

DURATION OF ACTION
Unknown.

DIETARY ADVICE
Nefazodone can be taken without regard to diet.

STORAGE
Store in a tightly sealed container away from moisture, heat, and direct light.

MISSED DOSE
Take it as soon as you remember. However, if it is near the time for the next dose, skip the missed dose and resume your regular dosage schedule. Do not double the next dose.

STOPPING THE DRUG
Take it as prescribed for the full treatment period, even if you begin to feel better before the scheduled end of therapy. The decision to stop taking the drug should be made in consultation with your doctor.

PROLONGED USE
The usual course of therapy lasts 6 months to 1 year; some patients benefit from additional therapy.

▼ PRECAUTIONS

Over 60: Adverse reactions may be more likely and more severe in older patients. A lower dose may be warranted.

Driving and Hazardous Work: Proceed with caution until you determine how the medicine affects you. Drowsiness may occur.

Alcohol: Avoid alcohol.

Pregnancy: Nefazodone has not been shown to cause birth defects in animals. Adequate human studies have not been done. Before you take this medication, tell your doctor if you are pregnant or plan to become pregnant.

Breast Feeding: Nefazodone may pass into breast milk; caution is advised.

Infants and Children: Safety and effectiveness of the drug in children under age 18 have not been established.

Special Concerns: Use sugarless gum or candy for relief of dry mouth.

OVERDOSE
Symptoms: Lightheadedness, dizziness, confusion, fainting, nausea, vomiting, drowsiness.

What to Do: Call your doctor, emergency medical services (EMS), or the nearest poison control center immediately.

▼ INTERACTIONS

DRUG INTERACTIONS
Do not take nefazodone if you are taking terfenadine or astemizole. Nefazodone and

MAO inhibitors should not be used within 14 days of each other. Very serious side effects such as myoclonus (uncontrolled muscle jerking), hyperthermia (excessive rise in body temperature), and extreme stiffness may result. For many patients, especially the elderly, the use of nefazodone in combination with triazolam is not recommended. Other drugs may also interact with nefazodone; consult your doctor if you are taking alprazolam, high blood pressure medication (antihypertensives), atorvastatin, simvastatin, central nervous system depressants (including cold medications, allergy drugs, narcotic pain relievers, and muscle relaxants), or tricyclic antidepressants.

FOOD INTERACTIONS
No known food interactions.

DISEASE INTERACTIONS
Consult your doctor if you have a history of drug or alcohol abuse, any heart condition, a history of seizures, any condition affecting blood vessels of the brain, symptoms of dehydration (such as confusion, irritability, flushed, dry skin, decreased urine output, extreme thirst), or a history of mental disorders.

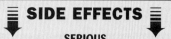

≣ SIDE EFFECTS ≣

SERIOUS
Blurred, partial loss of, or changes in vision, unsteadiness or clumsiness, skin rash, lightheadedness, ringing in the ears, prolonged or painful erection (lasting more than 4 hours). Call your doctor immediately.

COMMON
Drowsiness or dizziness, agitation, dry mouth, confusion, constipation or diarrhea, unusual dreams, heartburn, fever or chills, insomnia, loss of memory, headache, flushing, nausea or vomiting, increased appetite.

LESS COMMON
Joint pain, increased thirst, breast pain, cough, swelling of lower extremities, sore throat, trembling. Also unusual tingling, burning, or prickling sensations.

NEOMYCIN/POLYMYXIN B/HYDROCORTISONE OPHTHALMIC AND OTIC

Available in: Ophthalmic suspension, otic solution and suspension
Available OTC? No   **As Generic?** Yes
Drug Class: Antibiotic/corticosteroid combination

▼ USAGE INFORMATION

WHY IT'S PRESCRIBED
To treat or prevent bacterial infections of the eye or ear and to provide relief from eye or ear irritation and discomfort.

HOW IT WORKS
Ophthalmic and otic neomycin/polymyxin B/hydrocortisone kills bacteria by interfering with the genetic material of bacterial cells, preventing them from multiplying.

▼ DOSAGE GUIDELINES

RANGE AND FREQUENCY
Ophthalmic suspension—1 drop every 3 to 4 hours. Otic solution and suspension, for ear canal infection—Adults: 4 drops in the ear 3 to 4 times a day. Children: 3 drops in the ear 3 to 4 times a day.

ONSET OF EFFECT
Unknown.

DURATION OF ACTION
Unknown.

DIETARY ADVICE
No special restrictions.

STORAGE
Store in a tightly sealed container away from moisture, heat, and direct light. Do not allow it to freeze.

MISSED DOSE
Apply it as soon as you remember. However, if it is near the time for the next dose, skip the missed dose and resume your regular dosage schedule. Do not double the next dose.

STOPPING THE DRUG
Use this drug as prescribed for the full treatment period, even if you begin to feel better before the scheduled end of therapy.

PROLONGED USE
Do not use the ear medication for more than 10 days unless your doctor directs otherwise. If you use the eye medication for a prolonged period, you should see your doctor regularly for tests and examinations.

▼ PRECAUTIONS

Over 60: No special problems are expected.

Driving and Hazardous Work: Do not drive or engage in hazardous work until you determine how the medicine affects your vision.

Alcohol: No special precautions are necessary.

Pregnancy: This medication is not likely to cause problems unless absorbed into the bloodstream; consult your doctor for advice.

Breast Feeding: This combination medication has not been shown to cause problems in nursing babies.

Infants and Children: No special precautions.

Special Concerns: To use the eye drops, first wash your hands. Tilt your head back. Gently apply pressure to the inside corner of the eyelid and with the index finger of the same hand, pull downward on the lower eyelid to make a space. Drop the medicine into this space and close your eye. Apply pressure for 1 or 2 minutes while keeping the eye closed without blinking. To use the ear drops, lie down or tilt your head so the infected ear faces up. Gently pull the earlobe up and back for adults (down and back for children) to straighten the ear canal. Drop the medicine into the ear. Keep the ear facing upward for 5 minutes (2 minutes for children) after inserting the drops to allow the medicine to reach the infection. If necessary, insert a cotton ball to prevent the medicine from leaking out. Make sure the applicator for eye or ear drops does not touch your eye, ear, finger, or any other surface. If your symptoms do not improve in a few days or if they become worse, contact your doctor.

OVERDOSE
Symptoms: No specific ones have been reported.

What to Do: An overdose of this medication is unlikely to be life-threatening. If a large volume enters the eye, flush with water. If a large volume enters the ear or someone accidentally ingests the medicine, call your doctor, emergency medical services (EMS), or the nearest poison control center.

▼ INTERACTIONS

DRUG INTERACTIONS
Consult your doctor for specific advice if you are taking any other prescription or over-the-counter medication.

FOOD INTERACTIONS
No known food interactions.

DISEASE INTERACTIONS
Caution is advised when taking this combination antibiotic. Consult your doctor if you have any other eye or ear infection or medical problem.

▤ SIDE EFFECTS ▤

SERIOUS
Itching, rash, redness, swelling, or other eye or ear irritation that was not present before therapy. Call your doctor immediately.

COMMON
No common side effects have been reported with neomycin/polymyxin B/hydrocortisone.

LESS COMMON
Burning or stinging from the eye drops. There are no less common side effects associated with the ear preparation.

NIFEDIPINE

Available in: Extended-release tablets, capsules
Available OTC? No **As Generic?** Yes
Drug Class: Calcium channel blocker

▼ USAGE INFORMATION

WHY IT'S PRESCRIBED
To treat high blood pressure and to prevent attacks of angina pectoris (chest pain associated with coronary artery disease).

HOW IT WORKS
Nifedipine interferes with the movement of calcium into heart muscle cells and the smooth muscle cells in the walls of the arteries. This action relaxes blood vessels (causing them to widen), which lowers blood pressure, increases the blood supply to the heart, and decreases the heart's overall workload.

▼ DOSAGE GUIDELINES

RANGE AND FREQUENCY
Extended-release tablets: 30 or 60 mg once a day. The doses may be increased as determined by your doctor.

ONSET OF EFFECT
Within 20 minutes.

DURATION OF ACTION
Extended-release tablets: 12 to 24 hours.

DIETARY ADVICE
Nifedipine can be taken with or without food.

STORAGE
Store in a tightly sealed container away from heat and direct light.

MISSED DOSE
Take it as soon as you remember. If it is near the time for the next dose, skip the missed dose and resume your regular dosage schedule. Do not double the next dose.

STOPPING THE DRUG
Do not stop taking this drug suddenly, as this may cause potentially serious health problems. If therapy is to be discontinued, the dosage should be reduced gradually, according to your doctor's instructions.

PROLONGED USE
You should see your doctor regularly for examinations and tests if you take this medicine for an extended period. Remember that this medicine controls high blood pressure but does not cure it. You may have to take nifedipine for the rest of your life.

▼ PRECAUTIONS

Over 60: Adverse reactions may be more likely and more severe in older patients.

Driving and Hazardous Work: Do not drive or engage in hazardous work until you determine how the medicine affects you.

Alcohol: Avoid alcohol.

Pregnancy: In animal studies, large doses of nifedipine have been shown to cause birth defects. Human studies have not been done. Before you take nifedipine, tell your doctor if you are pregnant or plan to become pregnant.

Breast Feeding: Nifedipine passes into breast milk but has not been reported to cause problems; caution is advised. Consult your doctor for specific advice.

Infants and Children: While there is no specific information on the use of nifedipine in younger patients, the use of the capsule form is not recommended.

Special Concerns: In addition to taking nifedipine, be sure to follow all special instructions on weight control and diet. Your doctor will advise you which specific factors are most important for you. Check with your doctor before changing your diet.

OVERDOSE
Symptoms: Dizziness, slurred speech, confusion, weakness, drowsiness, nausea, abnormal heartbeat.

What to Do: Call your doctor, emergency medical services (EMS), or the nearest poison control center immediately.

▼ INTERACTIONS

DRUG INTERACTIONS
Consult your physician for specific advice if you are taking acetazolamide, amphotericin B, corticosteroids, dichlorphenamide, diuretics, methazolamide, beta-blockers, carbamazepine, cyclosporine, procainamide, quinidine, digitalis drugs, disopyramide or the following eye medicines: betaxolol, levobunolol, metipranolol, or timolol.

FOOD INTERACTIONS
Avoid foods high in sodium.

DISEASE INTERACTIONS
Caution is advised when taking nifedipine. Consult your doctor if you have any of the following: abnormal heart rhythm, other disorders of the heart and blood vessels, mental depression, or Parkinson's disease. Use of the drug may cause complications in patients with liver or kidney disease, since these organs work together to remove the medication from the body.

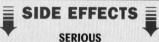

≡ SIDE EFFECTS ≡

SERIOUS
Breathing difficulty, coughing, or wheezing; irregular or pounding heartbeat; chest pain; fainting. Call your doctor immediately.

COMMON
Headache, dizziness, skin flushing and feeling of warmth, swelling in the feet, ankles, or calves, palpitations.

LESS COMMON
Constipation or diarrhea, nausea, unusual fatigue and weakness, skin rash, increased urination, vision problems.

NITROFURANTOIN

BRAND NAMES

Furadantin, Furalan, Furatoin, Macrobid, Macrodantin, Nitrofuracot

Available in: Capsules, oral suspension, tablets, extended-release capsules
Available OTC? No   **As Generic?** Yes
Drug Class: Anti-infective

▼ USAGE INFORMATION

WHY IT'S PRESCRIBED
To treat urinary tract infections (UTIs).

HOW IT WORKS
Nitrofurantoin interferes with bacterial metabolism and cell wall formation. Eventually the bacteria die out, bringing an end to the infection.

▼ DOSAGE GUIDELINES

RANGE AND FREQUENCY
Adults and teenagers–Capsules, oral suspension, tablets: 50 to 100 mg every 6 hours. Extended-release capsules: 100 mg every 12 hours. Children up to 12 years–Dosage must be determined by your doctor.

ONSET OF EFFECT
Within 1 hour.

DURATION OF ACTION
Capsules, oral suspension, tablets: 6 hours. Extended-release capsules: 24 hours.

DIETARY ADVICE
Nitrofurantoin should be taken with food or milk.

STORAGE
Store in a tightly sealed container away from heat and direct light. Keep the oral suspension from freezing.

MISSED DOSE
Take it as soon as you remember. If it is near the time for the next dose, skip the missed dose and resume your regular dosage schedule. Do not double the next dose.

STOPPING THE DRUG
Take as prescribed for the full treatment period, even if you begin to feel better before the scheduled end of therapy.

PROLONGED USE
See your doctor regularly if you must take this drug for a prolonged period.

▼ PRECAUTIONS

Over 60: Adverse reactions may be more likely and more severe in older patients.

Driving and Hazardous Work: Do not drive or engage in hazardous work until you determine how the medicine affects you.

Alcohol: Avoid alcohol.

Pregnancy: Nitrofurantoin should not be taken within several weeks of the delivery date or during labor.

Breast Feeding: Nitrofurantoin passes into breast milk; avoid use while breast feeding.

Infants and Children: Nitrofurantoin is not recommended for use by infants less than 1 month old.

Special Concerns: Nitrofurantoin may cause false results in some urine sugar tests for diabetes. If your symptoms do not improve or instead become worse within a few days, check with your doctor. When taking the oral suspension, be sure to shake the container forcefully before each dose. Use a specially marked measuring spoon or other device to dispense each dose. A household teaspoon might not hold the correct amount. Tell your doctor if you have ever had an allergic reaction to nitrofurantoin or any related medicine, such as furazolidone, or if you are allergic to any other substance. When taking the extended-release capsule, swallow it whole without chewing.

OVERDOSE
Symptoms: Severe nausea, vomiting, diarrhea, loss of appetite.

What to Do: An overdose of nitrofurantoin is unlikely to be life-threatening. However, if someone takes a much larger dose than prescribed, call your doctor, emergency medical services (EMS), or the nearest poison control center.

▼ INTERACTIONS

DRUG INTERACTIONS
Consult your doctor for specific advice if you are taking acetohydroxamine, oral diabetes medicine, dapsone, furazolidone, methyldopa, procainamide, quinidine, sulfonamides, vitamin K, carbamazepine, chloroquine, cisplatin, cytarabine, vaccine for diphtheria, tetanus, and pertussis (DTP), disulfiram, ethotoin, hydroxychloroquine, lindane, lithium, mephenytoin, mexiletine, pemoline, phenytoin, pyridoxine, vincristine, probenecid, sulfinpyrazone, quinine, or any other anti-infective agent.

FOOD INTERACTIONS
No known food interactions.

DISEASE INTERACTIONS
Consult your doctor if you have any of the following: glucose-6-phosphate dehydrogenase (G6PD) deficiency, kidney disease, lung disease, or nerve damage.

≡ SIDE EFFECTS ≡

SERIOUS
Chest pain, chills, cough, fever, troubled breathing, dizziness, drowsiness, tingling or burning of face or mouth, sore throat, unusual weakness, unusual fatigue. Call your doctor immediately.

COMMON
Abdominal pain or stomach upset, diarrhea, nausea, vomiting, loss of appetite.

LESS COMMON
Dark yellow or brownish urine.

NITROGLYCERIN

Available in: Capsules, tablets, ointment, skin patch, aerosol
Available OTC? No   **As Generic?** Yes
Drug Class: Nitrate

▼ USAGE INFORMATION

WHY IT'S PRESCRIBED
To prevent or relieve attacks of angina (chest pain associated with heart disease).

HOW IT WORKS
Nitroglycerin relaxes the smooth muscle surrounding blood vessels and increases the supply of blood and oxygen to the heart. It also reduces the heart's workload and demand for oxygen.

▼ DOSAGE GUIDELINES

RANGE AND FREQUENCY
Ointment: 15 to 30 mg applied to skin every 6 to 8 hours. Skin patch: 1 patch applied every day, left on for 12 to 14 hours. Aerosol: 1 or 2 doses on or under the tongue at 5-minute intervals to relieve angina attack. Extended-release capsules: 2.5, 6.5, or 9 mg every 12 hours; can be taken every 8 hours. Extended-release tablets: 1.3, 2.6, or 6.5 mg every 12 hours; can be taken every 8 hours. Sublingual (under tongue) or buccal (inside the cheek) tablets: 0.15 to 0.6 mg repeated at 5-minute intervals to treat angina attack. If 3 tablets do not relieve pain, call your doctor.

ONSET OF EFFECT
Sublingual: 2 to 4 minutes. Buccal: 3 minutes. Oral: 20 to 45 minutes. Ointment and skin patch: 30 minutes.

DURATION OF ACTION
Sublingual: 30 to 60 minutes. Buccal: 5 hours. Oral: 8 to 12 hours. Ointment: 4 to 8 hours. Skin patch: Up to 24 hours.

DIETARY ADVICE
Oral forms used as a preventive should be taken 30 minutes before or 1 to 2 hours after meals.

STORAGE
Store in a tightly sealed container away from moisture, heat, and direct light.

MISSED DOSE
Take it as soon as you remember you skipped a dose. If it is near the time for the next dose, skip the missed dose and resume your regular dosage schedule, as prescribed. Do not double the next dose.

STOPPING THE DRUG
The decision to stop taking nitroglycerin should be made by your doctor.

PROLONGED USE
You should see your doctor regularly for examinations and tests if you take this medicine for a prolonged period.

▼ PRECAUTIONS

Over 60: Adverse reactions may be more likely and more severe in older patients.

Driving and Hazardous Work: Do not drive or engage in hazardous work until you determine how the medicine affects you.

Alcohol: Avoid alcohol.

Pregnancy: Not recommended during pregnancy. Before taking nitroglycerin, be sure to tell your doctor if you are pregnant or plan to become pregnant.

Breast Feeding: Nitroglycerin may pass into breast milk; caution is advised. Consult your doctor for advice.

Infants and Children: No studies in infants and children have been done.

Special Concerns: Skin patch should be applied to different sites to prevent skin irritation.

OVERDOSE
Symptoms: Fast heartbeat, red and perspiring skin, headache, dizziness, palpitations, vision disturbances, nausea, vomiting, confusion, difficulty breathing.

What to Do: Call your doctor, emergency medical services (EMS), or the nearest poison control center immediately.

▼ INTERACTIONS

DRUG INTERACTIONS
Do not take nitroglycerin within 24 hours of taking sildenafil citrate. Sildenafil can enhance the action of nitrates (such as nitroglycerin), causing potentially dangerous decreases in blood pressure. Consult your doctor for specific advice if you are taking other heart medicines or drugs for hypertension.

FOOD INTERACTIONS
No known food interactions.

DISEASE INTERACTIONS
Consult your physician if you have any of the following: anemia, glaucoma, a recent head injury or stroke, a recent heart attack, or an overactive thyroid. Use of nitroglycerin may cause complications in patients with severe liver or kidney disease, since these organs work together to remove the medication from the body.

☰ SIDE EFFECTS ☰

SERIOUS
Blurred vision, severe or prolonged headache, skin rash, dry mouth. Call your doctor immediately.

COMMON
Flushing of face and neck, headache, nausea or vomiting, dizziness or lightheadedness when getting up, rapid heartbeat, restlessness.

LESS COMMON
Sore, reddened skin.

NIZATIDINE

Available in: Capsules, tablets
Available OTC? Yes **As Generic?** No
Drug Class: Histamine (H2) blocker

▼ USAGE INFORMATION

WHY IT'S PRESCRIBED
To treat and prevent return of ulcers of the stomach and duodenum, as well as conditions that cause increased stomach acid production (such as Zollinger-Ellison syndrome), gastroesophageal reflux (backwash of stomach acid into the esophagus that results in heartburn), and minor episodes of heartburn.

HOW IT WORKS
Nizatidine blocks the action of histamine (a compound produced in the body's cells), which in turn decreases the stomach's secretion of hydrochloric acid. Once stomach acid production has been decreased, the body is better able to heal itself.

▼ DOSAGE GUIDELINES

RANGE AND FREQUENCY
Adults and teenagers—To treat stomach ulcers: 300 mg once a day at bedtime, or 150 mg twice a day. To prevent the recurrence of duodenal ulcers: 150 mg once a day at bedtime. To treat gastroesophageal reflux: 150 mg, 2 times a day. To prevent minor cases of heartburn, acid indigestion, and sour stomach: 75 mg taken 30 to 60 minutes before a meal, once a day.

ONSET OF EFFECT
Within 30 minutes.

DURATION OF ACTION
Up to 12 hours.

DIETARY ADVICE
If you are taking two doses of nizatidine a day, the first dose can be taken after breakfast. Avoid foods that cause stomach irritation.

STORAGE
Store in a tightly sealed container away from heat and direct light.

MISSED DOSE
Take it as soon as you remember. If it is near the time for the next dose, skip the missed dose and resume your regular dosage schedule. Do not double the next dose.

STOPPING THE DRUG
Take the prescription-strength form for the full treatment period, even if you begin to feel better before the scheduled end of therapy.

PROLONGED USE
Do not take the maximum daily dosage continually for more than 2 weeks unless directed by your doctor.

▼ PRECAUTIONS

Over 60: Adverse reactions may be more likely and more severe in older patients.

Driving and Hazardous Work: Do not drive or engage in hazardous work until you determine how the medicine affects you.

Alcohol: Avoid alcohol.

Pregnancy: Risks vary, depending on patient and dosage. Consult your doctor.

Breast Feeding: Nizatidine passes into breast milk and may pose harm to the child; avoid or discontinue use while nursing.

Infants and Children: Nizatidine is not recommended for young patients, although it has not been shown to cause side effects or problems different from those in adults when used for short periods of time.

Special Concerns: Avoid cigarette smoking because it may increase stomach acid secretion and thus worsen the disease. Do not take the drug if you have ever had an allergic reaction to a histamine H2 blocker. If stomach pain becomes worse while using the drug, be sure to tell your doctor right away.

OVERDOSE
Symptoms: No cases of overdose have been reported.

What to Do: Although an overdose is unlikely, if someone takes a much larger dose than prescribed, call your doctor, emergency medical services (EMS), or the nearest poison control center right away.

▼ INTERACTIONS

DRUG INTERACTIONS
No significant drug interactions have been identified. However, nizatidine may increase blood levels of aspirin. Consult your doctor for specific advice if you are taking aspirin.

FOOD INTERACTIONS
Tomato-based vegetable juices, carbonated drinks, citrus fruits and juices, caffeine-containing beverages, and other acidic foods or liquids may irritate the stomach or interfere with the therapeutic action of nizatidine.

DISEASE INTERACTIONS
Patients with kidney disease should not use nizatidine or should use it in smaller, limited doses under careful supervision by a physician.

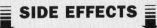

▤ SIDE EFFECTS ▤

SERIOUS
Irregular heart rhythm (palpitations), slowed heartbeat, severe blood problems, resulting in unusual bleeding, bruising, fever, chills, and increased susceptibility to infection. Call your doctor immediately.

COMMON
Headache, fatigue, drowsiness, dizziness, nausea, vomiting, abdominal pain, diarrhea, constipation.

LESS COMMON
Blurred vision, decreased sexual desire or function, swelling of breasts in males and females, temporary hair loss, hallucinations, depression, insomnia, skin rash, hives, or redness.

OLANZAPINE

Available in: Tablets
Available OTC? No   **As Generic?** No
Drug Class: Neuroleptic; antipsychotic

▼ USAGE INFORMATION

WHY IT'S PRESCRIBED
To treat psychotic conditions (severe mental disorders characterized by distorted thoughts and perceptions), such as schizophrenia.

HOW IT WORKS
While the exact mechanism of action of olanzapine is unknown, it appears to alter the activity of certain chemicals in the central nervous system to produce a tranquilizing and antipsychotic effect.

▼ DOSAGE GUIDELINES

RANGE AND FREQUENCY
Initial dose is 5 to 10 mg, once daily. Dose may be increased by your doctor to a maximum of 20 mg a day.

ONSET OF EFFECT
Sedation may occur within minutes, but onset of antipsychotic effect may take hours to occur or may not occur until days or weeks after the beginning of therapy.

DURATION OF ACTION
12 to 24 hours, but effects may persist for several days.

DIETARY ADVICE
No special restrictions.

STORAGE
Store in a tightly sealed container away from moisture, heat, and direct light.

MISSED DOSE
Take it as soon as you remember. However, if it is near the time for the next dose, skip the missed dose and resume your regular dosage schedule. Do not double the next dose.

STOPPING THE DRUG
The decision to stop taking the medication should be made in consultation with your physician.

PROLONGED USE
Consult your doctor about the need for follow-up evaluations and tests if you must take this drug for an extended period. Because olanzapine is a recently released drug, its risk of inducing potentially irreversible tardive dyskinesia (involuntary movements of the jaw, lips, tongue, and body) is unknown.

▼ PRECAUTIONS

Over 60: No special problems are expected.

Driving and Hazardous Work: Do not drive or engage in hazardous work until you determine how the medicine affects you.

Alcohol: Avoid alcohol.

Pregnancy: Large doses of olanzapine reduced fetal survival in animal tests. Before you take olanzapine, tell your doctor if you are pregnant or plan to become pregnant.

Breast Feeding: Olanzapine may pass into breast milk; avoid use while nursing.

Infants and Children: The safety and effectiveness of olanzapine in children under 18 have not been established.

Special Concerns: Avoid prolonged exposure to high temperatures or hot climates. Drink plenty of fluids and stay cool in the summertime. Avoid overexposure to sunlight until you determine if the drug heightens your skin's sensitivity to ultraviolet light.

OVERDOSE
Symptoms: Extreme drowsiness, slurred speech.

What to Do: Call your doctor, emergency medical services (EMS), or the nearest poison control center immediately.

▼ INTERACTIONS

DRUG INTERACTIONS
The following drugs may interact with olanzapine. Consult your doctor for specific advice if you are taking carbamazepine, omeprazole, rifampin, high blood pressure medication, or any drugs that depress the central nervous system, including antihistamines, antidepressants or other psychiatric medications, barbiturates, sedatives, cough medicines, decongestants, and painkillers. Be sure your doctor knows about any over-the-counter medication you may take.

FOOD INTERACTIONS
No known food interactions.

DISEASE INTERACTIONS
Consult your doctor if you have Parkinson's disease or any movement disorder, glaucoma, epilepsy, liver disease, or kidney disease.

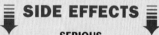
SIDE EFFECTS

SERIOUS
Stiffness; shuffling gait; difficulty swallowing or speaking; persistent, uncontrolled chewing, lip-smacking, or tongue movements; fever. Call your doctor immediately.

COMMON
Drowsiness, headache, dizziness, constipation, dry mouth, blurred vision, runny nose.

LESS COMMON
Stomach pain, unclear speech or stuttering, muscle tightness, faintness, increased appetite, increased cough, watering of mouth, insomnia, joint pain, nausea, vomiting, sore throat, rapid heartbeat, increased thirst, urinary incontinence, weight loss.

OMEPRAZOLE

Available in: Capsules
Available OTC? No   **As Generic?** No
Drug Class: Antacid/proton pump inhibitor

▼ USAGE INFORMATION

WHY IT'S PRESCRIBED
To treat duodenal (intestinal) ulcers, as well as conditions that cause increased stomach acid production (such as Zollinger-Ellison syndrome), erosive esophagitis (severe, chronic inflammation of the esophagus), and gastroesophageal reflux (backwash of stomach acid into the esophagus, resulting in heartburn).

HOW IT WORKS
Omeprazole blocks the action of a specific enzyme in the cells that line the stomach, thereby decreasing the production of stomach acid. Reduction of stomach acid promotes healing of ulcers.

▼ DOSAGE GUIDELINES

RANGE AND FREQUENCY
For duodenal ulcer, esophagitis, or gastroesophageal reflux: 20 mg per day.
For Zollinger-Ellison syndrome or similar conditions: 60 mg per day.

ONSET OF EFFECT
Within 1 to 3 hours.

DURATION OF ACTION
At least 72 hours.

DIETARY ADVICE
Take omeprazole immediately before a meal. Capsules should be swallowed whole.

STORAGE
Store in a tightly sealed container away from heat and direct light.

MISSED DOSE
Take it as soon as you remember. If it is near the time for the next dose, skip the missed dose and resume your regular dosage schedule. Do not double the next dose.

STOPPING THE DRUG
Take it as prescribed for the full treatment period, even if you begin to feel better before the scheduled end of therapy. The decision to stop taking the drug should be made in consultation with your doctor.

PROLONGED USE
Omeprazole should not be used indefinitely as maintenance therapy for duodenal ulcer or esophagitis; it is generally taken for a limited period of 4 to 8 weeks. Do not take it for a longer period unless instructed to do so by your doctor. See your doctor regularly for tests and examinations if you must take this drug for an extended period of time.

▼ PRECAUTIONS

Over 60: No specific problems for older people have been reported.

Driving and Hazardous Work: Do not drive or engage in hazardous activities until you determine how the drug affects you.

Alcohol: Avoid alcohol while taking this medication, as it may aggravate your condition.

Pregnancy: In animal tests, omeprazole has not caused problems. Human tests have not been done. Before you take omeprazole, tell your doctor if you are pregnant or plan to become pregnant.

Breast Feeding: Omeprazole may pass into breast milk; caution is advised. Consult your doctor for advice.

Infants and Children: Use and dose for anyone under 18 should be determined by your doctor or pediatrician.

Special Concerns: Tell any doctor or dentist whom you see for treatment that you are taking omeprazole. Do not chew the capsules. If you have trouble swallowing them, you may open them and sprinkle the contents on applesauce or similar food. If your doctor directs, you may take an antacid along with omeprazole.

OVERDOSE
Symptoms: Blurred vision, confusion, profuse sweating, drowsiness, dry mouth, flushing of the face, headache, nausea, palpitations or an unusually rapid heartbeat.

What to Do: Call your doctor, emergency medical services (EMS), or the nearest poison control center immediately.

▼ INTERACTIONS

DRUG INTERACTIONS
The following drugs may interact with omeprazole. Consult your doctor for specific advice if you are taking: ampicillin, sucralfate, iron salts or supplements, cyclosporine, diazepam, disulfiram, ketoconazole, phenytoin, or theophylline.

FOOD INTERACTIONS
No significant food interactions have been reported.

DISEASE INTERACTIONS
Caution is advised when taking omeprazole. Consult your doctor if you have liver disease, since it may increase the risk of side effects.

⇊ SIDE EFFECTS ⇊

SERIOUS
No serious side effects are associated with this medication.

COMMON
Diarrhea, constipation, vomiting, headache, dizziness, stomach pain. Consult your physician if such side effects persist or interfere with daily activities.

LESS COMMON
Bloody or cloudy urine, persistent or recurring sores or ulcers in the mouth, painful or very frequent urination, sore throat, fever, unusual bruising or bleeding, unusual weakness or tiredness, muscle pain, chest pain, nausea. Consult your doctor if such symptoms occur.

ORLISTAT

BRAND NAME

Xenical

Available in: Capsules
Available OTC? No   **As Generic?** No
Drug Class: Lipase inhibitor

▼ USAGE INFORMATION

WHY IT'S PRESCRIBED
To achieve weight loss and weight maintenance in the maintenance of obesity when used in conjunction with a reduced-calorie diet and appropriate physical activity. Orlistat is indicated for patients with an initial body mass index (BMI) of 30 or greater (see Special Concerns for information on BMI calculation) and for those with a BMI greater than 27 who also have other risk factors such as high blood pressure, high blood cholesterol, and diabetes.

HOW IT WORKS
Orlistat inhibits the activity of lipases, intestinal enzymes required for the digestion of dietary fats. Orlistat prevents the breakdown of a portion of ingested fat. The undigested fat cannot be absorbed and is excreted in the feces. At full dosage, orlistat can reduce the absorption of fat by about 30%.

▼ DOSAGE GUIDELINES

RANGE AND FREQUENCY
120 mg (one capsule) 3 times a day at mealtime.

ONSET OF EFFECT
Within 24 to 48 hours.

DURATION OF ACTION
48 to 72 hours.

DIETARY ADVICE
Take with liquid during or up to one hour after each main meal containing fat. Follow a balanced, reduced-calorie diet. The daily intake of fat (approximately 1/3 of the calories), carbohydrate, and protein should be spread out over the three meals. If a meal is missed or contains no fat, the dose of orlistat can be skipped. Since orlistat can also reduce the absorption of fat-soluble vitamins, a multivitamin supplement (containing vitamins A, D, and E and beta-carotene) should also be taken once a day at least two hours before or after ingesting orlistat.

STORAGE
Store in a tightly sealed container away from moisture, heat, and direct light.

MISSED DOSE
If you miss a dose, take it if you remember within 1 hour of eating. However, if more than 1 hour has passed, skip the missed dose and return to your regular schedule. Do not double the next dose.

STOPPING THE DRUG
The decision to stop taking the drug should be made in consultation with your doctor.

PROLONGED USE
The safety and effectiveness of this medication have not been determined beyond 2 years of use.

▼ PRECAUTIONS

Over 60: No specific studies using orlistat have been done on older patients.

Driving and Hazardous Work: The use of orlistat should not impair your ability to perform such tasks safely.

Alcohol: No special precautions are necessary.

Pregnancy: Adequate human studies have not been done. Before taking orlistat, tell your doctor if you are pregnant or plan to become pregnant.

Breast Feeding: It is unknown whether orlistat passes into breast milk. However, do not take the drug while nursing. Consult your doctor for advice.

Infants and Children: Safety and effectiveness have not been established for children under age 18.

Special Concerns: A medical cause for obesity (such as hypothyroidism) should be ruled out before taking orlistat. Consult your doctor or a nutritionist for information about a nutritionally balanced, reduced-calorie diet and an exercise program. The BMI can be calculated by dividing your weight in pounds by your height in inches squared, and then multiplying by 705.

OVERDOSE
Symptoms: No cases of overdose have been reported.

What to Do: An overdose with orlistat is unlikely. If someone takes a much larger dose than prescribed, call your doctor.

▼ INTERACTIONS

DRUG INTERACTIONS
The following drugs may interact with orlistat. Consult your doctor for specific advice if you are taking: statin (cholesterol-lowering) drugs, cyclosporine, warfarin, another weight-loss medication (such as sibutramine or phentermine), or any other prescription or over-the-counter medicines.

FOOD INTERACTIONS
Orlistat reduces the absorption of fat-soluble vitamins A, D, E, and K and beta-carotene. Gastrointestinal side effects may increase following the consumption of high-fat foods or with a diet high in fat (more than 30% of the day's total calories from fat).

DISEASE INTERACTIONS
This medication should not be used if you have chronic malabsorption or gallbladder problems. Consult your doctor if you have an eating disorder (anorexia or bulimia).

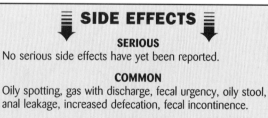

≣ SIDE EFFECTS ≣

SERIOUS
No serious side effects have yet been reported.

COMMON
Oily spotting, gas with discharge, fecal urgency, oily stool, anal leakage, increased defecation, fecal incontinence.

LESS COMMON
Abdominal pain or discomfort.

OSELTAMIVIR PHOSPHATE

Available in: Capsules, oral suspension
Available OTC? No **As Generic?** No
Drug Class: Antiviral

▼ USAGE INFORMATION

WHY IT'S PRESCRIBED
To treat and prevent infection from influenza type A or B. Oseltamivir can reduce the severity of symptoms and shorten the duration of flu episodes.

HOW IT WORKS
Oseltamivir is believed to interfere with the synthesis of the viral enzyme neuraminidase, which is needed in order for the virus to infect cells in the respiratory tract and elsewhere in the body. The drug affects only certain susceptible strains of the influenza type A or B viruses.

▼ DOSAGE GUIDELINES

RANGE AND FREQUENCY
For treatment—Adults and teenagers: 75 mg twice a day for 5 days. Treatment should be initiated as soon as possible, and no longer than 2 days after the onset of signs or symptoms of the flu. Children 12 and under: Consult your pediatrician. For prevention—Adults and teenagers: 75 mg once a day for 7 days. Therapy should be initiated within 2 days of exposure. For prevention during a community outbreak, 75 mg once a day for up to 6 weeks.

ONSET OF EFFECT
Unknown.

DURATION OF ACTION
Unknown.

DIETARY ADVICE
No special restrictions.

STORAGE
Store in a tightly sealed container away from moisture, heat, and direct light. Do not allow oral suspensions to freeze.

MISSED DOSE
Take it as soon as you remember. If it is near (within 2 hours) the time for the next dose, skip the missed dose and resume your regular dosage schedule. Do not double the next dose.

STOPPING THE DRUG
It is important to take oseltamivir for the full treatment period as prescribed. Do not stop taking the drug before the scheduled end of therapy even if you begin to feel better, as this may lead to a relapse.

PROLONGED USE
If your symptoms do not improve or if they become worse in a few days, consult your doctor.

▼ PRECAUTIONS

Over 60: No special problems are expected.

Driving and Hazardous Work: Do not drive or engage in hazardous work until you determine how the medicine affects you.

Alcohol: No special precautions are necessary.

Pregnancy: Adequate studies have not been completed. Discuss with your doctor the relative risks and benefits of using this medication while you are pregnant.

Breast Feeding: Oseltamivir may pass into breast milk, although it is unknown if this poses any risks to the nursing infant. Consult your doctor for specific advice.

Infants and Children: The safety and effectiveness of this drug for treatment have not been established for children under the age of 1. The safety and effectiveness of this drug for prevention have not been established for children under the age of 13.

Special Concerns: This medication is not a substitute for a flu shot. Continue to receive your annual flu shot. Shake the oral suspension well before use.

OVERDOSE
Symptoms: No cases have been reported. However, nausea and vomiting are likely symptoms.

What to Do: If you have any reason to suspect an overdose, call your doctor, emergency medical services (EMS), or the nearest poison control center.

▼ INTERACTIONS

DRUG INTERACTIONS
No known drug interactions.

FOOD INTERACTIONS
No known food interactions.

DISEASE INTERACTIONS
The dose of oseltamivir should be lowered in patients with significant kidney disease. Safety has not been determined in people with liver disease.

≣ SIDE EFFECTS ≣

SERIOUS
No serious side effects are associated with oseltamivir.

COMMON
Nausea and vomiting.

LESS COMMON
Bronchitis, insomnia, dizziness.

OXAPROZIN

Available in: Caplets
Available OTC? No   **As Generic?** No
Drug Class: Nonsteroidal anti-inflammatory drug (NSAID)

▼ USAGE INFORMATION

WHY IT'S PRESCRIBED
To treat mild to moderate pain and inflammation caused by tendinitis, arthritis, bursitis, gout, soft tissue injuries, migraine and other vascular headaches, menstrual cramps, and other conditions. When patients fail to respond to one NSAID, another may be tried. The greatest effectiveness often requires trial and error of several different NSAIDs.

HOW IT WORKS
NSAIDs work by interfering with the formation of prosta-glandins, naturally occurring substances in the body that cause inflammation and make nerves more sensitive to pain impulses. NSAIDs also have other modes of action that are less well understood.

▼ DOSAGE GUIDELINES

RANGE AND FREQUENCY
Adults: 1,200 mg once a day. The maximum daily dose is 1,800 mg divided into smaller amounts taken 2 or 3 times a day. Children: Consult your pediatrician.

ONSET OF EFFECT
From 30 minutes to several hours or longer.

DURATION OF ACTION
Varies.

DIETARY ADVICE
Take with food; maintain your usual food and fluid intake.

STORAGE
Store in a tightly sealed container away from moisture, heat, and direct light.

MISSED DOSE
Take it as soon as you remember. If it is near the time for the next dose, skip the missed dose and resume your regular dosage schedule. Do not double the next dose.

STOPPING THE DRUG
The decision to stop taking the drug should be made in consultation with your doctor.

PROLONGED USE
Prolonged use can cause gastrointestinal problems such as ulceration and bleeding, kidney dysfunction, and liver inflammation. Consult your doctor about the need for medical examinations and laboratory tests.

▼ PRECAUTIONS

Over 60: Because of the potentially greater consequences of gastrointestinal side effects, the dose of NSAIDs for older patients, especially those over age 70, is often cut in half.

Driving and Hazardous Work: Avoid such activities until you determine how the medicine affects you.

Alcohol: Avoid alcohol when using this medication because it increases the risk of stomach irritation.

Pregnancy: Avoid or discontinue using this drug if you are pregnant or if you plan to become pregnant.

Breast Feeding: Oxaprozin passes into breast milk; avoid use while nursing.

Infants and Children: May be used in exceptional circumstances; consult your doctor.

Special Concerns: Because NSAIDs can interfere with blood coagulation, this drug should be stopped at least 3 days prior to any surgery.

OVERDOSE
Symptoms: Severe nausea, vomiting, headache, seizures, confusion.

What to Do: Call your doctor, emergency medical services (EMS), or the nearest poison control center immediately.

▼ INTERACTIONS

DRUG INTERACTIONS
Do not take this drug with aspirin or any other NSAIDs without your doctor's approval. In addition, consult your doctor if you are taking antihypertensives, steroids, anticoagulants, antibiotics, itraconazole or ketoconazole, plicamycin, penicillamine, valproic acid, phenytoin, cyclosporine, digitalis drugs, lithium, methotrexate, probenecid, triamterene, or zidovudine.

FOOD INTERACTIONS
No known food interactions.

DISEASE INTERACTIONS
Consult your doctor if you have any of the following: bleeding problems, ulcers or inflammation of the stomach and intestines, diabetes, systemic lupus erythematosus (SLE, lupus), anemia, asthma, epilepsy, Parkinson's disease, kidney stones, or a history of heart disease or alcohol abuse. Use of oxaprozin may cause complications in patients with liver or kidney disease, since these organs work together to remove the medication from the body.

≡ SIDE EFFECTS ≡

SERIOUS
Shortness of breath or wheezing, with or without swelling of legs or other signs of heart failure; chest pain; peptic ulcer disease with vomiting of blood; black, tarry stools; decreasing kidney function. Call your doctor immediately.

COMMON
Nausea, vomiting, heartburn, diarrhea, constipation, headache, dizziness, sleepiness.

LESS COMMON
Ulcers or sores in mouth, depression, rashes or blistering of skin, ringing sound in the ears, unusual tingling or numbness of the hands or feet, seizures, blurred vision. Also elevated potassium levels, decreased blood counts; such problems can be detected by your doctor.

OXYCODONE HYDROCHLORIDE

Available in: Oral solution, tablets, controlled-release tablets
Available OTC? No   **As Generic?** No
Drug Class: Opioid (narcotic) analgesic

▼ USAGE INFORMATION

WHY IT'S PRESCRIBED
To relieve moderate to severe pain.

HOW IT WORKS
Opioid analgesics such as oxycodone relieve pain by acting on specific areas of the central nervous system (the brain and spinal cord) that process pain signals from nerves throughout the body.

▼ DOSAGE GUIDELINES

RANGE AND FREQUENCY
5 mg every 3 to 6 hours, or 10 mg, 3 to 4 times a day as needed. Children: Dosages must be determined by your pediatrician. Controlled-release tablets: Your doctor will determine the proper dosage for you.

ONSET OF EFFECT
10 to 15 minutes.

DURATION OF ACTION
3 to 6 hours.

DIETARY ADVICE
This medication can be taken with food or milk to lessen stomach upset.

STORAGE
Store in a tightly sealed container away from moisture, heat, and direct light. Do not freeze the liquid form.

MISSED DOSE
If you are taking oxycodone on a fixed schedule, take it as soon as you remember. If it is near the time for the next dose, skip the missed dose and resume your regular dosage schedule. Do not double the next dose.

STOPPING THE DRUG
The decision to stop taking the drug should be made by your doctor.

PROLONGED USE
You should see your doctor regularly for tests and physical examinations if you must take this medication for an extended period. Prolonged use of oxycodone can cause physical dependence.

▼ PRECAUTIONS

Over 60: Adverse reactions may be more likely and more severe in older patients.

Driving and Hazardous Work: Avoid such activities until you determine how the medicine affects you.

Alcohol: Avoid alcohol.

Pregnancy: Human studies have not been done. Before using this drug, tell your doctor if you are pregnant or plan to become pregnant. Overuse during pregnancy can cause drug dependence in the fetus.

Breast Feeding: Oxycodone may pass into breast milk; caution is advised. Consult your doctor for advice.

Infants and Children: Adverse reactions to oxycodone may be more likely and more severe in children. Consult your doctor.

Special Concerns: If you feel the medication is not working properly after a few weeks, do not increase the dose on your own. Consult your doctor. Before having any surgery, tell the doctor or dentist in charge that you are taking this drug. The controlled-release tablets are prescribed for use only in opioid-tolerant patients requiring daily doses of 160 mg or more.

OVERDOSE
Symptoms: Confusion; severe drowsiness, weakness, or dizziness; slurred speech; small, pinpoint pupils; cold, clammy skin; slow breathing; seizures; loss of consciousness.

What to Do: Call your doctor, emergency medical services (EMS), or the nearest poison control center immediately.

▼ INTERACTIONS

DRUG INTERACTIONS
Consult your doctor for specific advice if you are taking carbamazepine or other medicine for seizures, barbiturates, sedatives, cough medicines, decongestants, antidepressants, other prescription pain medications, MAO inhibitors, naltrexone, rifampin, or zidovudine.

FOOD INTERACTIONS
No known food interactions.

DISEASE INTERACTIONS
Consult your doctor if you have any of the following: a history of alcohol or drug abuse; emotional illness; brain disorders or head injury; seizures; lung disease; prostate problems or other problems with urination; gallstones; colitis; heart, kidney, liver, or thyroid disease.

≡ SIDE EFFECTS ≡

SERIOUS
Serious side effects of oxycodone are indistinguishable from those of overdose: Confusion; severe drowsiness, weakness, or dizziness; slurred speech; small, pinpoint pupils; cold, clammy skin; slow breathing; seizures; loss of consciousness.

COMMON
Dizziness or lightheadedness, nausea or vomiting, drowsiness, constipation, itching.

LESS COMMON
Swelling in the feet, sweating, false sense of well-being (euphoria), urinary retention.

OXYCODONE/ACETAMINOPHEN

BRAND NAMES
Endocet, Percocet, Roxicet, Roxicet 5/500, Roxilox, Tylox

Available in: Capsules, oral solution, tablets
Available OTC? No   **As Generic?** Yes
Drug Class: Opioid (narcotic) analgesic

▼ USAGE INFORMATION

WHY IT'S PRESCRIBED
To relieve moderate to severe pain when nonprescription pain relievers prove inadequate. A narcotic analgesic such as oxycodone, in combination with acetaminophen, may provide better pain relief than either medicine taken alone. Used together, relief may be achieved at lower doses of the two drugs.

HOW IT WORKS
Opioid medications such as oxycodone relieve pain by acting on specific areas of the central nervous system (the brain and the spinal cord) that process pain signals from nerves throughout the body. Acetaminophen appears to interfere with the action of prostaglandins, naturally occurring hormone-like substances in the body that cause inflammation and make nerves more sensitive to pain impulses.

▼ DOSAGE GUIDELINES

RANGE AND FREQUENCY
Adults: 1 capsule or tablet every 4 to 6 hours, or 1 teaspoon of the oral solution every 4 to 6 hours.

ONSET OF EFFECT
Unknown.

DURATION OF ACTION
Unknown.

DIETARY ADVICE
This medication can be taken with food or milk to lessen stomach irritation.

STORAGE
Store in a tightly sealed container away from moisture, heat, and direct light.

MISSED DOSE
If you are taking the drug on a fixed schedule, take it as soon as you remember. However, if it is near the time for the next dose, skip the missed dose and resume your regular dosage schedule. Do not double the next dose.

STOPPING THE DRUG
The decision to stop taking the drug should be made by your doctor.

PROLONGED USE
See your doctor regularly for examinations and laboratory tests if long-term therapy is required. Prolonged use of narcotic drugs such as oxycodone can cause physical dependence; prolonged use of acetaminophen at high doses can cause liver damage.

▼ PRECAUTIONS

Over 60: Adverse reactions may be more likely and more severe in older patients.

Driving and Hazardous Work: Do not drive or engage in hazardous work until you determine how the medicine affects you.

Alcohol: Avoid alcohol.

Pregnancy: Human studies have not been done. Before you use this drug, tell your doctor if you are pregnant or plan to become pregnant. Overuse of the medication while you are pregnant can cause drug dependence in the fetus.

Breast Feeding: It is not known whether this medication passes into breast milk; caution is advised. Consult your doctor for advice.

Infants and Children: Adverse reactions may be more likely and more severe in children.

Special Concerns: If you feel the medication is not working properly after a few weeks, do not increase the dose. Consult your doctor.

OVERDOSE
Symptoms: Severe dizziness or drowsiness; cold, clammy skin; difficult or slow breathing or shortness of breath; severe confusion; seizures; stomach cramps or pain; diarrhea; low blood pressure; constricted pupils of eyes; increased sweating; nausea or vomiting; irregular heartbeat; severe weakness.

What to Do: Call your doctor, emergency medical services (EMS), or the nearest poison control center immediately.

▼ INTERACTIONS

DRUG INTERACTIONS
Consult your doctor for specific advice if you are taking any prescription or over-the-counter drugs, especially drugs with acetaminophen; central nervous system depressants such as antihistamines or medicine for hay fever, allergies, or colds; barbiturates; seizure medications; muscle relaxants; anesthetics; tranquilizers, sedatives, or sleep aids.

FOOD INTERACTIONS
No known food interactions.

DISEASE INTERACTIONS
Consult your physician if you have a head injury or brain disease, an underactive thyroid, an enlarged prostate, seizures, kidney or liver disease, gallbladder problems, a blood disorder, or a history of alcohol or drug abuse.

≡ SIDE EFFECTS ≡

SERIOUS
Bloody, dark, or cloudy urine; severe pain in lower back or side; pale or black, tarry stools; yellowish tinge to the eyes or skin; hallucinations; frequent urge to urinate; painful or difficult urination; sudden decrease in amount of urine; unusual bleeding or bruising; irregular heartbeat; skin rash, hives, or itching; unusual excitement; swelling of face; confusion; trembling or uncontrolled muscle movements; redness or flushing of face. Call your doctor immediately.

COMMON
Dizziness, lightheadedness, nausea or vomiting, drowsiness, constipation.

LESS COMMON
Allergic reaction, false sense of well-being (euphoria), depression, loss of appetite, blurring or change in vision, headache, sweating.

PAROXETINE HYDROCHLORIDE

Paxil

Available in: Tablets, oral suspension
Available OTC? No   **As Generic?** No
Drug Class: Selective serotonin reuptake inhibitor (SSRI) antidepressant

▼ USAGE INFORMATION

WHY IT'S PRESCRIBED
To treat symptoms of major (classic) depression, and of obsessive-compulsive disorder, panic disorder, and social anxiety disorder.

HOW IT WORKS
Paroxetine affects levels of serotonin, an important brain chemical called a neurotransmitter, that is thought to be linked to mood, emotions, and mental state.

▼ DOSAGE GUIDELINES

RANGE AND FREQUENCY
Adults: To start, 20 mg once a day, usually taken in the morning; dose may be gradually increased by your doctor to 50 mg a day. Older adults: To start, 10 mg once a day; the dosage may be gradually increased by your doctor to 40 mg a day.

ONSET OF EFFECT
From 1 to 4 weeks.

DURATION OF ACTION
Unknown.

DIETARY ADVICE
This drug can be taken without regard to diet.

STORAGE
Store in a tightly sealed container away from moisture, heat, and direct light.

MISSED DOSE
Take it as soon as you remember. If it is near the time for the next dose, skip the missed dose and resume your regular dosage schedule. Do not double the next dose.

STOPPING THE DRUG
Take as prescribed for the full treatment period even if you begin to feel better. The decision to stop taking the drug should be made in consultation with your doctor. Dosage should be gradually tapered over 1 to 2 weeks.

PROLONGED USE
Usual course of therapy for depression lasts 6 months to 1 year; some patients may benefit from additional therapy.

▼ PRECAUTIONS

Over 60: Adverse reactions may be more likely and more severe in older patients. A lower dose may be warranted for people in this age group.

Driving and Hazardous Work: Use caution when driving or engaging in hazardous work until you determine how the medicine affects you.

Alcohol: Avoid alcohol.

Pregnancy: Adequate studies of paroxetine use during pregnancy have not been done. Before you take this medication, tell your doctor if you are pregnant or plan to become pregnant.

Breast Feeding: Paroxetine passes into breast milk; caution is advised. Consult your doctor for advice.

Infants and Children: The safety and effectiveness of paroxetine use in children have not been established.

Special Concerns: Take paroxetine at least 6 hours before bedtime to prevent insomnia, unless it causes drowsiness.

OVERDOSE
Symptoms: Agitation or irritability, severe drowsiness, dizziness, coma, dilated pupils, severe dry mouth, rapid heartbeat, trembling, severe nausea and vomiting.

What to Do: Call your doctor, emergency medical services (EMS), or the nearest poison control center immediately.

▼ INTERACTIONS

DRUG INTERACTIONS
Paroxetine and MAO inhibitors should not be used within 14 days of each other. Very serious side effects such as myoclonus (uncontrolled muscle spasms), hyperthermia (excessive rise in body temperature), and extreme stiffness may result. Do not take paroxetine with thioridazine; dangerous heart rhythm irregularities may result. Tryptophan, warfarin, sumatriptan, naratriptan, rizatriptan, and zolmitriptan may also interact with paroxetine; consult your doctor for advice.

FOOD INTERACTIONS
No known food interactions.

DISEASE INTERACTIONS
Caution is advised when taking paroxetine. Consult your doctor if you have a history of alcohol or drug abuse or a seizure disorder. Use of paroxetine may cause complications in patients with liver or kidney disease, because these organs work together to remove the medication from the body.

▼ SIDE EFFECTS

SERIOUS
Muscle pain or fatigue, lightheadedness or fainting, rash, agitation or irritability, severe drowsiness, dilated pupils, severe dry mouth, rapid heartbeat, trembling, severe nausea or vomiting. Call your doctor immediately.

COMMON
Insomnia, dizziness, sexual dysfunction, unusual fatigue, loss of initiative, nausea or vomiting, constipation, difficulty urinating, headache, trembling.

LESS COMMON
Decreased sexual desire, blurred vision, increased or decreased appetite, weight gain or loss, heartbeat irregularities, change in sense of taste. Also tingling, prickling, or burning feeling.

PENICILLIN V

Available in: Tablets, delayed-release tablets, liquid
Available OTC? No **As Generic?** Yes
Drug Class: Penicillin antibiotic

▼ USAGE INFORMATION

WHY IT'S PRESCRIBED
To treat a variety of bacterial infections, including those of the ear, nose, and throat, skin and soft tissues, genitourinary tract, and respiratory tract. It is also prescribed before surgery or dental work in patients at risk for endocarditis (infection of the lining of the heart, which may damage the heart's valves).

HOW IT WORKS
Penicillin V destroys susceptible bacteria by interfering with their ability to produce cell walls as they multiply.

▼ DOSAGE GUIDELINES

RANGE AND FREQUENCY
Adults: 500 to 2,000 mg a day for infections; 2,000 mg to prevent bacterial endocarditis; or as ordered by physician. Children: 15 to 50 mg per 2.2 lbs (1 kg) of body weight per day in divided doses to treat infections. To prevent infection after dental surgery, 2 g (1 g for children), 30 to 60 minutes before procedure, then 1 g (500 mg for children) 6 hours afterward.

ONSET OF EFFECT
Unknown.

DURATION OF ACTION
Up to 6 hours.

DIETARY ADVICE
Take it on an empty stomach, 1 to 2 hours before or 3 to 4 hours after a meal.

STORAGE
Store in a tightly sealed container away from heat and direct light.

MISSED DOSE
Take it as soon as you remember. If it is near the time for the next dose, skip the missed dose and resume your regular dosage schedule. Do not double the next dose.

STOPPING THE DRUG
It is very important to take this drug as prescribed for the full treatment period. Stopping the medicine prematurely may lead to serious complications.

PROLONGED USE
Prolonged use of any antibiotic increases the risk of superinfection (a more severe and drug-resistant infection); caution is advised.

▼ PRECAUTIONS

Over 60: No special problems are expected.

Driving and Hazardous Work: The use of penicillin should not impair your ability to perform such tasks safely.

Alcohol: No special precautions are necessary.

Pregnancy: Adequate studies of penicillin antibiotic use during pregnancy have not been done; however, no problems have been reported.

Breast Feeding: Penicillin V may pass into breast milk and cause problems in the nursing infant; avoid use while nursing.

Infants and Children: No special problems are expected.

Special Concerns: Penicillin V can cause false results on some urine sugar tests for patients with diabetes. If severe diarrhea occurs as a side effect of penicillin V, do not take antidiarrheal drugs; call your doctor. Oral contraceptives may not be effective while you are taking penicillin; consider other methods of birth control. Those who are prone to asthma, hay fever, hives, or allergies may be more likely to have an allergic reaction to a penicillin antibiotic medication.

OVERDOSE
Symptoms: Severe nausea, vomiting, diarrhea, seizures.

What to Do: An overdose of penicillin is unlikely to be life-threatening. However, if someone takes a much larger dose than prescribed, call your doctor or local emergency medical services (EMS) right away.

▼ INTERACTIONS

DRUG INTERACTIONS
Consult your physician for specific advice if you are taking aminoglycosides, ACE inhibitors, diuretics, potassium supplements or potassium-containing drugs, anticoagulants or other anticlotting drugs, nonsteroidal anti-inflammatory drugs, oral contraceptives, sulfinpyrazone, cholestyramine, colestipol, methotrexate, probenecid, or rifampin.

FOOD INTERACTIONS
Acidic foods or juices can reduce the antibiotic effect.

DISEASE INTERACTIONS
Consult your doctor if you have a history of allergies, asthma, congestive heart failure, gastrointestinal disorders (especially colitis associated with the use of antibiotics), or impaired kidney function.

≡ SIDE EFFECTS ≡

SERIOUS
Irregular, rapid, or labored breathing, lightheadedness or sudden fainting, joint pain, fever, severe abdominal pain and cramping with watery or bloody stools, severe allergic reaction (marked by sudden swelling of the lips, tongue, face, or throat; breathing difficulty; skin rash, itching, or hives), unusual bleeding or bruising, yellowish tinge to eyes or skin. Call your doctor immediately.

COMMON
Mild rash, mild diarrhea, nausea, vomiting, headache, vaginal discharge and itching, pain or white patches in the mouth or on the tongue.

LESS COMMON
Diminished urine output, chills, weakness, fatigue.

PHENYTOIN

BRAND NAMES

Di-Phen, Dilantin, Diphenylan, Phenytex

Available in: Prompt and extended capsules, chewable tablets, oral suspension
Available OTC? No   **As Generic?** Yes
Drug Class: Anticonvulsant

▼ USAGE INFORMATION

WHY IT'S PRESCRIBED
To prevent or control seizures in the treatment of certain types of epilepsy and other conditions.

HOW IT WORKS
Phenytoin is thought to depress the activity of certain parts of the brain and to suppress the irregular and uncontrolled firing of neurons that causes seizures.

▼ DOSAGE GUIDELINES

RANGE AND FREQUENCY
Adults: 200 to 500 mg a day, as a single dose or in 2 divided doses. Children: 5 to 300 mg a day, as a single dose or in 2 divided doses. Some patients require higher doses. A low dose is used to start, then gradually increased by your doctor.

ONSET OF EFFECT
Several hours.

DURATION OF ACTION
Maximum effect lasts for 24 hours or longer; effectiveness then gradually decreases.

DIETARY ADVICE
Take with food to minimize stomach upset. Tablets may be crushed, chewed, or swallowed whole.

STORAGE
Store in a tightly sealed container away from moisture, heat, and direct light.

MISSED DOSE
Take it as soon as you remember. Be especially attentive about not missing a dose if you are taking this drug only once daily.

STOPPING THE DRUG
This medication should never be stopped abruptly because this may cause seizures. The dose is typically tapered over a period of weeks under the supervision of your doctor.

PROLONGED USE
This drug is often taken for prolonged periods. See your doctor for periodic checkups.

▼ PRECAUTIONS

Over 60: Older patients may require lower doses to minimize side effects.

Driving and Hazardous Work: Do not drive or engage in hazardous work until you determine how the medicine affects you.

Alcohol: May contribute to excessive drowsiness.

Pregnancy: Anticonvulsant drugs are associated with an increased risk of birth defects. However, seizures during pregnancy can also increase the risks to the unborn child. Discuss with your doctor the potential risks and benefits of using this drug during pregnancy. Folate supplementation is recommended beginning 1 to 2 months before conception and throughout pregnancy.

Breast Feeding: Phenytoin passes into breast milk, although at low levels. Consult your doctor for advice.

Infants and Children: No special problems are expected.

Special Concerns: The generic version of this drug is not recommended. Do not change the brand of phenytoin you are taking without consulting your doctor. The suspension form of phenytoin should be shaken well before you take it. Your doctor may advise you to wear a medical bracelet or carry an identification card saying that you are taking this medication.

OVERDOSE
Symptoms: Blurred or double vision, difficulty walking, severe clumsiness or unsteadiness, severe confusion, dizziness or drowsiness.

What to Do: Call your doctor, emergency medical services (EMS), or the nearest poison control center immediately.

▼ INTERACTIONS

DRUG INTERACTIONS
Many other drugs may interact with phenytoin, including other anticonvulsants (carbamazepine, phenobarbital, primidone, valproic acid), allopurinol, amiodarone, anticancer drugs, chloramphenicol, chlorpheniramine, cimetidine, diazoxide, dicumarol, disulfiram, isoniazid, loxapine, phenylbutazone, rifampin, sulfonamides, trazodone, trimethoprim.

FOOD INTERACTIONS
No known food interactions.

DISEASE INTERACTIONS
Caution is advised in those with liver or kidney disease, since these organs work together to remove the medication from the body.

⇊ SIDE EFFECTS ⇊

SERIOUS
Fever, sore throat, swollen glands, point-like rash on the skin or mucous membranes, blistering or peeling, mouth sores or bleeding gums, easy bruising, pallor, weakness, confusion, or seizures may be a sign of a potentially fatal blood disorder or other complication. Call your doctor immediately.

COMMON
Sedation, lethargy, nervousness, dizziness, thickened gums, excessive growth of body and facial hair. High doses may cause abnormal movements of the eyes, mouth, tongue, or limbs. Prolonged use may cause mild nerve impairment in the arms or legs.

LESS COMMON
Constipation, acne, mild skin rash, incoordination. There are numerous additional possible side effects; consult your doctor if you are concerned about any adverse or unusual reactions.

POTASSIUM CHLORIDE

Available in: Liquid, soluble granules, powder, tablets, sustained-release capsules
Available OTC? No   **As Generic?** Yes
Drug Class: Electrolyte

▼ USAGE INFORMATION

WHY IT'S PRESCRIBED
To restore or maintain proper potassium levels in the body. Potassium is an electrolyte, a mineral that helps maintain proper fluid balance. It is also vital in the transmission of nerve impulses.

HOW IT WORKS
Potassium chloride is absorbed into body fluids and taken into the cells where it is part of a number of metabolic actions, especially those that involve the release of energy. It also aids in the conduction of nerve impulses responsible for muscle movement and heart contraction.

▼ DOSAGE GUIDELINES

RANGE AND FREQUENCY
20 milliequivalents (mEq) to 100 mEq daily in divided doses. A single dose should not exceed 20 mEq.

ONSET OF EFFECT
Unknown.

DURATION OF ACTION
Unknown.

DIETARY ADVICE
Must be taken after meals or with food and a glass of water or other liquid. Follow all special dietary guidelines as outlined by your doctor.

STORAGE
Store in a tightly sealed container away from heat and direct light. Keep liquid forms of potassium refrigerated, but do not allow to freeze.

MISSED DOSE
If you remember within 2 hours, take the missed dose with food or liquids and resume your regular dosage schedule. If you remember after 2 hours, skip the missed dose and return to your regular dosage schedule. Do not double the next dose.

STOPPING THE DRUG
Do not stop taking potassium without first consulting your physician. Be very careful not to stop taking potassium abruptly if you are also taking digitalis drugs (digoxin).

PROLONGED USE
Requires periodic testing of blood potassium levels by your doctor.

▼ PRECAUTIONS

Over 60: Elderly people may be at greater risk of retaining too much potassium because of age-related changes in the ability of the kidneys to excrete it. Older patients should have their potassium levels checked regularly.

Driving and Hazardous Work: No special problems are expected.

Alcohol: No special problems are expected.

Pregnancy: Potassium supplements are considered safe during pregnancy if used exactly as prescribed.

Breast Feeding: Potassium may pass into breast milk. Consult your doctor for specific advice.

Infants and Children: Although the safety and effectiveness of potassium use by children have not been established, no specific problems have been documented.

Special Concerns: Remember that the foods in your diet must also be considered when calculating your total intake of potassium. Be certain to read all labels carefully, especially on all products labeled "low-sodium," such as canned foods and some breads, many of which contain potassium. Do not crush sustained-release forms. Swallow tablets without chewing, sucking, or crushing. Be sure the powder form is completely dissolved before ingesting.

OVERDOSE

Symptoms: Irregular heartbeat; muscle weakness, which may progress to paralysis of the diaphragm and interfere with breathing.

What to Do: Call your doctor, emergency medical services (EMS), or the nearest poison control center immediately.

▼ INTERACTIONS

DRUG INTERACTIONS
The following drugs may interact adversely with potassium chloride. Consult your doctor for advice if you are taking digitalis drugs, potassium-sparing diuretics, thiazide diuretics, NSAIDs, beta-blockers, heparin, triamterene, anticholinergics, or ACE inhibitors.

FOOD INTERACTIONS
To prevent ingestion of too much potassium, discuss your diet with your doctor. Foods high in potassium include avocados, bananas, broccoli, dried fruits, grapefruit, beans, meats, nuts, spinach, low-salt milk, squash, melon, brussels sprouts, zucchini, frozen orange juice, and tomatoes.

DISEASE INTERACTIONS
Consult your doctor if you have any of the following medical conditions: intestinal obstruction, dehydration, severe diarrhea, compression of the esophagus, delayed gastric emptying, peptic ulcer, heart blockage, or a predisposition to retaining the mineral potassium.

≡ SIDE EFFECTS ≡

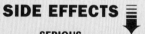

SERIOUS
Numbness or tingling in the hands, feet, or lips; slowed or irregular heartbeat; breathing difficulty; unusual fatigue or weakness; confusion. Stop taking the drug and consult your doctor at once.

COMMON
Diarrhea, abdominal discomfort, gas, nausea and vomiting.

LESS COMMON
Black or bloody stools, pain when swallowing. Consult your doctor if such symptoms persist.

PRAVASTATIN

Available in: Tablets
Available OTC? No   **As Generic?** No
Drug Class: Antilipidemic (cholesterol-lowering agent)

▼ USAGE INFORMATION

WHY IT'S PRESCRIBED
To treat high cholesterol. Usually prescribed after first lines of treatment–diet, weight loss, and exercise–fail to reduce total and low-density lipoprotein (LDL) cholesterol to acceptable levels.

HOW IT WORKS
Pravastatin blocks the action of an enzyme required for the manufacture of cholesterol, thereby interfering with its formation. By lowering the amount of cholesterol in the liver cells, the drug pravastatin increases the formation of receptors for LDL, and thereby reduces blood levels of total and LDL cholesterol. In addition to lowering LDL cholesterol, pravastatin also modestly reduces triglyceride levels and raises HDL (the so-called "good") cholesterol.

▼ DOSAGE GUIDELINES

RANGE AND FREQUENCY
Initial dose is 10 to 20 mg once a day. The dose may be increased to a maximum of 40 mg per day. The drug is most effective when taken in the evening.

ONSET OF EFFECT
2 to 4 weeks.

DURATION OF ACTION
The effect persists for the duration of therapy.

DIETARY ADVICE
Cholesterol-lowering drugs are only one part of a total program that should include regular exercise and a healthy diet. The American Heart Association publishes a "Healthy Heart" diet, which is recommended.

STORAGE
Store in a tightly sealed container away from heat and direct light.

MISSED DOSE
Take it as soon as you remember. Take the next scheduled dose at the proper time and resume your regular dosage schedule, as prescribed. Do not double the next dose.

STOPPING THE DRUG
The decision to stop taking the drug should be made in consultation with your doctor. Once the medication is discontinued, blood cholesterol is likely to return to original elevated levels.

PROLONGED USE
Side effects are more likely with prolonged use. As you continue with pravastatin, your doctor will periodically order blood tests to evaluate liver function.

▼ PRECAUTIONS

Over 60: No special problems are expected.

Driving and Hazardous Work: The use of pravastatin should not impair your ability to perform such tasks safely.

Alcohol: No special precautions are necessary.

Pregnancy: Pravastatin should not be used during pregnancy or by women who plan to become pregnant in the near future.

Breast Feeding: This drug is not recommended for women who are nursing.

Infants and Children: Long-term effects of pravastatin in children have not been determined. Rarely used in young patients; consult your doctor.

Special Concerns: Important elements of treatment for high cholesterol include proper diet, weight loss, regular moderate exercise, and the avoidance of certain medications that may increase cholesterol levels. Because pravastatin has potential side effects, it is important that you maintain a recommended healthy diet and cooperate with other treatments your physician may suggest.

OVERDOSE
Symptoms: Overdose is unlikely to occur.

What to Do: Emergency instructions not applicable.

▼ INTERACTIONS

DRUG INTERACTIONS
Consult your doctor if you are taking cyclosporine, gemfibrozil, niacin, antibiotics, especially erythromycin, or medications for fungus infections. All of these drugs may increase the risk of myositis (muscle inflammation) when taken with pravastatin and may lead to kidney failure.

FOOD INTERACTIONS
No known food interactions.

DISEASE INTERACTIONS
Consult your doctor if you have any of the following problems: liver, kidney, or muscle disease, or a medical history involving organ transplant or recent surgery.

≡ SIDE EFFECTS ≡

SERIOUS
Fever, unusual or unexplained muscle aches and tenderness. Call your doctor right away.

COMMON
Side effects occur in only 1% to 2% of patients. These include constipation or diarrhea, dizziness, gas, headache, heartburn, nausea, skin rash, stomach pain, rise in liver enzymes (detectable by your doctor).

LESS COMMON
Insomnia.

PREDNISONE

Available in: Oral suspension, syrup, tablets
Available OTC? No   **As Generic?** Yes
Drug Class: Corticosteroid

▼ USAGE INFORMATION

WHY IT'S PRESCRIBED
To treat numerous conditions that involve inflammation (a response by body tissues, producing redness, warmth, swelling, and pain). Such conditions include arthritis, allergic reactions, asthma, some skin diseases, multiple sclerosis flare-ups, and other autoimmune diseases. Also prescribed to treat deficiency of natural steroid hormones.

HOW IT WORKS
Prednisone mimics the effects of the body's natural corticosteroid hormones. It depresses the synthesis, release, and activity of inflammation-producing body chemicals. It also suppresses the activity of the immune system.

▼ DOSAGE GUIDELINES

RANGE AND FREQUENCY
Adults and teenagers—For severe inflammation or to suppress the immune system: 5 to 100 mg a day in divided doses. For multiple sclerosis: 200 mg daily for 1 week, then 80 mg every other day for 1 month. Children—Consult your pediatrician.

ONSET OF EFFECT
Variable.

DURATION OF ACTION
Variable.

DIETARY ADVICE
It can be taken with food or milk to minimize stomach upset. Your doctor may well suggest a low-salt, high-potassium, high-protein diet.

STORAGE
Store in a tightly sealed container away from moisture, heat, and direct light. Do not allow liquid forms to freeze.

MISSED DOSE
Take it as soon as you remember. If you take several doses a day and it is close to the next dose, double the next dose. If you take 1 dose a day and you do not remember until the next day, skip the missed dose and do not double the next dose.

STOPPING THE DRUG
With long-term therapy, do not stop taking the drug abruptly; the dosage should be decreased gradually.

PROLONGED USE
Long-term use may lead to cataracts, diabetes, hypertension, or osteoporosis; see your doctor for regular examinations.

▼ PRECAUTIONS

Over 60: Adverse reactions may be more likely and more severe.

Driving and Hazardous Work: Avoid such activities until you determine how the medicine affects you.

Alcohol: May cause stomach problems; avoid it unless your physician approves occasional moderate drinking.

Pregnancy: Overuse during pregnancy can retard the child's growth and cause other developmental problems. Consult your doctor.

Breast Feeding: Do not use this drug while nursing.

Infants and Children: Prednisone may retard the growth and development of bone and other tissues.

Special Concerns: This drug can lower resistance to infection. Avoid immunizations with live vaccines. Patients undergoing long-term therapy should wear a medical-alert bracelet. Call your doctor if you develop a fever.

OVERDOSE
Symptoms: Fever, muscle or joint pain, nausea, dizziness, fainting, difficulty breathing. Prolonged overuse: Moonface, obesity, unusual hair growth, acne, loss of sexual function, muscle wasting.

What to Do: Call your doctor, emergency medical services (EMS), or the nearest poison control center immediately.

▼ INTERACTIONS

DRUG INTERACTIONS
Consult your doctor for specific advice if you are taking aminoglutethimide, antacids, barbiturates, carbamazepine, griseofulvin, mitotane, phenylbutazone, phenytoin, primidone, rifampin, injectable amphotericin B, oral antidiabetes agents, insulin, digitalis drugs, diuretics, or medications containing potassium or sodium.

FOOD INTERACTIONS
Avoid excess sodium.

DISEASE INTERACTIONS
Consult your doctor if you have a history of bone disease, chicken pox, measles, gastrointestinal disorders, diabetes, recent serious infection, glaucoma, heart disease, hypertension, liver or kidney disorders, high blood cholesterol, thyroid problems, myasthenia gravis, or lupus.

≡ SIDE EFFECTS ≡

SERIOUS
Vision problems, frequent urination, increased thirst, rectal bleeding, blistering skin, confusion, hallucinations, paranoia, euphoria, depression, mood swings, redness and swelling at injection site. Call your doctor immediately.

COMMON
Increased appetite, indigestion, nervousness, insomnia, greater susceptibility to infections, increased blood pressure, slowed wound healing, weight gain, easy bruising, fluid retention.

LESS COMMON
Change in skin color, dizziness, headache, increased sweating, unusual growth of body or facial hair, increased blood sugar, peptic ulcers, adrenal insufficiency, muscle weakness, cataracts, glaucoma, osteoporosis.

PROMETHAZINE HYDROCHLORIDE

Available in: Tablets, syrup, injection, suppositories
Available OTC? No   **As Generic?** Yes
Drug Class: Antihistamine

▼ USAGE INFORMATION

WHY IT'S PRESCRIBED
To relieve the symptoms of hay fever and other allergies, to prevent motion sickness, and to treat nausea and vomiting. Promethazine may also be used in some patients for its sedative effect.

HOW IT WORKS
Promethazine interferes with, but does not block, the release and action of histamine, a naturally occurring substance in the body that causes swelling, itching, sneezing, watery eyes, hives, and other symptoms of allergic reaction. Promethazine also has an anticholinergic effect, meaning this medication blocks the transmission of certain nerve impulses, which in turn relaxes the smooth muscle tissue that controls activity in the bladder, stomach, intestine, lungs, and other organ systems. This effect thereby helps to ease the symptoms of motion sickness, nausea, gastrointestinal upset, and anxiety.

▼ DOSAGE GUIDELINES

RANGE AND FREQUENCY
Tablets or syrup—For allergies: Adults and teenagers: 10 to 12.5 mg, 4 times a day before meals and at bedtime, or 25 mg at bedtime. Children 2 and older: 5 to 12.5 mg, 3 times a day, or 25 mg at bedtime. For nausea and vomiting: Adults and teenagers: 25 mg for first dose, then 10 to 25 mg every 4 to 6 hours as needed. Children 2 and older: 10 to 25 mg every 4 to 6 hours. To prevent motion sickness: Adults and teenagers: 25 mg taken 30 to 60 minutes before traveling. Children 2 and older: 10 to 25 mg, 30 to 60 minutes before traveling. For dizziness: Adults and teenagers: 25 mg, 2 times a day. Children 2 and older: 10 to 25, mg 2 times a day. As a sedative: Adults and teenagers: 25 to 50 mg. Children 2 and older: 10 to 25 mg. Injection—For allergies: Adults and teenagers: 25 mg into a vein or muscle. Children 2 and older: 6.25 to 12.5 mg, 3 times a day into a muscle, or 25 mg at bedtime. For nausea and vomiting: Adults and teenagers: 12.5 to 25 mg every 4 hours into a vein or muscle. Children 2 and older: 12.5 to 25 mg every 4 to 6 hours into a muscle. As a sedative: Adults and teens: 25 to 50 mg injected into a vein or muscle. Children 2 and older: 12.5 to 25 mg into a muscle. Suppositories—For allergies: Adults and teens: 25 mg at first; 25 mg, 2 hours later if needed. Children 2 and older: 6.25 to 12.5 mg, 3 times a day, or 25 mg at bedtime. For nausea and vomiting: Adults and teenagers: 25 mg at first, then 12.5 to 25 mg every 4 to 6 hours if needed. Children 2 and older: 12.5 to 25 mg every 4 to 6 hours. For dizziness: Adults and teenagers: 25 mg, 2 times a day. Children 2 and older: 12.5 to 25 mg, 2 times a day. As a sedative: Adults and teenagers: 25 to 50 mg. Children 2 and older: 12.25 to 25 mg.

ONSET OF EFFECT
15 to 60 minutes orally or by suppository; 20 minutes after injection.

DURATION OF ACTION
Up to 12 hours.

DIETARY ADVICE
Take it with food or milk to lessen stomach irritation.

STORAGE
Store in a tightly sealed container away from heat and direct light at room temperature. Do not store the tablets in a place with excessive moisture, such as the bathroom medicine cabinet. Do not allow the syrup or injection to freeze.

MISSED DOSE
Take it as soon as you remember. If it is near the time for the next dose, skip the missed dose and resume your regular dosage schedule. Do not double the next dose.

STOPPING THE DRUG
You should take it as prescribed for the full treatment period, but you may stop taking the drug if you are feeling better before the scheduled end of therapy.

PROLONGED USE
See your doctor regularly if you take this medicine for a prolonged period. Prolonged use of this antihistamine may decrease salivary flow, which may lead to thrush (white, furry patches in the mouth caused by fungal infection), periodontal disease (disease and decay of the teeth, gums, jaw, and other supportive structures in the mouth), dental caries (cavities), and gingivitis (gum disease). Practice good oral hygiene to prevent these disorders.

▼ PRECAUTIONS

Over 60: Adverse reactions may be more likely and more severe in older patients.

≡ SIDE EFFECTS ≡

SERIOUS
Sore throat and fever, unusual fatigue, unusual bleeding or bruising. Call your doctor immediately.

COMMON
Drowsiness, thickening of mucus.

LESS COMMON
Blurred vision; confusion; difficult or painful urination; dizziness; dry mouth, nose, or throat; increased sensitivity of skin to sunlight; faintness; increased sweating; stinging or burning of rectum (suppository form); loss of appetite; ringing or buzzing in ears; skin rash; fast heartbeat; unusual excitement or irritability.

PROMETHAZINE HYDROCHLORIDE (continued)

Driving and Hazardous Work: Do not drive or engage in hazardous work until you determine how the medicine affects you.

Alcohol: Avoid alcohol.

Pregnancy: Promethazine has not been shown to cause birth defects in animals. Thorough human studies have not been done. However, if the mother takes the drug within 2 weeks of delivery, the baby may have jaundice or problems with blood clotting. Before you take it, tell your doctor if you are pregnant or plan to become pregnant.

Breast Feeding: Promethazine passes into breast milk; avoid or discontinue use while nursing. The flow of breast milk may be decreased as a result of the medication.

Infants and Children: Adverse reactions, such as seizures, may be more common and more severe in infants and children. It is not recommended for children with a history of breathing difficulty while sleeping or with a family history of sudden infant death syndrome (SIDS). Children and adolescents with signs of Reye's syndrome should not take this drug, especially by injection. Its side effects may be mistaken for symptoms of Reye's syndrome.

Special Concerns: If you have an allergy test, stop taking promethazine 4 days before the test and tell the doctor that you were taking promethazine.

OVERDOSE

Symptoms: Clumsiness; insomnia; seizures; severe dryness of mouth, nose, or throat; redness of face; hallucinations; muscle spasms; trouble breathing; jerky movements of head and face; dizziness; trembling and shaking of the hands.

What to Do: Call your doctor, emergency medical services (EMS), or the nearest poison control center immediately.

▼ INTERACTIONS

DRUG INTERACTIONS
Consult your doctor for specific advice if you are taking amoxapine, antipsychotics, medications containing alcohol, barbiturates, methyldopa, metoclopramide, metyrosine, epinephrine, metrizamide, pemoline, pimozide, rauwolfia alkaloids, anticholinergics, central nervous system depressants, maprotiline, other antihistamines, tricyclic antidepressants, levodopa, or MAO inhibitors.

FOOD INTERACTIONS
No known food interactions.

DISEASE INTERACTIONS
Consult your doctor if you have any of the following: blood disease, heart or blood vessel disease, enlarged prostate, urinary tract blockage, epilepsy, glaucoma, Reye's syndrome, jaundice, or liver disease.

PROPOXYPHENE/ACETAMINOPHEN

Available in: Tablets
Available OTC? No **As Generic?** Yes
Drug Class: Opioid (narcotic) analgesic

▼ USAGE INFORMATION

WHY IT'S PRESCRIBED
To relieve mild to moderate pain.

HOW IT WORKS
Opioids such as propoxyphene relieve pain by acting on specific areas of the spinal cord and of the brain that process pain signals from nerves throughout the body. Acetaminophen appears to interfere with the action of prostaglandins, naturally occurring substances in the body that cause inflammation and make nerves more sensitive to pain impulses.

▼ DOSAGE GUIDELINES

RANGE AND FREQUENCY
Adults: 1 or 2 tablets, depending on strength, every 4 to 6 hours. Children: Dose must be determined individually by your pediatrician.

ONSET OF EFFECT
Within 2 hours.

DURATION OF ACTION
Unknown.

DIETARY ADVICE
It can be taken with food to lessen stomach irritation.

STORAGE
Store in a tightly sealed container away from moisture, heat, and direct light.

MISSED DOSE
If you are taking the drug on a fixed schedule, take it as soon as you remember. If it is near the time for the next dose, skip the missed dose and resume your regular dosage schedule. Do not double the next dose.

STOPPING THE DRUG
The decision to stop taking this medication should be made only in consultation with your doctor.

PROLONGED USE
You should see your doctor regularly for tests and examinations if you take this medication for a prolonged period. Prolonged use can cause nerve damage as well as physical dependence.

▼ PRECAUTIONS

Over 60: Adverse reactions may be more likely and more severe in older patients.

Driving and Hazardous Work: Do not drive or engage in hazardous work until you determine how the medicine affects you.

Alcohol: Avoid alcohol.

Pregnancy: Propoxyphene has not caused birth defects in animals. Human studies have not been done. Before you use this medication, tell your doctor if you are pregnant or plan to become pregnant. Overuse of the medication during pregnancy can cause physical dependence in the newborn.

Breast Feeding: Propoxyphene and acetaminophen pass into breast milk and may cause sedation in the nursing infant. Consult your doctor for advice.

Infants and Children: Adverse reactions may be more likely and more severe in children. Consult your pediatrician for advice.

Special Concerns: If you feel the medication is not working properly after a few weeks, do not increase the dose on your own. Consult the doctor.

OVERDOSE

Symptoms: Severe dizziness or drowsiness; cold, clammy skin; difficult or slow breathing or shortness of breath; severe confusion; seizures; stomach cramps or pain; diarrhea; low blood pressure; increased sweating; constricted pupils; nausea or vomiting; irregular heartbeat; severe weakness.

What to Do: Call your doctor, emergency medical services (EMS), or the nearest poison control center immediately.

▼ INTERACTIONS

DRUG INTERACTIONS
Consult your doctor for specific advice if you are taking any prescription or over-the-counter drugs, especially other drugs containing acetaminophen, or central nervous system depressants which include: antihistamines or decongestants for hay fever, allergies, or colds; barbiturates; seizure medication; muscle relaxants; anesthetics; tranquilizers, sedatives, or sleep-inducing medications.

FOOD INTERACTIONS
No known food interactions.

DISEASE INTERACTIONS
Consult your doctor if you have a head injury or brain disease, an underactive thyroid, an enlarged prostate, seizures, kidney or liver disease, gall bladder problems, a blood disorder, or a history of alcohol or drug abuse.

≡ SIDE EFFECTS ≡

SERIOUS
Bloody, dark, or cloudy urine; severe pain in the lower back or side; pale or black, tarry stools; yellow discoloration of eyes or skin (jaundice); hallucinations; frequent urge to urinate; painful or difficult urination; sudden decrease in urine output; increased sweating; unusual bleeding or bruising; irregular heartbeat; skin rash, hives, or itching; excitability; ringing or buzzing in the ears; pinpoint red spots on skin; sore throat and fever; confusion; trembling or uncontrolled muscle movements; redness, flushing, or swelling of the face. Call your doctor immediately.

COMMON
Dizziness, lightheadedness, constipation, nausea, vomiting, drowsiness, unusual fatigue.

LESS COMMON
Stomach pain, false sense of well-being (euphoria), depression, loss of appetite, blurred vision, nightmares or unusual dreams, dry mouth, headache, nervousness, insomnia.

PROPRANOLOL HYDROCHLORIDE

Available in: Extended-release capsules, oral solution, tablets, injection
Available OTC? No   **As Generic?** Yes
Drug Class: Beta-blocker

▼ USAGE INFORMATION

WHY IT'S PRESCRIBED
To treat angina, mild to moderate high blood pressure, irregular heartbeat (cardiac arrhythmias), hypertrophic cardiomyopathy (weakness of the heart muscle), heart attack, pheochromocytoma, tremors, and migraine headaches.

HOW IT WORKS
Propranolol blocks nerve impulses to various parts of the body, which accounts for its many effects. For example, propranolol slows the heart's rate and force of the contraction (which helps lower blood pressure), decreases the heart's oxygen requirement (an action which helps prevent angina), and helps stabilize heart rhythm.

▼ DOSAGE GUIDELINES

RANGE AND FREQUENCY
Adults—For angina: 80 to 320 mg a day in 2, 3, or 4 doses. For high blood pressure: 40 mg, 2 times a day; may be increased up to 640 mg a day. For irregular heartbeat: 10 to 30 mg, 3 or 4 times a day. For cardiomyopathy: 20 to 40 mg, 3 or 4 times a day. For pheochromocytoma: 30 to 160 mg a day in divided doses. For preventing migraine headache: 20 mg, 4 times a day; may be increased to 240 mg a day. For trembling: 40 mg, 2 times a day; may be increased to 320 mg a day. Children—For high blood pressure: 0.5 mg to 4 mg per 2.2 lbs (1 kg) of body weight a day. For irregular heartbeat: 0.5 to 4 mg per 2.2 lbs of body weight a day in divided doses.

ONSET OF EFFECT
Within 30 minutes.

DURATION OF ACTION
Up to 12 hours.

DIETARY ADVICE
Mix the concentrated oral solution with water, juice, or a carbonated drink.

STORAGE
Store in a tightly sealed container away from heat and direct light.

MISSED DOSE
Take it as soon as you remember. If it is near the time for the next dose, skip the missed dose and resume your regular dosage schedule. Do not double the next dose.

STOPPING THE DRUG
Do not stop taking this drug suddenly; the dosage must be slowly tapered under your physician's close supervision.

PROLONGED USE
Lifelong therapy with propranolol may be necessary; prolonged use may be associated with a greater incidence of side effects. Regular monitoring and evaluation by your doctor is advised.

▼ PRECAUTIONS

Over 60: Adverse reactions may be more likely and more severe in older patients.

Driving and Hazardous Work: Avoid such activities until you determine how the drug affects you.

Alcohol: Avoid alcohol.

Pregnancy: Consult your doctor to weigh the risks and benefits of using propranolol during pregnancy.

Breast Feeding: Propranolol passes into breast milk; caution is advised.

Infants and Children: The correct dosage will be determined by your pediatrician.

Special Concerns: Take extra care during exercise or hot weather to avoid dizziness and fainting. Check your pulse often; if it is slower than usual or less than 50 beats a minute, call your doctor.

OVERDOSE
Symptoms: Unusually slow or rapid heartbeat, severe dizziness or fainting, poor circulation in the hands (bluish skin), breathing difficulty; seizures.

What to Do: Call your doctor, emergency medical services (EMS), or the nearest poison control center immediately.

▼ INTERACTIONS

DRUG INTERACTIONS
Consult your doctor for specific advice if you are taking allergy shots, aminophylline, caffeine, oxtriphylline, theophylline, oral antidiabetics, insulin, calcium channel blockers, clonidine, guanabenz, or MAO inhibitors.

FOOD INTERACTIONS
No known food interactions.

DISEASE INTERACTIONS
Must be used with caution in people with diabetes, especially for insulin-dependent diabetes, since the drug may mask symptoms of hypoglycemia. Consult a doctor if you have allergies, bronchitis, emphysema, heart or blood vessel disease (including congestive heart failure and peripheral vascular disease), mental depression, myasthenia gravis, psoriasis, hyperthyroidism, kidney disease, or liver disease.

≡ SIDE EFFECTS ≡

SERIOUS
Shortness of breath, wheezing; irregular or slow heartbeat (50 beats per minute or less); pain or feelings of tightness or pressure in the chest; swelling of the ankles, feet, and lower legs; depression. Call your doctor immediately.

COMMON
Dizziness or lightheadedness, especially when rising suddenly to a standing position; decreased sexual ability; unusual fatigue, weakness, or drowsiness; insomnia.

LESS COMMON
Anxiety, irritability; constipation; diarrhea; dry eyes; itching; nausea or vomiting; nightmares or intensely vivid dreams; numbness, tingling, or prickling in the fingers, toes, or scalp.

QUINAPRIL HYDROCHLORIDE

Available in: Tablets
Available OTC? No   **As Generic?** No
Drug Class: Angiotensin-converting enzyme (ACE) inhibitor

▼ USAGE INFORMATION

WHY IT'S PRESCRIBED
To control high blood pressure (hypertension); to treat congestive heart failure (CHF); to treat patients with left ventricular dysfunction (damage to the pumping chamber of the heart); and to minimize further kidney damage in diabetics with mild kidney disease.

HOW IT WORKS
Angiotensin-converting enzyme (ACE) inhibitors block an enzyme that produces angiotensin, a naturally occurring substance that causes blood vessels to constrict and stimulates production of the adrenal hormone, aldosterone, which promotes sodium retention in the body. As a result, ACE inhibitors relax blood vessels (causing them to widen) and reduces sodium retention, which lowers blood pressure and so decreases the workload of the heart.

▼ DOSAGE GUIDELINES

RANGE AND FREQUENCY
10 mg once a day. Dose may be increased to 20 to 80 mg a day, taken in 1 or 2 doses.

ONSET OF EFFECT
Within 1 hour.

DURATION OF ACTION
24 hours.

DIETARY ADVICE
Take quinapril on an empty stomach, about 1 hour before mealtime. Follow your doctor's dietary advice (such as low-salt or low-cholesterol restrictions) to improve control over high blood pressure and heart disease. Avoid high-potassium foods like bananas and citrus fruits and juices, unless you are also taking drugs such as diuretics that lower potassium levels.

STORAGE
Store in a tightly sealed container away from heat and direct light.

MISSED DOSE
Take it as soon as you remember. If it is near the time for the next dose, skip the missed dose and resume your regular dosage schedule. Do not double the next dose.

STOPPING THE DRUG
Do not stop taking this drug abruptly, as this may cause potentially serious health problems. Dosage should be reduced gradually, according to your doctor's instructions.

PROLONGED USE
Lifelong therapy may be necessary. See your doctor for regular evaluation.

▼ PRECAUTIONS

Over 60: No special advice.

Driving and Hazardous Work: Avoid such activities until you determine how the medicine affects you.

Alcohol: Consume alcohol only in moderation since it may increase the effect of the drug and cause an excessive drop in blood pressure.

Pregnancy: Use of quinapril during the last 6 months of pregnancy may cause severe defects, even death, to the fetus. The drug should be discontinued if you are pregnant or plan to become pregnant.

Breast Feeding: Quinapril may pass into breast milk; caution is advised. Consult your doctor for advice.

Infants and Children: The safety and efficacy of quinapril use by infants and children have not been established. Benefits must be weighed against potential risks; consult your pediatrician for specific advice.

OVERDOSE
Symptoms: None reported.

What to Do: While overdose is unlikely, call your doctor, emergency medical services (EMS), or the nearest poison control center immediately if you suspect that someone has taken a much larger dose than prescribed.

▼ INTERACTIONS

DRUG INTERACTIONS
Consult your doctor if you are taking diuretics (especially potassium-sparing diuretics), potassium supplements or drugs containing potassium (check ingredient labels), lithium, anticoagulants (such as warfarin), indomethacin or other anti-inflammatory drugs, or any over-the-counter medicines (especially cold remedies and diet pills).

FOOD INTERACTIONS
Avoid low-salt milk and salt substitutes. Many of these products contain potassium. Avoid large servings of high-potassium foods like bananas and citrus fruits or juices.

DISEASE INTERACTIONS
Consult your doctor if you have systemic lupus erythematosus (SLE) or if you have had a prior allergic reaction to ACE inhibitors. Quinapril should be used with caution by patients with severe kidney disease or renal artery stenosis (narrowing of one or both of the arteries that supply blood to the kidneys).

≡ SIDE EFFECTS ≡

SERIOUS
Fever and chills, sore throat and hoarseness, sudden difficulty breathing or swallowing, swelling of the face, mouth, or extremities, impaired kidney function (ankle swelling, decreased urination), confusion, yellow discoloration of the eyes or skin (indicating liver disorder), intense itching, chest pain or palpitations, abdominal pain. Serious side effects are very rare; contact your doctor immediately.

COMMON
Dry, persistent cough.

LESS COMMON
Dizziness or fainting, skin rash, numbness or tingling in the hands, feet, or lips, unusual fatigue or muscle weakness, nausea, drowsiness, loss of taste, headache.

RALOXIFENE HYDROCHLORIDE

Available in: Tablets
Available OTC? No   **As Generic?** No
Drug Class: Selective estrogen receptor modulator (SERM)

▼ USAGE INFORMATION

WHY IT'S PRESCRIBED
For the treatment and prevention of osteoporosis in postmenopausal women. Unlike estrogen, raloxifene does not stimulate overgrowth of the endometrium (the tissue lining the uterus) and thus does not increase the risk of uterine cancer.

HOW IT WORKS
Healthy bone tissue is continuously remodeled (broken down and then reformed); the minerals and other components of bone are reabsorbed by certain cells and then replaced by new bone formation. Raloxifene suppresses the activity of the cells that resorb bone; consequently, the breakdown of bone tissue occurs more slowly than the laying down of new bone. This action preserves bone density and strength.

▼ DOSAGE GUIDELINES

RANGE AND FREQUENCY
One 60 mg tablet a day.

ONSET OF EFFECT
Unknown.

DURATION OF ACTION
Unknown.

DIETARY ADVICE
Raloxifene may be taken at any time of day without regard to a meal schedule. Patients are generally advised to take calcium and vitamin D supplements to aid bone formation.

STORAGE
Store in a tightly sealed container away from moisture, heat, and direct light.

MISSED DOSE
If you miss a dose on one day, do not double the dose the next day.

STOPPING THE DRUG
The decision to stop taking this medication should be made in consultation with your doctor.

PROLONGED USE
Clinical research studies have not yet determined the drug's safety and effectiveness beyond three years of use.

▼ PRECAUTIONS

Over 60: No special advice.

Driving and Hazardous Work: No special warnings.

Alcohol: Alcohol should be restricted in high-risk women because it is a risk factor for osteoporosis.

Pregnancy: Raloxifene is normally not prescribed to premenopausal women. Raloxifene should not be given to pregnant women.

Breast Feeding: Raloxifene should not be used by nursing mothers.

Infants and Children: Not for use by children.

Special Concerns: Patients taking raloxifene are encouraged to engage in regular weight-bearing exercise and should avoid cigarettes and limit alcohol, which inhibit healthy bone production. Unlike estrogen replacement therapy, raloxifene does not reduce hot flashes in postmenopausal women.

OVERDOSE
Symptoms: No cases of overdose have been reported.

What to Do: An overdose with raloxifene is unlikely. If someone takes a much larger dose than prescribed, call your doctor.

▼ INTERACTIONS

DRUG INTERACTIONS
Estrogen should not be taken concurrently with raloxifene. Since cholestyramine reduces absorption of raloxifene, the two drugs should not be taken at the same time of day. Consult your doctor if you are taking any of the following medications that may interact with raloxifene: warfarin, indomethacin, clofibrate, naproxen, ibuprofen, diazepam, or diazoxide.

FOOD INTERACTIONS
No known food interactions.

DISEASE INTERACTIONS
You should not take raloxifene if you have any history of thromboembolic disease, including deep vein thrombosis, pulmonary embolism, and retinal vein thrombosis. Raloxifene must be used with caution by patients with impaired liver function; consult your doctor for specific advice about your own case.

≡ SIDE EFFECTS ≡

SERIOUS
No serious side effects have been reported.

COMMON
Increased incidence of infections, flu-like symptoms, hot flashes, joint pain, sinusitis, unexpected weight gain.

LESS COMMON
Leg cramps, mild chest pain, fever, migraine, indigestion, vomiting, flatulence, stomach upset, swelling of the legs and feet, muscle pain, insomnia, sore throat, increased cough, pneumonia, laryngitis, rash, sweating, yeast infection, urinary tract infection, white vaginal discharge.

RAMIPRIL

Available in: Tablets
Available OTC? No   **As Generic?** No
Drug Class: Angiotensin-converting enzyme (ACE) inhibitor

▼ USAGE INFORMATION

WHY IT'S PRESCRIBED
To control high blood pressure (hypertension); to treat congestive heart failure; to treat patients with left ventricular dysfunction (damage to the pumping chamber of the heart); to reduce risk of heart attack, stroke, and death from cardiovascular causes; and to minimize further kidney damage in diabetics with mild kidney disease.

HOW IT WORKS
Angiotensin-converting enzyme (ACE) inhibitors block an enzyme that produces angiotensin, a naturally occurring substance that causes blood vessels to constrict and stimulates production of the adrenal hormone, aldosterone, which promotes sodium retention in the body. As a result, ACE inhibitors relax blood vessels (causing them to widen) and reduces sodium retention, which lowers blood pressure and so decreases the workload of the heart.

▼ DOSAGE GUIDELINES

RANGE AND FREQUENCY
2.5 mg to 20 mg per day, taken in 1 or 2 doses.

ONSET OF EFFECT
Within 1 to 2 hours.

DURATION OF ACTION
24 hours.

DIETARY ADVICE
Take it on an empty stomach, about 1 hour before mealtime. Follow your doctor's dietary advice (such as low-salt or low-cholesterol restrictions) to improve control over high blood pressure and heart disease. Avoid high-potassium foods like bananas and citrus fruits and juices, unless you are also taking medications, such as diuretics, that lower potassium levels.

STORAGE
Store in a tightly sealed container away from heat and direct light. Avoid extremes in temperature.

MISSED DOSE
Take it as soon as you remember. If it is near the time for the next dose, skip the missed dose and resume your regular dosage schedule. Do not double the next dose.

STOPPING THE DRUG
Do not stop taking this drug abruptly, as this may cause potentially serious health problems. Dosage should be reduced gradually, according to your doctor's instructions.

PROLONGED USE
Lifelong therapy may be necessary. See your doctor for regular examinations and tests if you must take this medication for a prolonged period of time.

▼ PRECAUTIONS

Over 60: No special advice.

Driving and Hazardous Work: Do not drive or engage in hazardous work until you determine how the medicine affects you.

Alcohol: Consume alcohol only in moderation since it may increase the effect of the drug and cause an excessive drop in blood pressure. Consult your doctor for advice.

Pregnancy: Use of ramipril during the last 6 months of pregnancy may cause severe defects, even death, in the fetus. The drug should be discontinued if you are pregnant or plan to become pregnant.

Breast Feeding: Ramipril may pass into breast milk; caution is advised. Consult your doctor for advice.

Infants and Children: Children may be especially sensitive to the effects of ramipril. Benefits must be weighed against potential risks; consult your pediatrician for advice.

OVERDOSE
Symptoms: Dizziness or fainting due to extremely low blood pressure.

What to Do: Call your doctor, emergency medical services (EMS), or local hospital.

▼ INTERACTIONS

DRUG INTERACTIONS
Consult your doctor if you are taking diuretics (especially potassium-sparing diuretics), potassium supplements or drugs containing potassium (check ingredient labels), lithium, anticoagulants (such as warfarin), indomethacin or other anti-inflammatory drugs, or any over-the-counter medications (especially cold remedies and diet pills).

FOOD INTERACTIONS
Avoid low-salt milk and salt substitutes. Many of these products contain potassium. Avoid consuming large servings of high-potassium foods like bananas and citrus fruits or juices.

DISEASE INTERACTIONS
Consult your doctor if you have systemic lupus erythematosus (SLE) or if you have had a prior allergic reaction to ACE inhibitors. Ramipril should be used with caution by patients with severe kidney disease or renal artery stenosis (narrowing of one or both of the arteries that supply blood to the kidneys).

≡ SIDE EFFECTS ≡

SERIOUS
Fever and chills, sore throat and hoarseness, sudden difficulty breathing or swallowing, swelling of the face, mouth, or extremities, impaired kidney function (ankle swelling, decreased urination), confusion, yellow discoloration of the eyes or skin (indicating liver disorder), intense itching, chest pain or palpitations, abdominal pain. Serious side effects are very rare; contact your doctor immediately.

COMMON
Dry, persistent cough.

LESS COMMON
Dizziness or fainting, skin rash, numbness or tingling in the hands, feet, or lips, unusual fatigue or muscle weakness, nausea, drowsiness, loss of taste, headache.

RANITIDINE

BRAND NAMES

Zantac, Zantac 75

Available in: Capsules, tablets, injection, syrup, granules
Available OTC? Yes **As Generic?** Yes
Drug Class: Histamine (H2) blocker

▼ USAGE INFORMATION

WHY IT'S PRESCRIBED
To treat ulcers of the stomach and duodenum, conditions that cause increased stomach acid production (such as Zollinger-Ellison syndrome), erosive esopha-gitis (severe, chronic inflammation of the esophagus), and gastroesoph-ageal reflux (backwash of stomach acid into the esopha-gus, resulting in heartburn).

HOW IT WORKS
Ranitidine blocks the action of histamine (a compound produced in the body's cells), which in turn decreases the stomach's secretion of hydrochloric acid. Once stomach acid production is decreased, the body is better able to heal itself.

▼ DOSAGE GUIDELINES

RANGE AND FREQUENCY
Adults—Oral dose: 150 mg, 2 times a day, in the morning and at bedtime, or 300 mg once daily before bedtime.

Injection: 50 mg every 6 to 8 hours. Patients with Zollinger-Ellison syndrome may require up to 6 g per day, taken orally. For treatment of heart-burn with the over-the-counter form: 75 mg, as needed, not to exceed 150 mg a day. Children—Consult your pediatrician for appropri-ate individual dosage.

ONSET OF EFFECT
30 to 60 minutes.

DURATION OF ACTION
Up to 13 hours.

DIETARY ADVICE
Avoid foods that cause stom-ach irritation.

STORAGE
Store away from heat and direct light. Keep liquid form from freezing.

MISSED DOSE
Take it as soon as you remember. If it is near the time for the next dose, skip the missed dose and resume your regular dosage schedule. Do not double the next dose.

STOPPING THE DRUG
Take the prescription-strength medicine for the full treatment period, even if you begin to feel better before the sched-uled end of therapy.

PROLONGED USE
Do not take nonprescription-strength ranitidine for more than 2 weeks unless you have been otherwise instructed by your doctor.

▼ PRECAUTIONS

Over 60: Adverse reactions may be more likely and more severe in older patients.

Driving and Hazardous Work: Do not drive or engage in hazardous work until you determine how the medicine affects you.

Alcohol: Avoid drinking alco-hol. Ranitidine may increase blood alcohol levels.

Pregnancy: Risks vary, depending on the patient and dosage. Consult your doctor.

Breast Feeding: Ranitidine passes into breast milk and may pose harm to the child; avoid or discontinue use while nursing.

Infants and Children: Raniti-dine is not recommended for young patients, although it has not been shown to cause any side effects or problems different from those in adults when used for short periods of time.

Special Concerns: Avoid cig-arette smoking because it may increase stomach acid secretion and thus worsen

the disease. Do not take ranitidine if you have ever had an allergic reaction to a histamine (H2) blocker. If stomach pain becomes worse while using the drug, be sure to tell your doctor right away.

OVERDOSE
Symptoms: Vomiting, diar-rhea, breathing problems, slurred speech, rapid heart-beat, delirium.

What to Do: Call your doctor, emergency medical services (EMS), or the nearest poison control center immediately.

▼ INTERACTIONS

DRUG INTERACTIONS
Consult your doctor for spe-cific advice if you are taking antacids, antidepressants, aspirin, beta-blockers, caffeine, diazepam, glipizide, ketoconazole, lidocaine, phenytoin, procainamide, theophylline, or warfarin.

FOOD INTERACTIONS
Carbonated drinks, caffeine-containing beverages, citrus fruits and juices, and other acidic foods or liquids may irritate the stomach or inter-fere with the therapeutic action of ranitidine.

DISEASE INTERACTIONS
Patients with kidney disease should not use ranitidine or should use it in smaller, limited doses under careful supervision by a physician.

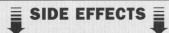

≡ SIDE EFFECTS ≡

SERIOUS
Irregular heart rhythm (palpitations), slowed heartbeat, severe blood problems resulting in unusual bleeding, bruis-ing, fever, chills, and increased susceptibility to infection. Call your doctor immediately.

COMMON
Headache, fatigue, drowsiness, dizziness, nausea, vomiting, abdominal pain, diarrhea, constipation.

LESS COMMON
Blurred vision, decreased sexual desire or function, swelling of breasts in males or females, temporary hair loss, hallucinations, depression, insomnia, skin rash, hives, or redness.

REPAGLINIDE

Available in: Tablets
Available OTC? No   **As Generic?** No
Drug Class: Antidiabetic agent

▼ USAGE INFORMATION

WHY IT'S PRESCRIBED
Used as an adjunct therapy to dietary measures and exercise to help control blood sugar levels in patients with type 2 diabetes mellitus. Repaglinide is the first in a new class of oral antidiabetic medications designed to control blood glucose levels following meals.

HOW IT WORKS
Repaglinide stimulates the pancreas to produce more insulin. Increased insulin levels reduce blood glucose by promoting the transport of glucose into muscle cells and other tissues, where it is used as a source of energy. The rapid onset and short duration of repaglinide's action make it effective in controlling glucose levels after a meal.

▼ DOSAGE GUIDELINES

RANGE AND FREQUENCY
Dosage must be determined for each patient individually, based on blood glucose levels and response to the drug. The recommended dosage range is 0.5 to 4 mg taken 15 to 30 minutes before meals. Repaglinide may be taken before meals 2, 3, or 4 times a day depending on the patient's meal pattern. The maximum recommended daily dose is 16 mg.

ONSET OF EFFECT
30 to 60 minutes.

DURATION OF ACTION
1 to 2 hours.

DIETARY ADVICE
Doses should be taken 15 to 30 minutes before meals.

STORAGE
Store in a tightly sealed container away from moisture, heat, and direct light.

MISSED DOSE
If you miss a dose, take it with the next meal. Do not double the next dose.

STOPPING THE DRUG
Do not stop taking the drug without the approval of your doctor.

≣ SIDE EFFECTS ≣

SERIOUS
Hypoglycemia (blood sugar levels that are too low), resulting in shakiness, headache, cold sweats, anxiety, and changes in mental state. Immediately ingest food or drink containing sugar. Inform your doctor about the frequency and timing of hypoglycemic events.

COMMON
Increased incidence of upper respiratory or sinus infection, headache, back pain, joint pain, diarrhea.

LESS COMMON
Constipation, indigestion, urinary tract infection, mild allergic reaction.

PROLONGED USE
Prolonged use increases the risk of adverse effects. Periodic physical examinations and blood tests to monitor glucose levels are needed.

▼ PRECAUTIONS

Over 60: Older patients may be more susceptible to adverse effects, especially hypoglycemia.

Driving and Hazardous Work: Caution is advised until you have reached a stable dosing regimen that does not produce episodes of hypoglycemia.

Alcohol: Limit alcohol intake; hypoglycemia is more likely to occur after the consumption of alcohol.

Pregnancy: Repaglinide is not usually given during pregnancy. Insulin is the treatment of choice for pregnant women with diabetes.

Breast Feeding: Repaglinide may pass into breast milk; consult your doctor for advice.

Infants and Children: Safety and effectiveness of repaglinide has not been established.

Special Concerns: Follow your doctor's advice about diet, exercise, and weight control carefully. These aspects of treatment are just as essential to the proper control of diabetes as taking the medication. Be sure to carry at all times some form of medical identification that indicates you have diabetes and that lists all of the drugs you are taking.

OVERDOSE
Symptoms: Excessive hunger, nausea, anxiety, cold sweats, drowsiness, rapid heartbeat, weakness, changes in mental state, loss of consciousness (indications of hypoglycemia). Overdose is most likely to occur when caloric intake is deficient, following or during more exercise than usual, or after consuming more than a small amount of alcohol.

What to Do: Call your doctor, emergency medical services (EMS), or local hospital immediately.

▼ INTERACTIONS

DRUG INTERACTIONS
Consult your doctor if you are taking antifungal agents such as ketoconazole or miconazole; also, antibiotics, rifampin, barbiturates, carbamazepine, aspirin or other NSAIDs, sulfonamides, chloramphenicol, probenecid, MAO inhibitors, beta-blockers, diuretics, corticosteroids, phenothiazines, estrogens, oral contraceptives, phenytoin, calcium channel blockers, sympathomimetics, or isoniazid.

FOOD INTERACTIONS
A special diet is essential for proper control of blood glucose levels.

DISEASE INTERACTIONS
Do not use repaglinide if you have type 1 diabetes mellitus. Use of repaglinide may cause complications in patients with impaired liver or kidney function, since these organs are both involved in removing the medication from the body.

RIMANTADINE HYDROCHLORIDE

Available in: Syrup, tablets
Available OTC? No   **As Generic?** No
Drug Class: Antiviral

▼ USAGE INFORMATION

WHY IT'S PRESCRIBED
To prevent or treat type A influenza.

HOW IT WORKS
Rimantadine interferes with the activity of the virus's genetic material, blocking an essential step in the the process of viral replication. The drug affects only certain susceptible strains of the influenza type A virus.

▼ DOSAGE GUIDELINES

RANGE AND FREQUENCY
Adults and children age 10 years and older: 100 mg, 2 times a day, or 200 mg once a day. Children up to age 10: 2.3 mg per lb of body weight, once a day; the dose should not exceed a total of 150 mg daily. Frail, older adults or those with impaired liver or kidney function: 100 mg once a day. The drug should be continued for about 7 days.

ONSET OF EFFECT
Unknown. For prevention of the flu, take rimantadine prior to or immediately after exposure to someone who has influenza.

DURATION OF ACTION
Unknown.

DIETARY ADVICE
Take it on an empty stomach at least 1 hour before or 2 hours after a meal.

STORAGE
Store in a tightly sealed container away from heat and direct light. Do not allow the syrup to freeze.

MISSED DOSE
Take it as soon as you remember. If it is near the time for the next dose, skip the missed dose and resume your regular dosage schedule. Do not double the next dose.

STOPPING THE DRUG
It is important to take rimantadine for the full treatment period as prescribed, whether for treatment or prevention of influenza. If you have the flu, do not stop taking the drug before the scheduled end of therapy even if you begin to feel better, as this may lead to a relapse.

PROLONGED USE
If your symptoms do not improve or if they become worse in a few days, you should consult your doctor. You should see your doctor regularly for tests and examinations if you take this medicine for a prolonged period.

▼ PRECAUTIONS

Over 60: Adverse reactions may be more likely and more severe; a smaller dose is commonly prescribed.

Driving and Hazardous Work: Do not drive or engage in hazardous work until you determine how the medicine affects you.

Alcohol: Avoid alcohol.

Pregnancy: Rimantadine has been shown to cause birth defects in animals. Human studies have not been done. Before you take rimantadine, tell your physician if you are pregnant or if you plan to become pregnant.

Breast Feeding: Rimantadine may pass into breast milk, although it is unknown if this poses any risks to the nursing infant. Consult your doctor for specific advice.

Infants and Children: In tests, rimantadine was not demonstrated to cause unusual side effects or problems in children over 1 year of age. Tests in children under 1 year of age have not been done. Consult your pediatrician for advice.

Special Concerns: Ask your doctor about receiving an influenza vaccine (flu shot) if you have not yet had one. If you are taking the syrup form of rimantadine, use a special measuring spoon to dispense the dose accurately. If the medicine causes insomnia, take it several hours before going to bed.

OVERDOSE
Symptoms: Agitation, heart rhythm abnormalities.

What to Do: An overdose of rimantadine is unlikely to be life-threatening. However, if someone takes a much larger dose than prescribed, call your doctor, emergency medical services (EMS), or the nearest poison control center.

▼ INTERACTIONS

DRUG INTERACTIONS
Other drugs may interact with rimantadine; consult your doctor for specific advice if you are taking any other prescription or over-the-counter medication.

FOOD INTERACTIONS
No known food interactions.

DISEASE INTERACTIONS
Consult your doctor if you have a history of epilepsy or other seizures. Use of the drug may cause complications in patients with liver or kidney disease, since these organs work together to remove the medication from the body.

≡ SIDE EFFECTS ≡

SERIOUS
No serious side effects are associated with rimantadine.

COMMON
Nausea and vomiting, mild diarrhea.

LESS COMMON
Dizziness, trouble concentrating, nervousness, dry mouth, loss of appetite, stomach pain, unusual fatigue, insomnia.

RISEDRONATE SODIUM

Available in: Tablets
Available OTC? No   **As Generic?** No
Drug Class: Bisphosphonate inhibitor of bone resorption

▼ USAGE INFORMATION

WHY IT'S PRESCRIBED
To treat and prevent osteoporosis in postmenopausal women. Also used to prevent and treat steroid-induced osteoporosis in men and women who are either beginning or continuing treatment with steroids (such as prednisone) for chronic diseases. To treat Paget's disease, a disorder characterized by rapid breakdown and reformation of bone, which can lead to fragility and malformation of bones.

HOW IT WORKS
Healthy bones are continuously remodeled (broken down and then reformed); the minerals and other bone components are reabsorbed by one set of cells (osteoclasts) and replaced by another set of cells to form new bone. Risedronate suppresses the activity of osteoclasts; consequently, the breakdown of bone tissue occurs more slowly than the laying down of new bone. As a result, bone density and strength are preserved.

▼ DOSAGE GUIDELINES

RANGE AND FREQUENCY
For treatment and prevention of osteoporosis (both postmenopausal and steroid-induced): 5 mg a day. For Paget's disease: 30 mg once a day for 2 months.

ONSET OF EFFECT
Unknown.

DURATION OF ACTION
Unknown.

DIETARY ADVICE
Take risedronate with a full glass of plain water. Taking the drug with any food or beverage (including mineral water) other than plain water is likely to reduce the absorption of the drug from the intestine. Take the tablets at least 30 minutes before the first food or drink of the day (other than plain water). The drug must be taken in an upright position. Maintain adequate vitamin D and calcium intake; however, vitamin or mineral supplements should be taken no sooner than 2 hours after taking risedronate.

STORAGE
Store in a tightly sealed container away from moisture, heat, and direct light.

MISSED DOSE
If you miss a dose on one day, do not double the dose the next day. Resume your regular dosage schedule.

STOPPING THE DRUG
Take it as prescribed for the full treatment period. The decision to stop taking the drug should be made in consultation with your physician.

PROLONGED USE
For Paget's disease: Risedronate is usually prescribed for a 2-month course of therapy. A second round of treatment may be considered after this 2 month period. Consult your doctor.

▼ PRECAUTIONS

Over 60: No special problems are expected.

Driving and Hazardous Work: Do not drive or engage in hazardous work until you determine how the medicine affects you.

Alcohol: No special precautions are necessary.

Pregnancy: Consult your doctor about whether the benefits of taking the medicine outweigh the potential risks to the unborn child.

Breast Feeding: Risedronate may pass into breast milk; caution is advised. Consult your doctor for specific advice about your particular situation.

Infants and Children: Safety and effectiveness have not been established for children under age 18.

Special Concerns: Remain upright for at least 30 minutes after taking this medication. If you develop symptoms of esophageal disease (such as difficulty or pain when swallowing; chest pain, specifically behind the sternum; or severe or persistent heartburn), contact your doctor before continuing risedronate.

OVERDOSE
Symptoms: No cases of overdose have been reported.

What to Do: If someone takes a much larger dose than prescribed, call your doctor, emergency medical services (EMS), or a poison control center.

▼ INTERACTIONS

DRUG INTERACTIONS
Antacids that contain calcium, aluminum, or magnesium, if needed, should be taken no sooner than 2 hours after taking risedronate.

FOOD INTERACTIONS
No known food interactions, although risedronate works best when taken on an empty stomach.

DISEASE INTERACTIONS
Kidney impairment or a gastrointestinal disease may increase the risk of side effects. Low blood calcium levels and vitamin D deficiency must be treated before using risedronate.

≡ SIDE EFFECTS ≡

SERIOUS
Serious side effects are rare and may include chest pain, swelling of the arms, legs, face, lips, tongue, or throat.

COMMON
Flu-like symptoms, diarrhea, abdominal pain, nausea, constipation, joint pain, headache, dizziness, skin rash.

LESS COMMON
Weakness, growth of tumors, belching, bone pain, leg cramps, muscle weakness, bronchitis, sinus infection, ringing in the ears, dry eye.

RISPERIDONE

Available in: Tablets, oral solution
Available OTC? No   **As Generic?** No
Drug Class: Antipsychotic

▼ USAGE INFORMATION

WHY IT'S PRESCRIBED
To treat psychotic conditions (severe mental disorders characterized by distorted thoughts, perceptions, and emotions), such as schizophrenia.

HOW IT WORKS
While the exact mechanism of action of risperidone is unknown, it appears to alter the activity of certain chemicals in the central nervous system to produce a tranquilizing and antipsychotic effect.

▼ DOSAGE GUIDELINES

RANGE AND FREQUENCY
Adults and teenagers–2 to 6 mg a day in 1 or 2 divided doses. Dosage may be adjusted by your doctor, if needed, at intervals of not less than one week. Older adults–To start, 0.5 mg, 2 times a day; may be increased to 3 mg a day.

ONSET OF EFFECT
Sedation may occur within minutes, but onset of antipsychotic effect may take hours to occur or may not occur until days or weeks after the beginning of therapy.

DURATION OF ACTION
At least 12 to 24 hours, although effects may persist for several days.

DIETARY ADVICE
No special restrictions.

STORAGE
Store in a tightly sealed container away from moisture, heat, and direct light.

MISSED DOSE
Take it as soon as you remember. However, if it is near the time for the next dose, skip the missed dose and resume your regular dosage schedule. Do not double the next dose.

STOPPING THE DRUG
The decision to stop taking the drug should be made in consultation with your doctor.

PROLONGED USE
Prolonged use may lead to tardive dyskinesia (involuntary movements of the jaw, lips, tongue, and, in rare cases, the arms, legs, hands, or body). Consult your doctor about the need for follow-up evaluations and tests if you must take this drug for an extended period.

▼ PRECAUTIONS

Over 60: Adverse reactions may be more likely and more severe in older patients.

Driving and Hazardous Work: Do not drive or engage in hazardous work until you determine how the medicine affects you.

Alcohol: Avoid alcohol.

Pregnancy: Adequate studies have not been done. Before you take risperidone, tell your doctor if you are pregnant or plan to become pregnant.

Breast Feeding: It is not known if risperidone passes into breast milk; caution is advised. Consult your doctor for specific advice.

Infants and Children: Risperidone is not commonly prescribed for patients under 18 years of age.

Special Concerns: Avoid prolonged exposure to high temperatures or hot climates. Drink plenty of fluids and stay cool in the summertime. Avoid overexposure to sunlight until you determine if the drug heightens your skin's sensitivity to ultraviolet light.

OVERDOSE
Symptoms: Drowsiness, rapid heartbeat, low blood pressure, seizures.

What to Do: Call your doctor, emergency medical services (EMS), or the nearest poison control center immediately.

▼ INTERACTIONS

DRUG INTERACTIONS
Other drugs may interact with risperidone. Consult your doctor for advice if you are taking an antidepressant, bromocriptine, carbamazepine, clozapine, high blood pressure medication, levodopa, pergolide, or any medications that depress the central nervous system, including antihistamines, cold remedies, decongestants, and tranquilizers.

FOOD INTERACTIONS
No known food interactions.

DISEASE INTERACTIONS
Consult your doctor if you have Parkinson's disease or any movement disorder, glaucoma, epilepsy, liver disease, kidney disease, heart disease.

☰ SIDE EFFECTS ☰

SERIOUS
Rapid heartbeat, profuse sweating, seizures, difficulty breathing, neck stiffness, swelling of the tongue, difficulty swallowing. Also a rare condition can develop called neuroleptic malignant syndrome, characterized by stiffness or spasms of the muscles, high fever, and confusion or disorientation. Call your doctor immediately.

COMMON
Nausea, reduced perspiration, dry mouth, blurred vision, drowsiness, shaking of the hands, muscle stiffness, stooped posture.

LESS COMMON
Difficult urination, menstrual irregularities, breast pain or swelling, unexpected weight gain, uncontrolled movements of the tongue, fever, chills, sore throat, unusual bruising or bleeding, heart palpitations, skin rash, itching, increased sensitivity of the skin to sunlight.

RIVASTIGMINE TARTRATE

Available in: Capsules, oral solution
Available OTC? No   **As Generic?** No
Drug Class: Reversible cholinesterase inhibitor

▼ USAGE INFORMATION

WHY IT'S PRESCRIBED
To treat mild to moderate Alzheimer's disease.

HOW IT WORKS
The exact mechanism of action is unknown. However, rivastigmine is believed to work by inhibiting acetyl-cholinesterase enzymes, which reduces the breakdown of acetylcholine, a brain chemical crucial to memory. An acetylcholine deficiency is thought to result in the severe memory loss associated with Alzheimer's disease.

▼ DOSAGE GUIDELINES

RANGE AND FREQUENCY
To start, 1.5 mg twice a day. After two weeks of treatment, your doctor may increase the dose to 3 mg twice a day. The dose may be further increased at no less than 2-week intervals to 4.5 mg twice a day and then to the maximum dose of 6 mg twice a day, if tolerated.

ONSET OF EFFECT
Unknown.

DURATION OF ACTION
Unknown.

DIETARY ADVICE
Rivastigmine should be taken with meals in the morning and evening. The oral solution may be swallowed directly from the syringe or mixed with a small glass of water, cold fruit juice, or soda.

STORAGE
Store in a tightly sealed container away from moisture, heat, and direct light. Do not freeze the oral solution.

MISSED DOSE
Take it as soon as you remember, unless the time for your next scheduled dose is within the next 2 hours. If so, do not take the missed dose. Take your next scheduled dose at the proper time and resume your regular dosage schedule. Do not double the next dose. If therapy has been interrupted for several days or longer, consult your doctor.

STOPPING THE DRUG
The decision to stop taking the drug should be made in consultation with your doctor.

PROLONGED USE
No problems are expected with long-term use.

▼ PRECAUTIONS

Over 60: No special advice.

Driving and Hazardous Work: Do not drive or engage in hazardous work until you determine how the medicine affects you.

Alcohol: Avoid alcohol while using this medication.

Pregnancy: In some animal studies, large doses of rivastigmine were shown to cause problems. Before you take rivastigmine, tell your doctor if you are pregnant or plan to become pregnant.

Breast Feeding: It is not known whether rivastigmine passes into breast milk; caution is advised. Consult your doctor for specific advice.

Infants and Children: Rivastigmine is not intended for use in children.

Special Concerns: Before you have any surgery or dental or emergency treatment, tell the doctor or dentist in charge that you are taking rivastigmine. Rivastigmine will not cure Alzheimer's disease and will not stop the disease from getting worse, but it will improve cognitive ability of some patients. Caretakers should be instructed in the correct way to administer the oral solution of rivastigmine.

OVERDOSE
Symptoms: Severe nausea, vomiting, increased salivation, sweating, slow heartbeat, low blood pressure, irregular breathing, unconsciousness, increased muscle weakness, and even death.

What to Do: Call your doctor, emergency medical services (EMS), or the nearest poison control center immediately.

▼ INTERACTIONS

DRUG INTERACTIONS
NSAIDs (nonsteroidal anti-inflammatory drugs) may increase the risk of peptic ulcer or gastrointestinal bleeding when taken with rivastigmine.

FOOD INTERACTIONS
No known food interactions.

DISEASE INTERACTIONS
Caution is advised when taking rivastigmine. Consult your doctor if you have asthma, epilepsy or a history of seizures, heart problems, intestinal blockage, stomach or duodenal ulcer, liver disease, or urinary problems.

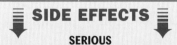

≡ SIDE EFFECTS ≡

SERIOUS
Possible gastrointestinal bleeding. No other serious side effects are associated with the use of rivastigmine.

COMMON
Significant nausea, vomiting, loss of appetite, and weight loss. Other common side effects include heartburn, weakness, dizziness, diarrhea, abdominal pain.

LESS COMMON
Increased sweating, fatigue, malaise, headache, drowsiness, tremor, flatulence, insomnia, depression, anxiety.

ROFECOXIB

Available in: Tablets, oral suspension
Available OTC? No   **As Generic?** No
Drug Class: Nonsteroidal anti-inflammatory drug (NSAID)/COX-2 inhibitor

▼ USAGE INFORMATION

WHY IT'S PRESCRIBED
For the management of chronic osteoarthritis pain. Rofecoxib is also used in the short-term relief of acute general and menstrual pain.

HOW IT WORKS
By inhibiting the activity of the enzyme cyclooxygenase-2 (COX-2), rofecoxib reduces the synthesis of prostaglandins that play a role in causing arthritis pain and inflammation. It does not inhibit the activity of COX-1, the enzyme involved in the synthesis of prostaglandins that help protect against stomach ulcers and other health problems.

▼ DOSAGE GUIDELINES

RANGE AND FREQUENCY
For osteoarthritis: To start, 12.5 mg once a day. Your doctor may increase the dose to 25 mg once a day if adequate relief is not achieved with the lower dose. For acute or menstrual pain: 50 mg once a day. To minimize potential gastrointestinal side effects, the lowest effective dose should be used for the shortest possible time. Use of rofecoxib for more than 5 days for relief of acute pain has not been studied.

ONSET OF EFFECT
For acute pain: Within 45 minutes. For osteoarthritis: Unknown.

DURATION OF ACTION
Unknown.

DIETARY ADVICE
Rofecoxib may be taken with or without food.

STORAGE
Store in a tightly sealed container away from moisture, heat, and direct light. Do not refrigerate the oral suspension.

MISSED DOSE
If you do not remember until the next day, skip the missed dose and resume your regular dosage schedule. Do not double the next dose.

STOPPING THE DRUG
The decision to stop taking the drug should be made in consultation with your doctor.

PROLONGED USE
The risk of gastrointestinal side effects may be increased with extended use.

▼ PRECAUTIONS

Over 60: No special problems are expected. Therapy should be started with the lowest recommended dose.

Driving and Hazardous Work: No special problems are expected.

Alcohol: Avoid alcohol when using this medication because it increases the risk of stomach irritation.

Pregnancy: Discuss with your doctor the relative risks and benefits of using this drug while you are pregnant. Do not use rofecoxib during the last trimester.

Breast Feeding: Rofecoxib may pass into breast milk; caution is advised. Consult your doctor for advice on whether to discontinue nursing or discontinue the drug.

Infants and Children: The safety and effectiveness of this drug have not been established for children under the age of 18.

OVERDOSE
Symptoms: No cases of overdose have been reported. Symptoms may include lethargy, drowsiness, nausea, vomiting, abdominal pain, black, tarry stools, breathing difficulty, and coma.

What to Do: If you suspect an overdose or if someone takes a much larger dose than prescribed, call your doctor, emergency medical services (EMS), or the nearest poison control immediately.

▼ INTERACTIONS

DRUG INTERACTIONS
Do not take this drug with aspirin or any other NSAIDs without your doctor's approval. In addition, consult your doctor if you are taking furosemide, ACE inhibitors, methotrexate, lithium, rifampin, or warfarin.

FOOD INTERACTIONS
No known food interactions.

DISEASE INTERACTIONS
Rofecoxib should not be taken by people who have experienced asthma, hives, or allergic-type reactions after taking aspirin or other NSAIDs. Consult your doctor if you have any of the following: bleeding problems, inflammation or ulcers of the stomach and intestines, asthma, high blood pressure, or heart failure. Use of the drug may cause complications in patients with liver or kidney disease, since these organs both work to remove the medication from the body.

≣ SIDE EFFECTS ≣

SERIOUS
Stomach ulcers. Black, tarry stools may signal stomach bleeding. Symptoms of liver disease (nausea, fatigue, lethargy, itching, yellowish discoloration of the eyes or skin, fluid retention). Call your doctor immediately.

COMMON
Indigestion, mild swelling, heartburn, nausea, increased blood pressure.

LESS COMMON
Flatulence, sore throat, upper respiratory tract infection, back pain, and mild abdominal pain.

ROSIGLITAZONE MALEATE

Available in: Tablets
Available OTC? No   **As Generic?** No
Drug Class: Thiazolidinedione/antidiabetic agent

▼ USAGE INFORMATION

WHY IT'S PRESCRIBED
As a single therapeutic agent or as an adjunct (supplemental) therapy to metformin to control blood glucose (sugar) levels in patients with type 2 (non-insulin-dependent) diabetes.

HOW IT WORKS
Rosiglitazone increases the body's sensitivity and response to its own insulin.

▼ DOSAGE GUIDELINES

RANGE AND FREQUENCY
To start, 4 mg, once a day (in the morning) or in two divided doses (in the morning and evening). Patients not responding adequately to 4 mg a day after 12 weeks may have their dose increased by their doctor to 8 mg once a day or in two divided doses.

ONSET OF EFFECT
Within 2 to 4 weeks.

DURATION OF ACTION
Unknown.

DIETARY ADVICE
Rosiglitazone may be taken with or without food.

STORAGE
Store in a tightly sealed container away from moisture, heat, and direct light.

MISSED DOSE
Take it as soon as you remember. If it is near the time for the next dose, skip the missed dose and resume your regular dosage schedule. Do not double the next dose.

STOPPING THE DRUG
The decision to stop taking the drug should be made in consultation with your doctor.

PROLONGED USE
See your doctor regularly for liver function tests if you take rosiglitazone for an extended period.

▼ PRECAUTIONS

Over 60:
No special problems are expected.

Driving and Hazardous Work:
The use of rosiglitazone should not impair your ability to perform such tasks safely.

Alcohol:
Drink alcohol only in moderation.

Pregnancy:
Adequate studies of rosiglitazone use during pregnancy have not been done. In general, insulin is the treatment of choice for controlling blood glucose levels during pregnancy. Rosiglitazone should not be used during pregnancy unless your doctor believes the potential benefit justifies the potential risk to the fetus. Rosiglitazone may stimulate ovulation in premenopausal women who have stopped ovulating. Contraception may be advised.

Breast Feeding:
Rosiglitazone may pass into breast milk; do not use it while nursing.

Infants and Children:
The safety and effectiveness of rosiglitazone have not been established in children.

Special Concerns:
Another thiazolidinedione drug, troglitazone, has been associated with rare, serious, and sometimes fatal, liver-related side effects. Although no similar side effects have been reported for rosiglitazone, liver function tests are often recommended just prior to treatment, every two months for the first year, and periodically thereafter. If you develop unexplained symptoms of liver dysfunction, such as nausea, vomiting, abdominal pain, fatigue, loss of appetite, or dark urine, call your doctor immediately. It is important to follow your doctor's advice on diet, exercise, and other measures to help control your diabetes.

OVERDOSE

Symptoms: No specific ones have been reported.

What to Do: While no cases of overdose have been reported, if someone takes a much larger dose than prescribed, call your doctor, emergency medical services (EMS), or the nearest poison control center immediately.

▼ INTERACTIONS

DRUG INTERACTIONS
No known drug interactions.

FOOD INTERACTIONS
No known food interactions.

DISEASE INTERACTIONS
Rosiglitazone should not be taken by those with type 1 diabetes or for the treatment of diabetic ketoacidosis. Caution is advised if you have edema or heart failure. Consult your doctor prior to using rosiglitazone if you have any type of liver abnormality.

⏬ SIDE EFFECTS ⏬

SERIOUS
No serious side effects have been associated with rosiglitazone.

COMMON
Weight gain.

LESS COMMON
Upper respiratory tract infection, headache, edema (swelling).

SALMETEROL XINAFOATE

Available in: Inhalation aerosol, inhalation powder
Available OTC? No **As Generic?** No
Drug Class: Bronchodilator/sympathomimetic

▼ USAGE INFORMATION

WHY IT'S PRESCRIBED
Salmeterol is used to dilate air passages in the lungs that have become narrowed as a result of disease or inflammation. This drug is used to treat asthma and chronic obstructive pulmonary disease.

HOW IT WORKS
Salmeterol widens constricted airways in the lungs by relaxing the smooth muscles that surround the bronchial passages.

▼ DOSAGE GUIDELINES

RANGE AND FREQUENCY
This drug may be used when needed to relieve breathing difficulty. Adults and teens— By inhalation aerosol: Two inhalations twice daily, approximately 12 hours apart. By inhalation powder: One inhalation twice a day, approximately 12 hours apart.

ONSET OF EFFECT
Within 15 minutes.

DURATION OF ACTION
Up to 12 hours.

DIETARY ADVICE
Maintain your usual food and fluid intake. Increase fluids if you have a fever or diarrhea, in hot weather, or during exercise.

STORAGE
Store in a tightly sealed container away from moisture, heat, and direct light.

MISSED DOSE
Take it as soon as you remember. If it is near the time for the next dose, skip the missed dose and resume your regular dosage schedule. Do not double the next dose.

STOPPING THE DRUG
The decision to stop taking the drug should be made by your doctor.

PROLONGED USE
It may not be necessary to finish the recommended course of therapy. Consult your doctor.

▼ PRECAUTIONS

Over 60: Adverse reactions may be more likely and more severe in older patients.

Driving and Hazardous Work: Do not drive or engage in hazardous work until you determine how the medicine affects you.

Alcohol: No special warnings.

Pregnancy: Safety of use during pregnancy has not been established. Consult your doctor.

Breast Feeding: It is not known if salmeterol passes into breast milk. Mothers who wish to breast-feed while taking this drug should discuss the matter with their doctor.

Infants and Children: Use of salmeterol inhalation aerosol is not recommended for children younger than 12.

Special Concerns: This medication takes 15 minutes to work. Do not use salmeterol for acute or sudden attacks, or for worsening asthma. Pay heed to any asthma attack or other breathing difficulty that does not improve after your usual rescue treatment. Seek help immediately if you feel your lungs are persistently constricted, if you are using more than the recommended number of treatments or puffs per day, or if you feel a recent attack is somehow different from others. Do not wash the device for the inhalation powder. Keep it dry.

OVERDOSE
Symptoms: Chest pain or heaviness; irregular, fluttering, racing, or pounding heartbeat; dizziness; lightheadedness; severe weakness; fainting; severe headache; muscle tremors or shaking.

What to Do: Call your doctor, emergency medical services (EMS), or the nearest poison control center immediately.

▼ INTERACTIONS

DRUG INTERACTIONS
Consult your doctor for specific advice if you are taking beta-blockers.

FOOD INTERACTIONS
No known food interactions.

DISEASE INTERACTIONS
Consult your doctor if you have a history of any of the following: heart disease or heartbeat irregularities, high blood pressure, anxiety disorders, or a thyroid condition.

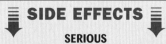 **SIDE EFFECTS**

SERIOUS
Salmeterol may become ineffective if used too often, resulting in more-severe breathing difficulty that does not improve. Signs include persistent wheezing, coughing, or shortness of breath; confusion; bluish color to lips or fingernails; inability to speak. Other side effects include chest pain or heaviness; irregular, racing, fluttering, or pounding heartbeat; lightheadedness; fainting; severe weakness; severe headache.

COMMON
Headache, sore throat, runny or stuffy nose.

LESS COMMON
Abdominal pain, diarrhea, nausea, cough, muscle aches.

SAQUINAVIR

Available in: Capsules
Available OTC? No   **As Generic?** No
Drug Class: Antiviral/protease inhibitor

▼ USAGE INFORMATION

WHY IT'S PRESCRIBED
To treat HIV (human immuno-deficiency virus) infection in combination with other drugs. While not a cure for HIV infection, saquinavir may suppress replication of the virus and delay progression of the disease.

HOW IT WORKS
Saquinavir blocks the activity of a viral protease, an enzyme that is needed by HIV to reproduce. Blocking the protease causes HIV to make copies that cannot infect new cells.

▼ DOSAGE GUIDELINES

RANGE AND FREQUENCY
Adults and teenagers 16 and over: 600 mg, 3 times a day, in combination with other antiretroviral drugs. Higher doses (up to 1,200 mg, 3 times a day) are sometimes used. Lower doses (400 mg,

2 times a day) are used when saquinavir is combined with ritonavir, a similar drug.

ONSET OF EFFECT
Unknown. With most anti-retroviral drugs, an early response can be seen within the first few days of therapy, but the maximum effect may take 12 to 16 weeks.

DURATION OF ACTION
Unknown.

DIETARY ADVICE
It should be taken within 2 hours after a full meal.

STORAGE
Capsules should be refrigerated. If brought to room temperature, store in a tightly sealed container away from heat and direct light and use within 3 months.

MISSED DOSE
Take it as soon as you remember. However, if it is

near the time for the next dose, skip the missed dose and resume your regular dosage schedule. Do not double the next dose.

STOPPING THE DRUG
The decision to stop taking the drug should be made in consultation with your doctor.

PROLONGED USE
See your doctor regularly for tests and examinations.

▼ PRECAUTIONS

Over 60: No special studies have been done.

Driving and Hazardous Work: Avoid such activities until you determine how the medicine affects you.

Alcohol: Avoid alcohol if liver function is impaired.

Pregnancy: Human studies have not been done. Nevertheless, the drug is being used increasingly in combination with other antiretroviral drugs to treat pregnant HIV-infected women.

Breast Feeding: It is unknown whether saquinavir passes into breast milk; however, women with HIV should not breast-feed, to avoid transmitting the virus to an uninfected child.

Infants and Children: The safety and effectiveness in children under the age of 16 have not been established.

Special Concerns: Use of saquinavir does not eliminate the risk of passing the AIDS virus to other persons. You should take appropriate pre-

ventive measures. If saquinavir increases skin sensitivity to sunlight, wear tightly woven clothing and use sunscreen. Do not substitute one brand of saquinavir for another without consulting your doctor. They are not equal in strength.

OVERDOSE
Symptoms: No cases of overdose have been reported.

What to Do: If you have reason to suspect an overdose, call your doctor, emergency medical services (EMS), or the nearest poison control.

▼ INTERACTIONS

DRUG INTERACTIONS
Saquinavir should not be used at the same time as triazolam, midazolam, "statins" (cholesterol-lowering drugs), or ergotamine/belladonna alkaloids. Consult your doctor if you are taking any other medication, especially rifampin, rifabutin, nevirapine, or sildenafil. Some drugs, such as ketoconazole, delavirdine, ritonavir, and nelfinavir, are used in combination with saquinavir because they increase its blood levels and, possibly, its effectiveness.

FOOD INTERACTIONS
Fatty foods and grapefruit juice enhance the body's absorption of saquinavir. Food may reduce side effects.

DISEASE INTERACTIONS
Consult your doctor if you have any other medical condition. Use of saquinavir may cause complications in patients with liver disease, because this organ works to remove the medication from the body.

≡ SIDE EFFECTS ≡

SERIOUS
High blood sugar (diabetes) has occurred in patients taking drugs of this class, although a cause-and-effect relationship has not been established. Contact your doctor if you develop increased thirst or excessive urination. Other side effects include: psychosis, thoughts of suicide, and lung disease.

COMMON
Burning, prickling, numbness, or tingling sensations in various parts of the body, confusion, seizures, headache, loss of muscle coordination, diarrhea, abdominal discomfort, nausea, skin rash, increased skin sensitivity to light, general weakness.

LESS COMMON
Loss of appetite, kidney stones, urinary tract bleeding, hair loss, swelling of the eyelid, nail problems, night sweats, small bump-like growths on the skin, impotence, anxiety attack, leg cramps.

SERTRALINE HYDROCHLORIDE

Available in: Capsules, tablets
Available OTC? No   **As Generic?** No
Drug Class: Selective serotonin reuptake inhibitor (SSRI) antidepressant

▼ USAGE INFORMATION

WHY IT'S PRESCRIBED
To treat symptoms of major depression, obsessive-compulsive disorder, and panic disorder.

HOW IT WORKS
Sertraline affects levels of serotonin, a hormone-like brain chemical that is thought to be linked to changes in a person's mood, emotions, and mental state.

▼ DOSAGE GUIDELINES

RANGE AND FREQUENCY
Adults: To start, 50 mg once a day, in the morning or in the evening. Dose may be gradually increased by your doctor to 200 mg a day. Older adults: To start, 12.5 to 25 mg once a day. Dose may be gradually increased by your doctor to 200 mg a day. Children ages 6 to 12: To start, 25 mg once a day. Children ages 13 to 17: To start, 50 mg once a day. Dose may be gradually increased by your pediatrician.

ONSET OF EFFECT
1 to 4 weeks.

DURATION OF ACTION
Unknown.

DIETARY ADVICE
No special restrictions.

STORAGE
Store in a tightly sealed container away from moisture, heat, and direct light.

MISSED DOSE
Take it as soon as you remember. If it is near the time for the next dose, skip the missed dose and resume your regular dosage schedule. Do not double the next dose.

STOPPING THE DRUG
Take it as prescribed for the full treatment period. When it is time to stop therapy, your dosage will be tapered gradually by your doctor.

PROLONGED USE
Usual course of therapy lasts 6 months to 1 year; some patients benefit from additional therapy.

▼ PRECAUTIONS

Over 60: No special problems have been reported.

Driving and Hazardous Work: Use caution when driving or engaging in hazardous work until you determine how the medicine affects you.

Alcohol: Avoid alcohol.

Pregnancy: Adequate studies of sertraline use during pregnancy have not been done. Before you take sertraline, tell your doctor if you are currently pregnant or if you plan to become pregnant.

Breast Feeding: It is not known whether sertraline passes into breast milk; caution is advised. Consult your doctor for specific advice.

Infants and Children: The safety and effectiveness of the use of sertraline in children under age 6 have not been established.

Special Concerns: Take sertraline at least 6 hours before bedtime to prevent insomnia, unless it causes drowsiness.

OVERDOSE

Symptoms: Sleepiness, nausea, vomiting, rapid heartbeat, anxiety, dilated pupils.

What to Do: Call your doctor, emergency medical services (EMS), or the nearest poison control center immediately.

▼ INTERACTIONS

DRUG INTERACTIONS
Sertraline and MAO inhibitors should not be used within 14 days of each other. Very serious side effects such as myoclonus (uncontrolled muscle spasms), hyperthermia (excessive rise in body temperature), and extreme stiffness may result. The following drugs may also interact with sertraline; consult your doctor for advice if you are taking cimetidine, digitoxin, warfarin, sumatriptan, naratriptan, zolmitriptan, oral antidiabetic agents (such as tolbutamide), tricyclic antidepressants, or any prescription or over-the-counter drugs that depress the central nervous system (including antihistamines, barbiturates, sedatives, cough medicines, and decongestants).

FOOD INTERACTIONS
No known food interactions.

DISEASE INTERACTIONS
Consult your doctor if you have a history of alcohol or drug abuse. Use of sertraline may cause complications in patients with liver or kidney disease, since these organs work together to remove the medication from the body.

≣ SIDE EFFECTS ≣

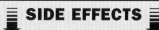

SERIOUS
Skin rash, hives, or itching; unusually fast speech, fever, extreme agitation. Call your doctor immediately.

COMMON
Insomnia, diarrhea, sexual dysfunction, decrease in appetite, weight loss, drowsiness, headache, dry mouth, stomach cramps, abdominal pain, gas, trembling, fatigue, loss of initiative.

LESS COMMON
Anxiety, agitation, increased appetite, blurred or altered vision, constipation, heartbeat irregularities, flushing, unusual feeling of warmth, vomiting.

SIBUTRAMINE HYDROCHLORIDE MONOHYDRATE

BRAND NAME
Meridia

Available in: Capsules
Available OTC? No   **As Generic?** No
Drug Class: Inhibitor of neurotransmitter reuptake

▼ USAGE INFORMATION

WHY IT'S PRESCRIBED
To aid in the medical management of obesity in conjunction with a carefully supervised diet and exercise program. Sibutramine is only recommended for overweight people with a body mass index (BMI) greater than 30 or greater than 27 in people with other medical risk factors such as diabetes or high blood pressure.

HOW IT WORKS
Sibutramine affects the appetite control center in the brain by inhibiting the reuptake of neurotransmitters like serotonin. The resulting increase in their availability suppresses appetite.

▼ DOSAGE GUIDELINES

RANGE AND FREQUENCY
To start, 10 mg once a day. Dose may be increased up to 15 mg once a day.

ONSET OF EFFECT
Significant weight changes may take several weeks or months to develop.

DURATION OF ACTION
When taking sibutramine regularly, most people lose weight within the first six months. Weight loss is maintained for duration of therapy.

DIETARY ADVICE
Can be taken with a meal or on an empty stomach.

STORAGE
Store in a tightly sealed container away from moisture, heat, and direct light.

MISSED DOSE
If you miss a dose one day, do not double the dose the next day. Resume your regular dosage schedule.

STOPPING THE DRUG
The decision to stop taking the drug should be made in consultation with your doctor.

PROLONGED USE
The safety and effectiveness have not been determined beyond 2 years of use.

▼ PRECAUTIONS

Over 60: No specific studies have been done.

Driving and Hazardous Work: Do not drive or engage in hazardous work until you determine how the medicine affects you.

Alcohol: Sibutramine may increase the sedative effects of alcohol. Consult you doctor for specific advice.

Pregnancy: Sibutramine should not be used by pregnant women. Before taking sibutramine, tell your doctor if you are pregnant or plan to become pregnant.

Breast Feeding: Sibutramine should not be used by nursing mothers.

Infants and Children: Children under the age of 16 should not use sibutramine.

Special Concerns: Although no serious adverse reactions have been reported with sibutramine (at the time of publication), other diet drugs have been associated with an increased risk of potentially grave cardiovascular and cardiopulmonary problems. If you experience any unusual or disturbing adverse effects, stop taking sibutramine and call your doctor immediately.

OVERDOSE
Symptoms: No cases of overdose have been reported.

What to Do: If someone takes a much larger dose than prescribed or a child swallows the drug, call your doctor, emergency medical services (EMS), or the nearest poison control immediately.

▼ INTERACTIONS

DRUG INTERACTIONS
You should not take sibutramine if you take MAO inhibitors, other weight loss medications, medications for depression, migraine medications, dihydroergotamine, meperidine, fentanyl, pentazocine, dextromethorphan (found in many cough medicines), lithium, or tryptophan. Sibutramine may interact with ketoconazole, erythromycin, over-the-counter cough and cold medications, allergy medicines, and decongestants. Consult your doctor for specific advice.

FOOD INTERACTIONS
No known food interactions.

DISEASE INTERACTIONS
You should not take sibutramine if you have coronary artery disease, angina, cardiac arrhythmia, history of heart attack, congestive heart failure, history of stroke, anorexia nervosa, history of seizures, or narrow angle glaucoma. Sibutramine can substantially raise blood pressure in some patients. Use of sibutramine may cause complications in patients with liver or kidney disease, since these organs work together to remove the medication from the body. Consult your doctor if you have a history of migraines, mental depression, Parkinson's disease, thyroid disorders, osteoporosis, gallbladder disease, a major eating disorder (such as bulimia nervosa), or any other medical problem.

⬇ SIDE EFFECTS ⬇

SERIOUS
No serious side effects have yet been reported. However, if you experience symptoms such as shortness of breath or chest pain that were not present before taking the medication, call your doctor.

COMMON
Dry mouth, constipation, insomnia.

LESS COMMON
Headache, increased sweating, increased blood pressure and heart rate.

SILDENAFIL CITRATE

Available in: Tablets
Available OTC? No **As Generic?** No
Drug Class: Phosphodiesterase type 5 inhibitor

▼ USAGE INFORMATION

WHY IT'S PRESCRIBED
To treat erectile dysfunction (impotence), which may occur in association with athero-sclerosis, vascular disease or other circulatory problems, diabetes, kidney disease, hormonal abnormalities, neurological disease or injury, severe depression or other psychological difficulties.

HOW IT WORKS
Sildenafil selectively inhibits the action of an enzyme (phosphodiesterase type 5) that breaks down a substance that relaxes smooth muscles and permits blood flow that engorges the columns of erectile tissue in the penis. Unlike other treatments for erectile dysfunction, which produce erections with or without sexual arousal, silde-nafil allows the patient to respond naturally to sexual stimulation.

▼ DOSAGE GUIDELINES

RANGE AND FREQUENCY
The recommended dose for most patients is 50 mg, taken approximately 1 hour before sexual activity. The dose may be increased to no more than 100 mg, or decreased to 25 mg. Your doctor will help to determine the correct dose. Do not take the drug more than once in a 24-hour period.

ONSET OF EFFECT
Within 30 minutes to 4 hours.

DURATION OF ACTION
Unknown.

DIETARY ADVICE
No special recommendations.

STORAGE
Store in a tightly sealed container away from moisture, heat, and direct light.

MISSED DOSE
Not applicable.

STOPPING THE DRUG
Not applicable.

PROLONGED USE
Sildenafil treats but does not cure erectile dysfunction. Patients must continue using sildenafil to maintain its bene-fit; lifelong therapy may be warranted.

▼ PRECAUTIONS

Over 60: No special prob-lems are expected.

Driving and Hazardous Work: This drug should not impair your ability to perform such tasks safely.

Alcohol: No special precau-tions are necessary. However, alcohol is known to decrease sexual function.

Pregnancy: Not applicable; sildenafil is not approved for use by women.

Breast Feeding: Not applica-ble; sildenafil is not approved for use by women.

Infants and Children: Not applicable; sildenafil is not to be used by children.

Special Concerns: Sildenafil does not offer any protection against sexually transmitted dis-eases. Appropriate measures (for example, using condoms) should be taken to ensure adequate protection against sexually transmitted diseases, including infection with the human immunodeficiency virus (HIV). Sildenafil should be taken only by men who have been clinically evaluated for and diagnosed with erec-tile dysfunction by a doctor.

OVERDOSE
Symptoms: No cases of over-dose have been reported.

What to Do: An overdose with sildenafil is unlikely. If someone takes a much larger dose than prescribed, call your doctor.

▼ INTERACTIONS

DRUG INTERACTIONS
Sildenafil can enhance the action of nitrates (such as nitroglycerin, which is used to treat episodes of angina), causing potentially dangerous decreases in blood pressure. Therefore, sildenafil should not be used by patients taking nitrates of any kind. Use of sildenafil in conjunc-tion with other erectile-dysfunction medications is not recommended. Consult your doctor if you are taking protease inhibitors such as ritonavir and saquinavir, which may affect levels of sildenafil in the blood.

FOOD INTERACTIONS
No known food interactions.

DISEASE INTERACTIONS
Caution is advised when tak-ing sildenafil. Consult your doctor if you have a history of any of the following: high or very low blood pressure; structural deformity of the penis; a bleeding disorder; heart attack, stroke, or life-threatening arrhythmia within the past six months; heart failure; coronary heart dis-ease; retinitis pigmentosa; peptic ulcer; sickle cell anemia; multiple myeloma; or leukemia.

⬇ SIDE EFFECTS ⬇

SERIOUS
Rarely, a painful or prolonged erection (lasting more than 4 hours) may occur. If erection does not resolve on its own in a reasonable amount of time, seek medical help promptly. If erection does resolve on its own, consult your doctor for specific guidelines. Serious cardiovascular events such as heart attack, cardiac arrhythmias, cerebral hemorrhage, and transient ischemic attack have been reported following the use of sildenafil. However, it is unclear whether these events are due to sildenafil, the presence of preexisting cardiovascular risk factors, to sexual activity, or a combination of these factors.

COMMON
Headache, flushing, indigestion. Such side effects are generally mild to moderate and usually short-lived.

LESS COMMON
Nasal congestion, vision abnormalities, bloodshot or burning eyes, diarrhea, blood in the urine.

SIMVASTATIN

Available in: Tablets
Available OTC? No   **As Generic?** No
Drug Class: Antilipidemic (cholesterol-lowering agent)

▼ USAGE INFORMATION

WHY IT'S PRESCRIBED
To treat high cholesterol. Also used to reduce the risk of stroke or transient ischemic attack ("mini-stroke") in patients with high cholesterol and coronary artery disease. Usually prescribed after the first lines of treatment—diet, weight loss, and exercise—fail to reduce total cholesterol and low-density lipoprotein (LDL) cholesterol to acceptable levels.

HOW IT WORKS
Simvastatin blocks the action of an enzyme required for the manufacture of cholesterol, thereby interfering with its formation. By lowering the amount of cholesterol in the liver cells, simvastatin increases the formation of receptors for low-density lipoprotein (LDL) cholesterol, and thereby reduces blood levels of total and LDL cholesterol. In addition to lowering LDL cholesterol, simvastatin also modestly reduces triglyceride levels and raises HDL (the so-called "good") cholesterol levels in the blood.

▼ DOSAGE GUIDELINES

RANGE AND FREQUENCY
Initial dose is 10 to 40 mg once a day. It may be increased to a maximum of 80 mg per day. Simvastatin is most effective when taken in the evening.

ONSET OF EFFECT
2 to 4 weeks.

DURATION OF ACTION
The effect persists for the duration of therapy.

DIETARY ADVICE
Cholesterol-lowering drugs are only one part of a total program that should include regular exercise and a healthy diet. The American Heart Association publishes a "Healthy Heart" diet, which is recommended.

STORAGE
Store in a tightly sealed container away from heat and direct light.

MISSED DOSE
Take it as soon as you remember. Take your next dose at the proper time and resume your regular dosage

schedule. Do not double the next dose.

STOPPING THE DRUG
The decision to stop taking the drug should be made in consultation with your doctor. Once the medication is discontinued, blood cholesterol is likely to return to original elevated levels.

PROLONGED USE
Side effects are more likely with prolonged use. As you continue with simvastatin, your doctor will periodically order blood tests to evaluate liver function.

▼ PRECAUTIONS

Over 60: No special problems are expected in older patients.

Driving and Hazardous Work: The use of simvastatin should not impair your ability to perform such tasks safely.

Alcohol: No special precautions are necessary.

Pregnancy: Should not be used during pregnancy or by women who plan to become pregnant in the near future.

Breast Feeding: This drug is not recommended for women who are nursing.

Infants and Children: The long-term effects of simvastatin in children have not been determined. It is rarely used in children; consult your pediatrician.

Special Concerns: Important elements of treatment for high cholesterol include

proper diet, weight loss, regular moderate exercise, and the avoidance of certain medications that may increase cholesterol levels. Because simvastatin has potential side effects, it is important that you maintain a recommended healthy diet and cooperate with other treatments your physician may suggest.

OVERDOSE
Symptoms: No specific ones have been reported; overdose is unlikely.

What to Do: Emergency instructions not applicable.

▼ INTERACTIONS

DRUG INTERACTIONS
Consult your doctor if you are taking cyclosporine, gemfibrozil, niacin, antibiotics, especially erythromycin, HIV protease inhibitors, or medications for fungus infections. All of these drugs may increase the risk of myositis (muscle inflammation) when taken with simvastatin and may lead to kidney failure.

FOOD INTERACTIONS
No known food interactions.

DISEASE INTERACTIONS
Consult your doctor if you have liver, kidney, or muscle disease, or a medical history involving organ transplant or recent surgery.

≡ SIDE EFFECTS ≡

⬇ SERIOUS ⬇
Fever, unusual or unexplained muscle aches and tenderness. Call your doctor right away.

COMMON
Side effects occur in only 1% to 2% of patients. They may include constipation or diarrhea, dizziness or lightheadedness, bloating or gas, heartburn, nausea, skin rash, stomach pain, rise in liver enzymes.

LESS COMMON
Insomnia.

SUMATRIPTAN SUCCINATE

Available in: Tablets, injection, nasal spray
Available OTC? No   **As Generic?** No
Drug Class: Antimigraine/antiheadache drug

▼ USAGE INFORMATION

WHY IT'S PRESCRIBED
To treat severe, acute migraine headaches (sumatriptan is not effective against any other kinds of pain or headache). Because of the risk of side effects, sumatriptan is generally used only when other treatments prove ineffective.

HOW IT WORKS
Sumatriptan appears to activate chemical messengers that cause blood vessels in the brain to constrict, thus lessening the effects of a migraine. It not only relieves the pain, but also nausea, vomiting, sensitivity to sound and light, and other symptoms associated with migraines.

▼ DOSAGE GUIDELINES

RANGE AND FREQUENCY
Tablets—A single dose of 25 to 100 mg taken with fluid is generally effective. If the headache returns or there is only partial relief, additional single doses of up to 50 mg may be given at intervals of least 2 hours, but no more than 200 mg should be taken in a 24-hour period. Injection—Initial dose: 6 mg injection. Additional doses: Another 6 mg injection separated by at least one hour. Nasal spray—A single dose of 5, 10, or 20 mg into one nostril. A 10-mg dose may be achieved by administering a 5-mg dose in each nostril. If the headache returns or there is only partial relief, an additional single dose of up to 20 mg may be given at an interval of least 2 hours, but no more than 40 mg should be taken in a 24-hour period.

ONSET OF EFFECT
Tablets: Within 30 minutes. Injection: Within 10 to 20 minutes. Nasal spray: Within 15 to 30 minutes.

DURATION OF ACTION
Unknown, but peak effect occurs within 1 to 4 hours.

DIETARY ADVICE
No special recommendations.

STORAGE
Keep away from heat and direct light; do not allow solution to freeze.

MISSED DOSE
Not applicable.

STOPPING THE DRUG
Consult your doctor before discontinuing sumatriptan.

PROLONGED USE
Consult your doctor if you have used sumatriptan for three migraine episodes and have not had relief, there is no improvement in symptoms after several weeks of use, or migraines increase in severity or frequency.

▼ PRECAUTIONS

Over 60: Sumatriptan is not recommended for use in older patients.

Driving and Hazardous Work: Sumatriptan may cause drowsiness or dizziness. Avoid such activities until you determine how it affects you.

Alcohol: No special warnings; alcohol may trigger or exacerbate migraine headaches.

Pregnancy: Do not use this drug while pregnant.

Breast Feeding: Do not use this drug while nursing.

Infants and Children: Not recommended for children.

Special Concerns: Rare but serious heart-related problems may occur after sumatriptan use. Anyone at risk for unrecognized coronary artery disease—such as postmenopausal women, men over age 40, or those with heart disease risk factors—should have the first dose of sumatriptan administered in a doctor's office. It should not be used by anyone with any symptoms of active heart disease (chest pain or tightness, shortness of breath).

OVERDOSE
Symptoms: No overdoses have been reported.

What to Do: Although overdose is unlikely, if you take a much larger dose than prescribed, call your doctor, emergency medical services (EMS), or the nearest poison control center immediately.

▼ INTERACTIONS

DRUG INTERACTIONS
Do not take sumatriptan within 24 hours of taking any other migraine drug. Consult your doctor for advice if you are taking antidepressants, selective serotonin reuptake inhibitors (SSRIs), or lithium.

FOOD INTERACTIONS
See Dietary Advice.

DISEASE INTERACTIONS
You should not take sumatriptan if you have a history of coronary artery disease, especially angina, heart attack, Prinzmetal's angina, or uncontrolled hypertension. It should be used with caution in patients with liver disease or severe kidney dysfunction.

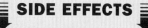 **SIDE EFFECTS**

SERIOUS
Chest pain (mild to severe) or feeling of heaviness or pressure in the chest; wheezing or shortness of breath, and rapid, shallow, or irregular breathing; puffiness or swelling of the eyelids, face or, lips; hives; intense itching. Seek emergency medical assistance immediately.

COMMON
Pain, burning, or redness at injection site; a general feeling of warmth or heat; a feeling of numbness, tightness, or tingling; mild pain of the jaw, mouth, tongue, throat, nose, or sinuses; dizziness; drowsiness; feeling cold or weak; feeling flushed or lightheaded; muscle aches, cramps, or stiffness; nausea or vomiting.

LESS COMMON
Mild chest pain; heaviness or pressure in the chest or neck; anxiety; feeling tired or ill; vision changes.

TACRINE

Cognex

Available in: Capsules
Available OTC? No   **As Generic?** No
Drug Class: Psychotherapeutic; antidementia agent

▼ USAGE INFORMATION

WHY IT'S PRESCRIBED
To treat mild to moderate Alzheimer's disease.

HOW IT WORKS
Tacrine prevents the breakdown of acetylcholine, a brain chemical that is crucial to memory. Acetylcholine deficiency is thought to result in memory loss associated with Alzheimer's disease.

▼ DOSAGE GUIDELINES

RANGE AND FREQUENCY
To start, 10 mg, 4 times a day. The dose may be raised to 40 mg, 4 times a day.

ONSET OF EFFECT
Unknown.

DURATION OF ACTION
Unknown.

DIETARY ADVICE
Best taken on an empty stomach, at least 1 hour before or 2 hours after eating.

Tacrine can be taken with food to minimize stomach upset, but this will decrease the absorption and effectiveness of the drug.

STORAGE
Store in a tightly sealed container away from moisture, heat, and direct light.

MISSED DOSE
Take it as soon as you remember, unless the time for your next scheduled dose is within the next 2 hours. If so, do not take the missed dose. Take your next scheduled dose at the proper time and resume your regular dosage schedule. Do not double the next dose.

STOPPING THE DRUG
The decision to stop taking the drug should be made in consultation with your doctor.

PROLONGED USE
You should see your doctor regularly for tests and examinations if you must take this drug for a prolonged period.

≡ SIDE EFFECTS ≡

SERIOUS
Clumsiness or unsteadiness, severe vomiting, rapid or pounding heartbeat, slow heartbeat, seizures, elevated liver function tests (detectable by your doctor). Call your doctor right away.

COMMON
Nausea and vomiting, stomach pain or cramps, indigestion, muscle aches or pains, headache, dizziness, loss of appetite, diarrhea.

LESS COMMON
Belching, general feeling of discomfort or illness, rapid breathing, flushed skin, increased urination, increased sweating, watering of the eyes and mouth, insomnia, runny nose, swelling of the feet or lower legs.

▼ PRECAUTIONS

Over 60: No special problems are expected.

Driving and Hazardous Work: Do not drive or engage in hazardous work until you determine how the medicine affects you.

Alcohol: Avoid alcohol.

Pregnancy: Adequate studies on the use of tacrine during pregnancy have not been done. Consult your doctor for specific advice.

Breast Feeding: Tacrine may pass into breast milk and be harmful to the nursing infant; do not use the medication while nursing.

Infants and Children: Tacrine is not intended for use by infants and children.

Special Concerns: Have your blood tested every other week for at least 16 weeks when you start taking tacrine, to see if it is affecting your liver. Do not smoke tobacco products while taking tacrine. Smoking will decrease the effects of tacrine.

OVERDOSE
Symptoms: Sweating and watering of mouth, seizures, increased muscle weakness, low blood pressure, severe nausea or vomiting, fast and weak pulse, large pupils, irregular breathing, slow heartbeat.

What to Do: Call your doctor, emergency medical services (EMS), or the nearest poison control center immediately.

▼ INTERACTIONS

DRUG INTERACTIONS
The following drugs may interact with tacrine. Consult your doctor for advice if you are taking cimetidine, medicine for inflammation or pain, or theophylline.

FOOD INTERACTIONS
No known food interactions.

DISEASE INTERACTIONS
Caution is advised when taking tacrine. Consult your doctor if you have any of the following: asthma, epilepsy or a history of seizures, heart problems, intestinal blockage, stomach or duodenal ulcer, liver disease, Parkinson's disease, urinary problems, brain disease, or history of a head injury that involved a loss of consciousness.

TAMOXIFEN CITRATE

Available in: Tablets
Available OTC? No **As Generic?** Yes
Drug Class: Antiestrogen; antineoplastic (anticancer) agent

▼ USAGE INFORMATION

WHY IT'S PRESCRIBED
To treat breast cancer in women and men; to help reduce the incidence of breast cancer in women at high risk.

HOW IT WORKS
Tamoxifen blocks the effects of the hormone estrogen on certain organs in the body. Because the growth of some types of breast cancer is stimulated by estrogen, tamoxifen interferes with the growth of such tumors.

▼ DOSAGE GUIDELINES

RANGE AND FREQUENCY
For treatment and prevention: 20 mg a day.

ONSET OF EFFECT
Several weeks.

DURATION OF ACTION
Several weeks.

DIETARY ADVICE
It is recommended that tamoxifen be taken after breakfast and after dinner. Swallow the tablet whole with a glass of water.

STORAGE
Store in a tightly sealed container away from moisture, heat, and direct light.

MISSED DOSE
Take it as soon as you remember and resume your regular dosage schedule.

STOPPING THE DRUG
The decision to stop taking the drug should be made by your doctor.

PROLONGED USE
See your doctor regularly for tests and examinations if you take this drug for a prolonged period. Tamoxifen does not prevent all breast cancers, so women taking the drug for prevention should continue to have regular breast exams and mammograms.

▼ PRECAUTIONS

Over 60: No different side effects or problems are expected in older patients.

Driving and Hazardous Work: No special precautions.

Alcohol: No special problems are expected, but you should consult your doctor.

Pregnancy: Tamoxifen may cause miscarriage, birth defects, fetal death, and unexpected vaginal bleeding, and so should not be taken during pregnancy. Avoid becoming pregnant for at least two months after stopping tamoxifen. Notify your doctor and stop taking tamoxifen immediately if pregnancy occurs.

Breast Feeding: Tamoxifen may pass into breast milk; do not nurse while taking it.

Infants and Children: Tamoxifen is not prescribed for infants and children.

Special Concerns: Women should have regular gynecological examinations while taking tamoxifen and for months or years after discontinuing it, because the medication may increase the long-term risk of uterine cancer. Tamoxifen may change or stop a woman's normal menstrual cycle, but she may still be fertile. A reliable birth control method other than oral contraceptives (barrier method) should therefore be used while taking this drug. Tamoxifen for breast cancer risk reduction has not been studied in women under the age of 35. Risk factors for breast cancer include: early age at first menstruation, late age at first pregnancy, no pregnancies, breast cancer in a first-degree relative, history of previous breast biopsies, or high-risk changes seen on a biopsy.

OVERDOSE
Symptoms: Nausea, vomiting, irregular heartbeat, tremor, dizziness, seizures, exaggerated reflexes.

What to Do: Call your doctor, emergency medical services (EMS), or the nearest poison control center immediately.

▼ INTERACTIONS

DRUG INTERACTIONS
You should not take tamoxifen to prevent breast cancer if you are taking anticoagulants (such as warfarin). Consult your doctor for advice if you are taking antacids, cimetidine, famotidine, ranitidine, birth control pills.

FOOD INTERACTIONS
No known food interactions.

DISEASE INTERACTIONS
Consult your doctor if you have a medical history that includes any of the following: cataracts or other vision disturbances, high blood levels of cholesterol or triglycerides, blood clots, low white blood cell and/or platelet counts. Tamoxifen should not be taken to prevent breast cancer by women with a history of deep vein thrombosis or pulmonary embolism.

⬇ SIDE EFFECTS ⬇

SERIOUS
Endometrial cancer (menstrual irregularities, abnormal nonmenstrual vaginal bleeding, changes in vaginal discharge, pelvic pain or pressure); deep vein thrombosis and pulmonary embolism (pain or swelling in legs, shortness of breath, sudden chest pain, coughing up blood); cataracts; new breast lumps; confusion, weakness, or drowsiness; yellowish tinge to eyes or skin. Call your doctor promptly.

COMMON
Hot flashes, weight gain.

LESS COMMON
Bone pain, headache, nausea or vomiting, skin dryness or rash, changes in menstrual period, vaginal discharge, itching in genital area of women, depression, erectile dysfunction (impotence) or decreased sexual interest in men. Other side effects include high blood calcium levels and liver dysfunction; such problems can be detected by your doctor.

TAMSULOSIN HYDROCHLORIDE

BRAND NAME

Flomax

Available in: Capsules
Available OTC? No   **As Generic?** No
Drug Class: BPH therapy agent

▼ USAGE INFORMATION

WHY IT'S PRESCRIBED
To treat symptoms of urinary difficulty that occur with benign prostatic hyperplasia (BPH)—a noncancerous enlargement of the prostate gland. BPH is extremely common among men over the age of 50.

HOW IT WORKS
By blocking a specific (alpha) receptor, tamsulosin relaxes muscle tissue in the prostate and the opening of the bladder. Note that tamsulosin will not shrink the prostate; symptoms may worsen and surgery may eventually be required. Unlike other alpha receptor blockers used to treat BPH, tamsulosin is not used to treat hypertension.

▼ DOSAGE GUIDELINES

RANGE AND FREQUENCY
0.4 mg once a day. It should be taken 30 minutes following the same meal each day. If patients fail to respond to the 0.4 mg dose after 2 to 4 weeks of therapy, they may increase the dose to 0.8 mg once a day.

ONSET OF EFFECT
Unknown.

DURATION OF ACTION
Unknown.

DIETARY ADVICE
There are no dietary restrictions. However, tamsulosin should be taken 30 minutes after the same meal every day. Do not chew, crush, or open the capsules.

STORAGE
Store in a tightly sealed container away from moisture, heat, and direct light.

MISSED DOSE
If therapy is discontinued or interrupted for several days at either the 0.4 mg dose or the 0.8 mg dose, therapy should be started again with the 0.4 mg once daily dose.

STOPPING THE DRUG
Take tamsulosin as prescribed for the full treatment period.

PROLONGED USE
If you take this drug for an extended period, see your doctor regularly so that changes in prostate size can be monitored.

▼ PRECAUTIONS

Over 60: No special problems are expected.

Driving and Hazardous Work: Tamsulosin may impair mental functioning, causing drowsiness, lightheadedness, or dizziness, especially when you take the medication for the first time. Caution is advised; for 24 hours after the initial dose, avoid driving or other activities requiring mental alertness. Effects should diminish after taking several doses.

Alcohol: May increase effects of dizziness or fainting; drink in moderation.

Pregnancy: Tamsulosin is not indicated for use by women.

Breast Feeding: Tamsulosin is not indicated for use by women.

Infants and Children: Tamsulosin is not indicated for use by children.

Special Concerns: The first dose is likely to cause dizziness or lightheadedness. Take the drug at night and get out of bed slowly the next day. Be cautious while exercising and during hot weather. Tell your primary care physician if you are planning to have surgery requiring general anesthesia, including dental surgery. Do not chew, crush, or open the capsules.

OVERDOSE
Symptoms: An overdose is unlikely to occur. Possible symptoms after an excessive dose may include severe headache or orthostatic hypotension (see Less Common Side Effects).

What to Do: If someone takes a much larger dose than prescribed, keep the patient lying down and call your doctor, emergency medical services (EMS), or the nearest poison control center immediately.

▼ INTERACTIONS

DRUG INTERACTIONS
Tamsulosin should not be used in conjunction with other BPH therapy agents. Consult your doctor if you are taking either cimetidine or warfarin, which may interact with tamsulosin.

FOOD INTERACTIONS
None reported.

DISEASE INTERACTIONS
None reported.

≡ SIDE EFFECTS ≡

▼ SERIOUS
No serious side effects have been reported.

COMMON
Headache, increased susceptibility to infection, joint pain, back pain, muscle pain, dizziness, runny nose, diarrhea, abnormal ejaculation.

LESS COMMON
Mild chest pain, drowsiness, insomnia, decreased libido, sore throat, cough, sinus infection, nausea, mouth pain, vision problems. The drug may also promote orthostatic hypotension (episodes of low blood pressure most likely to occur when getting up quickly from a seated or lying position), which produces symptoms of lightheadedness, dizziness, confusion, or fainting.

TEMAZEPAM

Available in: Capsules, tablets
Available OTC? No   **As Generic?** Yes
Drug Class: Benzodiazepine tranquilizer

▼ USAGE INFORMATION

WHY IT'S PRESCRIBED
To treat insomnia.

HOW IT WORKS
Temazepam generally produces mild sedation by depressing activity in the central nervous system. In particular, temazepam appears to enhance the effect of gamma-aminobutyric acid (GABA), a natural chemical that inhibits the firing of neurons and dampens nerve-signal transmission, thus decreasing nervous excitation.

▼ DOSAGE GUIDELINES

RANGE AND FREQUENCY
Adults: 15 mg, taken at bedtime. Older adults: To start, 7.5 mg, taken at bedtime. The dose may be increased. Use and dose for children under 18 must be determined by your doctor.

ONSET OF EFFECT
Unknown.

DURATION OF ACTION
Unknown. It may take more than 2 hours.

DIETARY ADVICE
Take it 30 minutes before bedtime with a full glass of water. Temazepam can be taken with food to prevent gastrointestinal upset.

STORAGE
Store in a tightly sealed container away from heat and direct light.

MISSED DOSE
Take it as soon as you remember, unless it is late at night. Do not take the medicine unless your schedule allows a full night's sleep.

STOPPING THE DRUG
Discontinuing the drug abruptly may produce withdrawal symptoms (sleep

disruption, nervousness, irritability, diarrhea, abdominal cramps, muscle aches, memory impairment). The dosage should be reduced gradually according to your doctor's instructions.

PROLONGED USE
This medication may slowly lose its effectiveness, and adverse reactions are more likely to occur with prolonged use. You should see your doctor for periodic evaluation if you must take it for an extended time.

▼ PRECAUTIONS

Over 60: Adverse reactions may be more likely and more severe. A lower dose may be warranted.

Driving and Hazardous Work: Do not drive or engage in hazardous work until you determine how the medicine affects you.

Alcohol: Avoid alcohol.

Pregnancy: Use during pregnancy should be avoided if possible. Be sure to tell your doctor if you are pregnant or plan to become pregnant.

Breast Feeding: Temazepam passes into breast milk; do not take it while nursing.

Infants and Children: Safety and effectiveness have not been established for children under age 18.

Special Concerns: Temazepam use can lead to psychological or physical dependence if the drug is not taken in strict accordance

with your doctor's instructions. Never take more than the prescribed daily dose.

OVERDOSE
Symptoms: Extreme drowsiness, confusion, slurred speech, slow reflexes, poor coordination, staggering gait, tremor, slowed breathing, loss of consciousness.

What to Do: Call your doctor, emergency medical services (EMS), or the nearest poison control center immediately.

▼ INTERACTIONS

DRUG INTERACTIONS
Consult your physician for advice if you are taking drugs that depress the central nervous system; these include antihistamines, antidepressants or other psychiatric medications, barbiturates, sedatives, cough medicines, decongestants, and painkillers. Be sure your doctor knows about any over-the-counter drug you may take.

FOOD INTERACTIONS
None reported.

DISEASE INTERACTIONS
Consult your doctor if you have a history of alcohol or drug abuse, stroke or other brain disease, any chronic lung disease, glaucoma, hyperactivity, depression or other mental illness, sleep apnea, myasthenia gravis, epilepsy, porphyria, kidney disease, or liver disease.

≡ SIDE EFFECTS ≡

▼ SERIOUS ▼
Difficulty concentrating, outbursts of anger, other behavior problems, depression, convulsions, hallucinations, low blood pressure (causing faintness or confusion), memory impairment, muscle weakness, skin rash or itching, sore throat, fever and chills, sores or ulcers in throat or mouth, unusual bruising or bleeding, extreme fatigue, yellowish tinge to eyes or skin. Call your doctor immediately.

COMMON
Loss of coordination, unsteady gait, lightheadedness, dizziness, drowsiness, slurred speech.

LESS COMMON
Stomach cramps or pain, vision disturbances, change in sexual desire or ability, constipation or diarrhea, dry mouth or watering mouth, false sense of well-being, rapid or pounding heartbeat, headache, muscle spasms, nausea and vomiting, urinary problems, trembling.

TERAZOSIN

Available in: Tablets, capsules
Available OTC? No **As Generic?** Yes
Drug Class: Antihypertensive; BPH therapy agent

▼ USAGE INFORMATION

WHY IT'S PRESCRIBED
To lower and control high blood pressure (hypertension). It is also used to treat symptoms of urinary difficulty that occur with benign prostatic hyperplasia (BPH).

HOW IT WORKS
Terazosin helps to control hypertension by relaxing blood vessels and permitting them to expand, an action that decreases blood pressure in the process. When used for BPH, the medication helps relax the muscles in the prostate gland and the opening of the bladder, improving the passage of urine.

▼ DOSAGE GUIDELINES

RANGE AND FREQUENCY
For high blood pressure: Initially, 1 mg taken at bedtime, then 1 to 5 mg once daily. For children, the dose and frequency must be determined by your pediatrician. For BPH: Initially, 1 mg taken at bedtime, then 5 to 10 mg once daily.

ONSET OF EFFECT
Within 15 minutes, with peak blood pressure effect within 2 to 3 hours. When the drug is used to treat urinary difficulty associated with BPH, the full effect may not be seen for 4 to 6 weeks.

DURATION OF ACTION
24 hours.

DIETARY ADVICE
Terazosin can be taken before, with, or after meals.

STORAGE
Store in a tightly sealed container away from moisture, heat, and direct light.

MISSED DOSE
Take it as soon as possible the same day. If it is the next day, skip the missed dose. Do not double the dose. Resume your regular dosage schedule.

STOPPING THE DRUG
Do not discontinue taking the medication suddenly, even if you start to experience unpleasant side effects. Consult your physician. If terazosin is discontinued for several days, you may need to start therapy over, using the initial dosing regimen.

PROLONGED USE
When taking the medication for hypertension, blood pressure measurement is recommended at regular intervals.

▼ PRECAUTIONS

Over 60: Older persons are generally more sensitive to terazosin and more likely to experience adverse side effects, especially when getting up from a lying or seated position. Rise slowly to minimize symptoms.

Driving and Hazardous Work: Terazosin may impair mental ability, causing drowsiness, lightheadedness, or dizziness, especially when you take the medication for the first time. Caution is advised; for 24 hours after the initial dose, avoid driving or other activities requiring mental alertness. Effects should diminish after several doses.

Alcohol: May increase effects of dizziness or fainting; drink in strict moderation, if at all.

Pregnancy: Well-controlled studies have not been done. Consult your physician if you are pregnant or if you plan to become pregnant.

Breast Feeding: It is not known whether terazosin passes into breast milk. Consult your physician for specific advice.

Infants and Children: Adequate studies of terazosin use in this age group have not been performed. Discuss the risks and benefits with your pediatrician.

Special Concerns: Be sure to notify your doctor if you are taking nonprescription medications for asthma, colds, cough, allergy, or appetite suppression. These drugs can increase blood pressure and cause other complications if they are taken with terazosin.

OVERDOSE
Symptoms: Extremely low blood pressure (hypotension), with accompanying fatigue, weakness, head-ache, palpitations, fainting, or dizziness.

What to Do: Call your doctor, emergency medical services (EMS), or the nearest poison control center immediately.

▼ INTERACTIONS

DRUG INTERACTIONS
Several drugs may interact with terazosin, including anti-inflammatory medications, especially indomethacin, which can cause fluid and sodium retention, and estrogen, which can reduce the antihypertensive effects of the drug. Consult your doctor.

FOOD INTERACTIONS
None are expected.

DISEASE INTERACTIONS
Consult your physician if you have kidney disease, severe heart disease, or chest pain caused by angina pectoris. Terazosin may aggravate these conditions.

≋ SIDE EFFECTS ≋

SERIOUS
No serious side effects have been reported.

COMMON
Dizziness.

LESS COMMON
Chest pain; lightheadedness or fainting, especially when getting up quickly from a seated or lying position. Such symptoms are typically more common when you first take the medication, and generally diminish over time. These symptoms tend to recur when the dosage is increased. Take it at bedtime to minimize such problems.

TERBINAFINE HYDROCHLORIDE

Available in: Tablets, topical cream
Available OTC? Yes   **As Generic?** No
Drug Class: Antifungal

▼ USAGE INFORMATION

WHY IT'S PRESCRIBED
The tablets are used only to treat fungal infections of the fingernails and toenails (tinea unguium). The cream is used to treat fungal infections of the skin, such as tinea corporis (ringworm), tinea cruris (jock itch), and tinea pedis (athlete's foot).

HOW IT WORKS
Terbinafine inhibits an enzyme essential for the production of substances vital for the reproduction and survival of some types of fungal organisms.

▼ DOSAGE GUIDELINES

RANGE AND FREQUENCY
Tablets: 250 mg once a day for 6 weeks for fingernail fungus; 250 mg once a day for 12 weeks for toenail fungus. Cream: Apply a thin film of medicine to the affected area 1 to 2 times a day for ring-worm or jock itch; 2 times a day for athlete's foot. Apply the cream for at least 1 week, but no longer than 4 weeks.

ONSET OF EFFECT
Tablets: The optimal effect is seen several months after the completion of treatment. Cream: Unknown.

DURATION OF ACTION
Unknown.

DIETARY ADVICE
Terbinafine can be taken or applied without regard to meals.

STORAGE
Store in a tightly sealed container away from moisture, heat, and direct light. Do not allow the cream to freeze.

MISSED DOSE
It is important to not miss any doses. Take or apply as soon as you remember. If you do not remember until the next day, skip the missed dose and resume your regular dosage schedule. Do not double the next dose and do not use excessive amounts of the cream.

STOPPING THE DRUG
Take terbinafine tablets as prescribed for the full treatment period.

PROLONGED USE
Side effects are more likely to occur with prolonged use. Tests of liver function are recommended if the tablets are used for longer than 6 weeks.

▼ PRECAUTIONS

Over 60: No special advice.

Driving and Hazardous Work: No special precautions.

Alcohol: No special warnings.

Pregnancy: Terbinafine tablets are not recommended for pregnant women.

Breast Feeding: Avoid use of the tablets while nursing.

Infants and Children: Terbinafine is not recommended for children under the age of 18.

Special Concerns: Wash your hands before and after applying the cream. Avoid allowing topical terbinafine to come into contact with the eyes, nose, and mouth. If using terbinafine for ringworm, wear loose-fitting, well-ventilated clothing and avoid excess heat and humidity. It is also recommended to use a bland, absorbent powder like talcum once or twice a day after the cream has been applied and absorbed by the skin. If using the medication for jock itch, do not wear underwear that is tight or made from synthetic materials; wear loose-fitting cotton underwear. If using terbinafine for athlete's foot, dry your feet carefully after bathing and wear clean cotton socks with sandals or well-ventilated shoes. Before applying the medication, wash the affected area with soap and warm water and dry thoroughly.

OVERDOSE
Symptoms: Tablets: nausea, vomiting, abdominal pain, dizziness, rash, frequent urination, and headache.

What to Do: Call your doctor as soon as possible.

▼ INTERACTIONS

DRUG INTERACTIONS
Consult your doctor if you are taking rifampin, cimetidine, or any other preparation that is to be applied to the same area of skin as terbinafine cream.

FOOD INTERACTIONS
No known food interactions.

DISEASE INTERACTIONS
Use of terbinafine tablets may cause complications in patients with liver or kidney disease, since these organs work together to remove the medication from the body. Consult your doctor if you have a history of alcohol abuse (a potential cause of liver disease).

≡ SIDE EFFECTS ≡

SERIOUS
Serious side effects with terbinafine are rare. However, terbinafine tablets may cause liver dysfunction; severe skin reactions such as Stevens-Johnson syndrome; severe blood disorders, potentially resulting in increased susceptibility to infection, uncontrolled bleeding or other problems; or severe allergic reactions. Seek emergency medical assistance immediately.

COMMON
Headache, diarrhea, rash, stomach pain, indigestion, nausea.

LESS COMMON
Tablets may cause flatulence, itching, skin eruptions, loss of taste, weakness, fatigue, vomiting, joint and muscle pain, or hair loss. Terbinafine cream may cause redness, itching, burning, blistering, swelling, oozing, or other signs of skin irritation not present before using the drug.

TETRACYCLINE HYDROCHLORIDE

BRAND NAMES

Achromycin,
Achromycin V,
Panmycin, Robitet,
Sumycin, Tetracyn

Available in: Capsules, tablets, liquid, topical forms, ophthalmic forms, injection
Available OTC? No   **As Generic?** Yes
Drug Class: Tetracycline antibiotic

▼ USAGE INFORMATION

WHY IT'S PRESCRIBED
To treat infections caused by bacteria or protozoa (tiny single-celled organisms); also, to treat acne.

HOW IT WORKS
Tetracycline kills bacteria and protozoa by inhibiting the manufacture of specific proteins needed by the organisms to survive.

▼ DOSAGE GUIDELINES

RANGE AND FREQUENCY
Oral forms (capsules, tablets, liquid), for bacterial and protozoal infections: 500 to 2,000 mg,1 to 4 times a day, as determined by your doctor. Topical forms (cream, topical ointment, topical solution), for acne or skin infections: Apply 1 or 2 times a day to affected areas. Ophthalmic forms (opthalmic ointment, ophthalmic solution) for eye infections: Apply once every 2 to 12 hours as determined by your doctor.

ONSET OF EFFECT
Unknown.

DURATION OF ACTION
Unknown.

DIETARY ADVICE
Oral forms are best taken on an empty stomach with a full glass of water.

STORAGE
Store in a tightly sealed container away from heat and direct light. Refrigerate liquid forms but do not freeze.

MISSED DOSE
Take it as soon as you remember. If it is near the time for the next dose, skip the missed dose and resume your regular dosage schedule. Do not double the next dose.

STOPPING THE DRUG
Take as prescribed for the full treatment period, even if you begin to feel better before the scheduled end of therapy.

PROLONGED USE
May increase susceptibility to infections by microorganisms resistant to antibiotics.

▼ PRECAUTIONS

Over 60: It is not known whether tetracycline causes different or more severe adverse reactions in older patients than it does in younger persons.

Driving and Hazardous Work: Do not drive or engage in hazardous work until you determine how the medicine affects you.

Alcohol: It is advisable to abstain from alcohol when fighting an infection.

Pregnancy: Tetracycline should not be used during pregnancy.

Breast Feeding: Tetracycline passes into breast milk and may be harmful to the nursing infant. The patient must choose between using the drug or breast feeding.

Infants and Children: Tetracycline should be used by children younger than 8 years of age only if other antibiotics are unlikely to be effective, since it can cause permanent tooth staining.

Special Concerns: If tetracycline causes increased sensitivity of your skin to sunlight, wear protective clothing, use a sunscreen with an SPF (sun protection factor) of 15 or higher, and try to avoid direct exposure to sunlight, especially between 10 am and 3 pm. Before having surgery, tell the doctor or dentist in charge that you are taking tetracycline. If you use makeup, it is best to apply only water-based cosmetics and to keep the amount to a minimum during tetracycline therapy for the skin. The drug can reduce the effectiveness of oral contraceptives. You should use a different method of birth control while taking this antibiotic. Absorption of tetracycline may be altered if you take antacids.

OVERDOSE
Symptoms: Severe nausea, vomiting, diarrhea, difficulty swallowing.

What to Do: An overdose is unlikely to be life-threatening. However, if someone takes a much larger dose than prescribed, call your doctor, emergency medical services (EMS), or the nearest poison control center immediately.

▼ INTERACTIONS

DRUG INTERACTIONS
Consult your physician for advice if you are taking antacids, calcium supplements, cholestyramine, choline and magnesium salicylates, medicines containing iron, laxatives containing magnesium, or oral contraceptives.

FOOD INTERACTIONS
Avoid dairy products while taking tetracycline.

DISEASE INTERACTIONS
Consult your doctor if you have a history of kidney disease or liver disease.

≡ SIDE EFFECTS ≡

SERIOUS
Increased frequency of urination, increased thirst, unusual fatigue, discoloration of skin and mucous membranes. Call your doctor immediately.

COMMON
Stomach cramps and discomfort, diarrhea, nausea, vomiting, increased sensitivity of skin to sunlight, itching in genital or rectal area, sore mouth or tongue, dizziness, lightheadedness, or unsteadiness.

LESS COMMON
No less-common side effects have been reported.

THEOPHYLLINE

Available in: Tablets, capsules, extended release forms, elixir, syrup, oral solution
Available OTC? No   **As Generic?** Yes
Drug Class: Bronchodilator/xanthine

▼ USAGE INFORMATION

WHY IT'S PRESCRIBED
Theophylline is used to reduce the frequency and severity of breathing problems in people with asthma, emphysema, bronchitis, and other lung disorders.

HOW IT WORKS
An asthma attack occurs when the smooth muscles in the bronchial passages of the lungs go into a spasm (bronchospasm). Theophylline relaxes these muscles, helping to widen the constricted airways and restore normal breathing.

▼ DOSAGE GUIDELINES

RANGE AND FREQUENCY
Adults not currently taking any theophylline medications: Your physician will prescribe a "loading dose," which is based on your weight and taken only once. This is followed by a daily maintenance dose, usually 300 to 600 mg per day, taken in 1 or 2 doses. Patients given extended-release capsules: After the loading dose, take one-half of the total daily dose at 12-hour intervals, unless otherwise directed by your doctor. Adults currently taking theophylline: Dose is determined by blood level of theophylline. Children: Consult a pediatrician.

ONSET OF EFFECT
Variable.

DURATION OF ACTION
Variable.

DIETARY ADVICE
Avoid large amounts of caffeine-containing foods or beverages, including colas. Otherwise, maintain your usual food and fluid intake.

STORAGE
Store in a tightly sealed container away from heat and direct light. Keep away from moisture and extremes in temperature.

MISSED DOSE
Take it as soon as you remember. If it is near the time for the next dose, skip the missed dose and resume your regular dosage schedule. Do not double the next dose.

STOPPING THE DRUG
The decision to stop taking the drug should be made by your doctor.

PROLONGED USE
Therapy with this medication may require months or years.

▼ PRECAUTIONS

Over 60: Adverse reactions may be more likely and more severe in older patients.

Driving and Hazardous Work: Do not drive or engage in hazardous work until you determine how the medicine affects you.

Alcohol: Avoid alcohol.

Pregnancy: Discuss the relative risks with your doctor. Generally, this drug should be used only if necessary and if a substitute cannot be prescribed.

Breast Feeding: Theophylline passes into breast milk and may be toxic to nursing infants; avoid or discontinue use while breast feeding.

Infants and Children: Theophylline has been used in children of all ages. Consult your pediatrician for specific dosages. Theophylline elixir contains alcohol and should not be used by children.

Special Concerns: You will need periodic blood tests to determine theophylline levels. Do not switch between different brands of theophylline, and especially do not switch between extended-release forms and other forms without notifying your doctor. Inform your doctor if you have stopped smoking; tobacco affects the level of theophylline in the blood.

OVERDOSE
Symptoms: Abdominal pain; bloody vomiting; disorientation, extreme anxiety, or unusual behavior; seizures; twitching, trembling, or shaking; rapid, pounding, or irregular heartbeat; dizziness, lightheadedness, or fainting.

What to Do: Call your doctor, emergency medical services (EMS), or the nearest poison control center immediately.

▼ INTERACTIONS

DRUG INTERACTIONS
Consult your doctor for specific advice if you are taking beta-blockers, cimetidine, ciprofloxacin, clarithromycin, enoxacin, erythromycin, fluvoxamine, mexiletine, pentoxifylline, propranolol, tacrine, thiabendazole, ticlopidine, troleandomycin; moricizine, phenytoin, or rifampin.

FOOD INTERACTIONS
Your doctor may suggest that you restrict caffeine intake.

DISEASE INTERACTIONS
Consult your doctor if you have a history of convulsions, heart failure, liver disease, or underactive thyroid.

≡ SIDE EFFECTS ≡
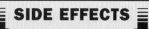

SERIOUS
Vomiting, trembling, confusion, rapid, irregular, or pounding pulse, chest pain, dizziness, convulsions, skin rashes.

COMMON
Restlessness, insomnia, loss of appetite, nervousness, irritability, nausea.

LESS COMMON
Heartburn, diarrhea.

TOLTERODINE TARTRATE

Available in: Tablets
Available OTC? No   **As Generic?** No
Drug Class: Anticholinergic

▼ USAGE INFORMATION

WHY IT'S PRESCRIBED
To treat overactive bladder with symptoms of urinary frequency, urgency, or urge incontinence.

HOW IT WORKS
Tolterodine decreases the urge to urinate by blocking nerve receptors that trigger contractions of the bladder.

▼ DOSAGE GUIDELINES

RANGE AND FREQUENCY
Adults: 2 mg, twice a day. Dose may be lowered by your doctor to 1 mg, twice a day, depending upon response to the medication. Adults with impaired liver function: no more than 1 mg, twice a day.

ONSET OF EFFECT
Unknown.

DURATION OF ACTION
Unknown.

DIETARY ADVICE
Tolterodine can be taken with or without food. It's best to maintain your usual food and fluid intake.

STORAGE
Store in a tightly sealed container away from moisture, heat, and direct light.

MISSED DOSE
Take it as soon as you remember. If it is near the time for the next dose, skip the missed dose and resume your regular dosage schedule. Do not double the next dose.

STOPPING THE DRUG
The decision to stop taking the drug should be made in consultation with your physician.

PROLONGED USE
See your doctor periodically if you must take this drug for a prolonged period.

▼ PRECAUTIONS

Over 60: No special problems are expected in older patients.

Driving and Hazardous Work: The use of tolterodine should not impair your ability to perform such tasks safely.

Alcohol: No special problems are expected.

Pregnancy: No human studies have been done with tolterodine. Before taking this medication, tell your doctor if you are pregnant or plan to become pregnant.

Breast Feeding: Tolterodine may pass into breast milk; avoid use while nursing. Consult your doctor for specific advice.

Infants and Children: Not recommended for use by children under the age of 18.

OVERDOSE
Symptoms: Drowsiness, mental confusion, dizziness, loss of coordination, dry mouth.

What to Do: Few cases of overdose have been reported. However, if someone takes a much larger dose than prescribed, call your doctor, emergency medical services (EMS), or the nearest poison control center immediately.

▼ INTERACTIONS

DRUG INTERACTIONS
The following drugs may interact with tolterodine. Consult your doctor for specific advice if you are taking fluoxetine, macrolide antibiotics, or antifungal drugs.

FOOD INTERACTIONS
There are no known food interactions.

DISEASE INTERACTIONS
You should not take tolterodine if you have urinary retention, gastric retention, or uncontrolled narrow-angle glaucoma. Tolterodine should be used with caution in patients with liver or kidney disease, since these organs work together to remove the medication from the body.

≡ SIDE EFFECTS ≡

SERIOUS
Chest pain. Consult your doctor immediately.

COMMON
Headache, constipation, indigestion, dry eye, dry mouth.

LESS COMMON
Numbness, tingling or prickling sensation, abdominal pain, flatulence, nausea or vomiting, bronchitis, cough, dry skin, nervousness, drowsiness, blurred vision.

TRAMADOL HYDROCHLORIDE

BRAND NAME

Ultram

Available in: Tablets
Available OTC? No **As Generic?** No
Drug Class: Analgesic

▼ USAGE INFORMATION

WHY IT'S PRESCRIBED
To help manage moderate to somewhat severe pain, such as that which occurs following joint surgery and certain gynecological procedures (for example, cesarean section).

HOW IT WORKS
Tramadol acts on the central nervous system to block pain transmission signals. The drug works like narcotic analgesics, and while it is not a narcotic, it can be habit-forming, leading to mental and physical drug dependence.

▼ DOSAGE GUIDELINES

RANGE AND FREQUENCY
1 or 2 tablets (50 mg each) every 6 hours as needed. For severe pain, your doctor may prescribe 2 tablets for the first dose.

ONSET OF EFFECT
Usually within 1 hour, with a peak effect at 2 hours.

DURATION OF ACTION
6 to 7 hours.

DIETARY ADVICE
Tramadol can be taken with or without food.

STORAGE
Store in a tightly sealed container away from heat and direct light.

MISSED DOSE
Take it as soon as you remember. However, if it is near the time for the next dose, skip the missed dose and resume your regular dosage schedule. Do not double the next dose.

STOPPING THE DRUG
The decision to stop taking the drug should be made by your doctor.

PROLONGED USE
You should see your doctor regularly for tests and examinations if you take this drug for a prolonged period.

▼ PRECAUTIONS

Over 60: Tramadol stays longer in the body of older patients than younger ones; your doctor may adjust the dose accordingly.

Driving and Hazardous Work: Do not drive or engage in hazardous work until you determine how the medicine affects you.

Alcohol: Do not consume alcohol while taking tramadol because this medication may compound the drug's sedative effect on the central nervous system.

Pregnancy: Tramadol has caused birth defects and other problems in animals. Human studies have not been done. Before you take the drug, tell your doctor if you are pregnant or are planning to become pregnant.

Breast Feeding: Tramadol passes into breast milk; avoid or discontinue use while breast feeding.

Infants and Children: Safety and effectiveness have not been established for the use of tramadol in children under 16 years old.

Special Concerns: Before undergoing any kind of surgery, including dental surgery, be sure your doctor or dentist knows that you are taking tramadol.

OVERDOSE
Symptoms: Breathing difficulty, seizures, vomiting.

What to Do: Call your doctor, emergency medical services (EMS), or the nearest poison control center immediately.

▼ INTERACTIONS

DRUG INTERACTIONS
Consult your doctor for specific advice if you are taking carbamazepine, anesthetics, MAO inhibitors, or any drugs known to depress the central nervous system, including sedatives, tranquilizers, sleeping pills, antihistamines, other prescription pain medicines, barbiturates, medications for seizures, or muscle relaxants.

FOOD INTERACTIONS
No known food interactions.

DISEASE INTERACTIONS
Caution is advised when taking tramadol. Consult your doctor if you have severe abdominal or stomach conditions, or a history of alcohol abuse, drug abuse, head injury, or seizure disorders. Use of tramadol may cause complications in patients with liver or kidney disease, since these organs work together to remove the medication from the body.

≡ SIDE EFFECTS ≡

SERIOUS
Blurred vision, difficulty urinating, frequent urge to urinate, blisters under the skin, change in walking balance, dizziness or lightheadedness when getting up, fainting, fast heartbeat, memory loss, hallucinations, shortness of breath. Also numbness, tingling, pain, or weakness in hands or feet; redness, swelling, and itching of skin; trembling and shaking of hands or feet; trouble performing routine tasks. Call your doctor immediately.

COMMON
Dizziness, vertigo, headache, drowsiness, nausea, vomiting, constipation.

LESS COMMON
Weakness, lack of energy, anxiety, confusion, euphoria, nervousness, insomnia, visual disturbances, stomach upset, dry mouth, diarrhea, abdominal pain, loss of appetite, gas, menopausal symptoms, sweating, muscle spasm, rash.

TRAZODONE

Available in: Tablets
Available OTC? No   **As Generic?** Yes
Drug Class: Antidepressant

▼ USAGE INFORMATION

WHY IT'S PRESCRIBED
To treat symptoms of major depression. It may be taken with selective serotonin reuptake inhibitor (SSRI) antidepressants such as fluoxetine, sertraline, and paroxetine when these drugs cause insomnia.

HOW IT WORKS
Trazodone helps to balance levels of serotonin, a brain chemical that is profoundly linked to mood, emotions, and mental state.

▼ DOSAGE GUIDELINES

RANGE AND FREQUENCY
Adults: To start, 50 mg, 3 times a day, or 75 mg, 2 times a day, or 100 mg at bedtime. The dose may be gradually increased by your doctor to 400 mg a day. Older adults: To start, 25 mg, 3 times a day, or 50 mg at bedtime. The dose may be increased by your doctor.

ONSET OF EFFECT
1 to 4 weeks.

DURATION OF ACTION
Unknown.

DIETARY ADVICE
It can be taken with a meal or light snack to reduce the chance of dizziness and to increase the absorption of the drug by the body.

STORAGE
Store in a tightly sealed container away from moisture, heat, and direct light.

MISSED DOSE
Take it as soon as you remember, unless the time for your next scheduled dose is within the next 4 hours. If so, do not take the missed dose. Take your next scheduled dose at the proper time and resume your regular dosage schedule. Do not double the next dose.

STOPPING THE DRUG
Take as prescribed for the full treatment period, even if you begin to feel better before the scheduled end of therapy. The decision to stop taking the drug should be made in consultation with your doctor.

PROLONGED USE
The usual course of therapy lasts for 6 months to 1 year; some patients benefit from additional therapy beyond that period.

▼ PRECAUTIONS

Over 60: Adverse reactions may be more likely and more severe in older patients. Lower doses may be needed.

Driving and Hazardous Work: Use caution when driving or engaging in hazardous work until you determine how the medicine affects you. Drowsiness may occur.

Alcohol: Avoid alcohol.

Pregnancy: Adequate studies of trazodone use during pregnancy have not been done. Before you take trazodone, tell your doctor if you are pregnant or plan to become pregnant.

Breast Feeding: Trazodone passes into breast milk; caution is advised. Consult your doctor for specific advice.

Infants and Children: The safety and effectiveness have not been established for infants and children.

OVERDOSE
Symptoms: Severe nausea and vomiting, loss of coordination, drowsiness.

What to Do: Call your doctor, emergency medical services (EMS), or the nearest poison control center immediately.

▼ INTERACTIONS

DRUG INTERACTIONS
The following drugs may interact with trazodone. Consult your doctor for specific advice if you are taking high blood pressure medication, central nervous system depressants (including cold and allergy drugs, narcotic pain relievers, and muscle relaxants), fluoxetine, or tricyclic antidepressants.

FOOD INTERACTIONS
No known food interactions.

DISEASE INTERACTIONS
Caution is advised when taking trazodone. Consult your doctor if you have a history of alcohol abuse or any heart condition. Use of trazodone may cause complications in patients with liver or kidney disease, since these organs work together to remove the medication from the body.

▤ SIDE EFFECTS ▤

SERIOUS
Muscle twitching, confusion. Call your doctor immediately.

COMMON
Drowsiness, dry mouth, dizziness, lightheadedness, unpleasant taste in mouth, nausea and vomiting, headache.

LESS COMMON
Blurred vision, muscle pains, diarrhea, constipation, unusual fatigue.

TRETINOIN

Available in: Cream, gel, liquid
Available OTC? No   **As Generic?** Yes
Drug Class: Acne drug

▼ USAGE INFORMATION

WHY IT'S PRESCRIBED
Tretinoin is used to treat mild to moderate acne.

HOW IT WORKS
Although the exact mechanism of action of tretinoin is unknown, the drug appears to affect skin cells so that they are shed in a more normal fashion, therefore "unplugging" blackheads and whiteheads (comedones), the initial changes in acne formation.

▼ DOSAGE GUIDELINES

RANGE AND FREQUENCY
Adults: Apply once daily at bedtime.

ONSET OF EFFECT
Variable, usually within 2 to 6 weeks after starting therapy.

DURATION OF ACTION
The effect of tretinoin typically persists for as long as the medication continues to be applied.

DIETARY ADVICE
No special restrictions.

STORAGE
Store in a tightly sealed container away from heat and direct light. Keep away from moisture and extremes in temperature. The gel form of this medication is flammable; keep away from heat and open flame.

MISSED DOSE
This drug is applied once every 24 hours, at night. If you miss a day, resume your regular dosage schedule the next day. There is no need to apply extra medication with the next dose to compensate for the missed dose.

STOPPING THE DRUG
Use as prescribed for the full treatment period, even if you show signs of improvement before the scheduled end of therapy.

PROLONGED USE
Therapy with this medication is frequently long-term.

▼ PRECAUTIONS

Over 60: No special problems are expected.

Driving and Hazardous Work: No special precautions are necessary.

Alcohol: No special precautions are necessary.

Pregnancy: Avoid or discontinue tretinoin if you are pregnant or if you are trying to become pregnant.

Breast Feeding: Tretinoin may pass into breast milk; caution is advised. Consult your doctor for advice.

Infants and Children: The drug is not recommended for children.

Special Concerns: People with a history of allergy to tretinoin or any other ingredients in the medication should not use the product. Do not apply large amounts of tretinoin to your skin in expectation of better or faster results. This will only lead to unnecessary irritation of affected skin and surrounding areas. Sunburned skin is more susceptible to irritation from tretinoin, and application should be avoided. Avoid excessive exposure to sunlight or use of sunlamps. Keep this medication away from your eyes, mouth, and nostrils. Severe irritation and redness may result. Do not apply tretinoin to inflamed skin. If your skin becomes reddened and painful while using tretinoin, discontinue use of the medication and call your doctor. If you are using cosmetics, gently cleanse skin to be treated before applying the medication.

OVERDOSE
Symptoms: Excessive application of tretinoin may lead to severe irritation of the skin.

What to Do: If tretinoin is ingested, call your doctor, emergency medical services (EMS), or the nearest poison control center.

▼ INTERACTIONS

DRUG INTERACTIONS
Consult your doctor for specific advice if you are taking other acne medications that are applied to the same area of skin, including prescription and nonprescription treatments containing sulfur, resorcinol, alpha hydroxy acids, or salicylic acid; medicated soaps, abrasives, cleansers, or cosmetics; topical preparations with a high concentration of alcohol, astringents, extract of lime, or spices; and medications used for a drying effect.

FOOD INTERACTIONS
No known food interactions.

DISEASE INTERACTIONS
Caution is advised when using tretinoin. Consult your doctor if you have eczema.

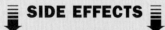
≡ SIDE EFFECTS ≡

SERIOUS
No serious side effects are associated with regular applications of of tretinoin when used as directed.

COMMON
Mild redness and peeling, or excessive dryness, at the site of application.

LESS COMMON
Irritation or allergy with severe redness, swelling, blistering, pain, rash, or crusting at sites of application; changes in pigment (either lightening or darkening of skin color). These problems generally improve when the medication is stopped or reduced in dosage or frequency of application. Consult your doctor.

TRIAMCINOLONE INHALANT AND NASAL

Available in: Nasal spray, oral inhalation
Available OTC? No   **As Generic?** No
Drug Class: Respiratory corticosteroid

▼ USAGE INFORMATION

WHY IT'S PRESCRIBED
Oral inhalation: To treat bronchial asthma. Nasal spray: To treat allergic rhinitis (seasonal or perennial allergies such as hay fever), and to prevent recurrence of nasal polyps after surgical removal.

HOW IT WORKS
Respiratory corticosteroids such as triamcinolone primarily reduce or prevent inflammation of the lining of the airways (the underlying cause of asthma), reduce the allergic response to inhaled allergens, and inhibit the secretion of mucus within the airways.

▼ DOSAGE GUIDELINES

RANGE AND FREQUENCY
Adults and children ages 12 and older—Oral inhalation: 2 inhalations of 100 micrograms (mcg) each, 3 or 4 times a day. Maximum dose is 16 inhalations a day. In some patients maintenance can be achieved when the total daily dose is given 2 times a day. Nasal spray: 2 sprays (55 mcg each) in each nostril once a day. It can be increased to 440 mcg per day in 1 or up to 4 doses. After relief is achieved, it can be decreased to as little as 1 spray (55 mcg) in each nostril once a day.

ONSET OF EFFECT
Usually within 1 week; it may take 3 weeks for the full effect to occur.

DURATION OF ACTION
Several days.

DIETARY ADVICE
No special restrictions.

STORAGE
Store in a tightly sealed container away from heat and direct light.

MISSED DOSE
Take it as soon as you remember. However, if it is near the time for the next dose, skip the missed dose and resume your regular dosage schedule. Do not double the next dose.

STOPPING THE DRUG
The decision to stop taking the drug should be made only after consultation with your doctor.

≡ SIDE EFFECTS ≡

SERIOUS
No serious side effects have been reported.

COMMON
Oral inhalation: Sore throat, white patches in mouth or throat, hoarseness. Nasal spray: Nosebleeds or bloody nasal secretions, nasal burning or irritation, sore throat.

LESS COMMON
Eye pain, watering eyes, gradual decrease of vision, stomach pain and digestive disturbances.

PROLONGED USE
Consult your doctor about the need for regular periodic medical tests and examinations if you must take this drug for a prolonged period.

▼ PRECAUTIONS

Over 60: No special problems are expected with older patients.

Driving and Hazardous Work: The use of triamcinolone should not impair your ability to perform such tasks safely.

Alcohol: No special precautions are necessary.

Pregnancy: Inhaled or nasal steroids have not been reported to cause birth defects if taken during pregnancy. Before using such drugs, tell your doctor if you are or if you are planning to become pregnant.

Breast Feeding: Triamcinolone may pass into breast milk; caution is advised. Consult your doctor for advice.

Infants and Children: No special problems are expected in children, but the lowest possible dose should be used.

Special Concerns: Inhaled steroids will not help an asthma attack in progress. Inhaled steroids can lower resistance to yeast infections of the mouth, throat, or voice box. To prevent yeast infections, gargle or rinse your mouth with water after each use; do not swallow the water. Know how to use the spray properly; read and follow the directions that come with the device. Before you have surgery, tell the doctor or dentist that you are using a steroid.

OVERDOSE
Symptoms: No specific ones have been reported.

What to Do: Call your doctor, emergency medical services (EMS), or the nearest poison control center if you have any reason to suspect an overdose.

▼ INTERACTIONS

DRUG INTERACTIONS
Consult your physician for advice if you are taking systemic corticosteroids, other inhaled corticosteroids, or any drugs that suppress the immune system.

FOOD INTERACTIONS
No known food interactions.

DISEASE INTERACTIONS
Consult your physician if you have any of the following: nasal septal ulcers, ocular herpes simplex, or any fungal, bacterial, or systemic viral infection. If you are exposed to chicken pox or measles, tell your doctor at once.

TRIMETHOPRIM/SULFAMETHOXAZOLE

Available in: Tablets, injection
Available OTC? No   **As Generic?** Yes
Drug Class: Anti-infective

▼ USAGE INFORMATION

WHY IT'S PRESCRIBED
To treat urinary tract infections, ear infections, chronic bronchitis, Pneumocystis carinii pneumonia (a lung infection commonly seen in patients with compromised immune systems), traveler's diarrhea, and other types of diarrheal disease.

HOW IT WORKS
This drug is a combination of two active ingredients. Both trimethoprim and sulfamethoxazole kill or inhibit growth of bacteria by disrupting their ability to make necessary proteins.

▼ DOSAGE GUIDELINES

RANGE AND FREQUENCY
For common bacterial infections—Adults: The usual dose is 1 double strength (DS) tablet 2 times a day. Duration of therapy depends on the type of infection and will be determined by your doctor. For alternative dosages and for treatment of children, consult your pediatrician, as dosages can vary considerably depending on age, weight, and kidney function.

ONSET OF EFFECT
Unknown.

DURATION OF ACTION
Unknown.

DIETARY ADVICE
Tablets should be taken with a full glass of water and can be taken with food to lessen stomach upset.

STORAGE
Store in a tightly sealed container away from heat and direct light.

MISSED DOSE
Take it as soon as you remember. However, if it is near the time for the next dose, skip the missed dose and resume your regular dosage schedule. Do not double the next dose.

STOPPING THE DRUG
Take the drug as prescribed for the full treatment period, even if you begin to feel better before the scheduled end of therapy.

PROLONGED USE
See your doctor regularly for tests and examinations if you must take this medicine for an extended period.

▼ PRECAUTIONS

Over 60: Adverse reactions may be more likely and more severe in older patients.

Driving and Hazardous Work: Do not drive or engage in hazardous work until you determine how the medicine affects you.

Alcohol: No special problems are expected, although it is generally advisable to abstain from alcohol when fighting an infection.

Pregnancy: Trimethoprim with sulfamethoxazole has caused birth defects in animals. Human studies have not been done. It should be used during pregnancy only if the benefits clearly outweigh the possible risks. Before you take this medication, tell your doctor if you are pregnant or plan to become pregnant.

Breast Feeding: Trimethoprim with sulfamethoxazole passes into breast milk; avoid or discontinue use while nursing.

Infants and Children: This medication is not recommended for use by children under the age of 2 months.

Special Concerns: Some patients experience increased sensitivity to sunlight, so take preventive measures: use sunscreens, wear protective clothing, and avoid exposure to the sun. Patients with acquired immunodeficiency syndrome (AIDS) may have a higher incidence of side effects, especially rash. Nonetheless, trimethoprim with sulfamethoxazole remains valuable for treating a number of problems associated with this disease.

OVERDOSE
Symptoms: Loss of appetite, nausea, vomiting, dizziness, headache, drowsiness, depression, confusion, altered mental status, fever, blood in urine, yellow skin or eyes.

What to Do: Call your doctor, emergency medical services (EMS), or the nearest poison control center immediately.

▼ INTERACTIONS

DRUG INTERACTIONS
The following drugs may interact with trimethoprim with sulfamethoxazole. Consult your doctor for specific advice if you are taking cyclosporine, methotrexate, phenytoin, procainamide, sulfonylureas, or warfarin.

FOOD INTERACTIONS
No known food interactions.

DISEASE INTERACTIONS
Use of sulfamethoxazole may cause complications in patients with liver or kidney disease, since these organs work together to remove the medication from the body. This drug can also cause complications in patients with certain types of anemia. Consult your doctor for specific advice if you have any other medical condition.

≡ SIDE EFFECTS ≡

SERIOUS
Skin rash, sore throat, fever, joint pain, shortness of breath, pale skin, reddish spots on skin, unusual bleeding or bruising. Call your doctor immediately.

COMMON
Nausea, vomiting, loss of appetite, allergic skin reactions, itching, hives.

LESS COMMON
Abdominal pain, diarrhea, seizures, dizziness, ringing in ears, headache, hallucinations, depression, unusual sensitivity to sunlight.

VALPROIC ACID (VALPROATE; DIVALPROEX SODIUM)

Available in: Capsules, syrup
Available OTC? No   **As Generic?** Yes
Drug Class: Anticonvulsant

▼ USAGE INFORMATION

WHY IT'S PRESCRIBED
To control certain types of seizures in the treatment of epilepsy and other disorders. Also used to treat acute mania in the treatment of bipolar disorder.

HOW IT WORKS
Valproic acid is thought to depress the activity of certain parts of the brain and suppress the abnormal firing of neurons that causes seizures.

▼ DOSAGE GUIDELINES

RANGE AND FREQUENCY
Adults and children: 7 to 27 mg per lb of body weight, in 3 or 4 divided doses. Higher doses may be required. A low dose is used to start; it may be gradually increased by your doctor to achieve maximum therapeutic benefit with a minimum of side effects.

ONSET OF EFFECT
Within several hours.

DURATION OF ACTION
Maximum effect lasts for 12 hours or longer. Effectiveness then gradually decreases.

DIETARY ADVICE
Take it with food to minimize stomach upset. The syrup can be taken with liquids, but avoid carbonated beverages because the combination can irritate the mouth and throat.

STORAGE
Store in a tightly sealed container away from moisture, heat, and direct light. Do not allow the syrup to freeze.

MISSED DOSE
Take it as soon as you remember. If it is almost time for the next dose, skip the missed dose and resume your regular dosage schedule. Do not double the next dose without doctor's approval.

STOPPING THE DRUG
Abruptly stopping this drug may cause seizures. Your doctor will taper the dose over a period of weeks.

PROLONGED USE
See your doctor regularly for tests if you must take this drug for a prolonged period.

▼ PRECAUTIONS

Over 60: Older patients may require lower doses to minimize side effects.

Driving and Hazardous Work: This drug may cause drowsiness or dizziness. Do not drive or engage in hazardous work until you determine how it affects you.

Alcohol: May contribute to excessive drowsiness.

Pregnancy: Valproic acid is associated with an increased risk of birth defects when taken during pregnancy. However, seizures during pregnancy can also increase the risks to the fetus. Discuss with your doctor the potential risks and benefits of using this drug during pregnancy. Folate supplementation is recommended starting 1 to 2 months before conception and throughout pregnancy.

Breast Feeding: Valproic acid passes into breast milk, although at low levels. Consult your doctor for specific advice before nursing.

Infants and Children: Adverse reactions may be more likely and more severe in children.

Special Concerns: The generic version of this drug is not recommended. Your doctor may advise you to wear a medical bracelet or carry an identification card saying that you are taking this drug.

OVERDOSE
Symptoms: Restlessness, sleepiness, hallucinations, trembling arms and hands, loss of consciousness.

What to Do: Call your doctor, emergency medical services (EMS), or the nearest poison control center immediately.

▼ INTERACTIONS

DRUG INTERACTIONS
Valproic acid can interact with many drugs, including other anticonvulsants (carbamazepine, clonazepam, ethosuximide, felbamate, lamotrigine, phenobarbital, phenytoin, primidone), antacids, aspirin and other NSAIDs, barbiturates, cholestyramine, haloperidol, heparin, isoniazid, loxapine, MAO inhibitors, maprotiline, phenobarbital, tricyclic antidepressants, and warfarin.

FOOD INTERACTIONS
No known food interactions.

DISEASE INTERACTIONS
Special caution is advised if you have a history of blood disease, brain disease, or kidney or liver disease.

≡ SIDE EFFECTS ≡

SERIOUS
Severe abdominal pain and vomiting, muscle weakness and lethargy, yellow discoloration of the skin or eyes, facial swelling, abnormal bleeding or bruising, or seizures may be a sign of liver failure or other potentially fatal complications. Call your doctor immediately.

COMMON
Nausea and vomiting, heartburn, diarrhea, cramps, loss of appetite and weight loss, increased appetite and weight gain, hair loss, tremor, dizziness, confusion, clumsiness or unsteadiness, sedation.

LESS COMMON
Drowsiness, restlessness, constipation, unusual excitability, skin rash, headache, blurred or double vision, irritability or other changes in mental state. There are numerous additional side effects; consult your doctor if you are concerned about any adverse or unusual reactions.

VALSARTAN

Available in: Capsules
Available OTC? No   **As Generic?** No
Drug Class: Antihypertensive/angiotensin II antagonist

▼ USAGE INFORMATION

WHY IT'S PRESCRIBED
To control high blood pressure. This drug appears to have the same benefits as the class of antihypertensive drugs known as ACE inhibitors, without producing the common side effect (experienced by as many as 30% of patients) of a dry cough. Your doctor may prescribe valsartan to be used by itself or in conjunction with other antihypertensive medications.

HOW IT WORKS
Valsartan blocks the effects of angiotensin II, a naturally occurring substance that causes blood vessels to narrow. Valsartan causes the blood vessels to dilate, thereby lowering blood pressure and decreasing the workload of the heart.

▼ DOSAGE GUIDELINES

RANGE AND FREQUENCY
To start, 80 mg once a day. The dose may be increased by your doctor to a maximum dose of 320 mg per day.

ONSET OF EFFECT
Within 2 to 4 weeks.

DURATION OF ACTION
Unknown.

DIETARY ADVICE
Follow a healthy diet (low-salt, low-fat, low-cholesterol) as advised by your doctor to help control blood pressure and prevent heart disease.

STORAGE
Store in a tightly sealed container away from moisture, heat, and direct light.

MISSED DOSE
Take it as soon as you remember. If it is near the time for the next dose, skip the missed dose and resume your regular dosage schedule. Do not double the next dose.

STOPPING THE DRUG
Take it as prescribed for the full treatment period. The decision to stop taking the drug should be made in consultation with your physician.

PROLONGED USE
Lifelong therapy may be necessary. If you change certain health habits (for example, increasing exercise or losing weight), a reduced dose may be possible under a doctor's supervision.

▼ PRECAUTIONS

Over 60: No special problems are expected.

Driving and Hazardous Work: Do not drive or engage in hazardous work until you determine how the medicine affects you.

Alcohol: No special precautions are necessary.

Pregnancy: In certain ways valsartan is similar to a class of drugs that have caused damage to the unborn child when taken in the second or third trimester of pregnancy. Because safer, more effective medications can lower blood pressure during pregnancy, and because adequate studies on the use of valsartan during pregnancy have not been done, women who are pregnant or planning to become pregnant should not take it.

Breast Feeding: Valsartan may pass into breast milk; caution is advised. Consult your doctor for advice.

Infants and Children: The safety and effectiveness of use in children have not been established.

Special Concerns: Valsartan may cause dizziness or lightheadedness, which is most noticeable when you change position. This may lead to fainting, falls, and injury. Sit or lie down immediately if you feel dizzy or lightheaded.

This side effect may be worsened by alcohol, hot weather, dehydration, fever, prolonged standing, prolonged sitting, or exercise.

OVERDOSE
Symptoms: Fainting, dizziness, weak pulse that might be very slow or very fast, nausea, vomiting, confusion, chest pain.

What to Do: An overdose of valsartan is unlikely to be life-threatening. However, if someone takes a much larger dose than prescribed, call your doctor, emergency medical services (EMS), or the nearest poison control center immediately.

▼ INTERACTIONS

DRUG INTERACTIONS
No drug interactions have yet been observed with valsartan. Consult your doctor for specific advice if you are taking any other medication, including other high blood pressure drugs. Valsartan can be taken together with diuretics or other medications for high blood pressure, if your doctor approves.

FOOD INTERACTIONS
No known food interactions.

DISEASE INTERACTIONS
Caution is advised when taking valsartan. Use of valsartan may cause complications in patients with liver or kidney disease, since these organs work together to remove the medication from the body.

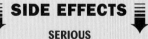

≡ SIDE EFFECTS ≡

SERIOUS
No serious side effects have been reported.

COMMON
No common side effects have been reported.

LESS COMMON
Headache, dizziness, upper respiratory infection, cough, diarrhea, rhinitis, sinusitis, nausea, viral infection, abdominal pain, fatigue, edema, joint pains, heart palpitations, skin rash, constipation, dry mouth, gas, anxiety, insomnia, erectile dysfunction (impotence) in men.

VENLAFAXINE

Available in: Tablets, extended-release capsules
Available OTC? No   **As Generic?** No
Drug Class: Antidepressant

▼ USAGE INFORMATION

WHY IT'S PRESCRIBED
To treat symptoms of major depression and generalized anxiety disorder (GAD).

HOW IT WORKS
Venlafaxine helps to balance levels of serotonin and norepinephrine, which are brain chemicals that are profoundly linked to mood, emotions, and mental state.

▼ DOSAGE GUIDELINES

RANGE AND FREQUENCY
Tablets: Adults: 75 mg a day in 2 or 3 divided doses. The dose may be gradually increased by your doctor to 375 mg a day. Extended-release capsules: 75 mg, once a day. The dose may be increased by up to 75 mg at a time at intervals of not less than 4 days, up to a maximum dose of 225 mg a day.

ONSET OF EFFECT
2 weeks or more.

DURATION OF ACTION
Unknown.

DIETARY ADVICE
Venlafaxine should be taken with meals.

STORAGE
Store in a tightly sealed container away from moisture, heat, and direct light.

MISSED DOSE
Tablets: Take it as soon as you remember, unless the time for your next scheduled dose is within the next 2 hours. If so, skip the missed dose, take the next scheduled dose, and resume your regular schedule. Do not double the next dose. Extended-release capsules: If you miss a dose on one day, do not double the dose the next day.

STOPPING THE DRUG
Take as prescribed for the full treatment period.

PROLONGED USE
See your doctor regularly for tests and examinations if you must take this medicine for an extended period.

▼ PRECAUTIONS

Over 60: No special problems are expected.

Driving and Hazardous Work: Do not drive or engage in hazardous work until you determine how the medicine affects you.

Alcohol: Avoid alcohol.

Pregnancy: Adequate studies of venlafaxine use during pregnancy have not been done. Before you take venlafaxine, tell your doctor if you are pregnant or plan to become pregnant.

Breast Feeding: It is not known whether venlafaxine passes into breast milk; caution is advised. Consult your doctor for specific advice.

Infants and Children: The safety and effectiveness of venlafaxine use by children have not been established.

Special Concerns: Venlafaxine can cause an elevation in blood pressure. Therefore, blood pressure should be monitored regularly, especially in the first several months of drug therapy.

OVERDOSE
Symptoms: Extreme drowsiness or fatigue.

What to Do: Call your doctor, emergency medical services (EMS), or the nearest poison control center immediately.

▼ INTERACTIONS

DRUG INTERACTIONS
Venlafaxine and MAO inhibitors should not be used within 14 days of each other. Serious side effects such as myoclonus (uncontrolled muscle spasms), hyperthermia (excessive rise in body temperature), and extreme stiffness may result. Consult your doctor for specific advice if you are taking any other prescription or over-the-counter medication.

FOOD INTERACTIONS
No known food interactions.

DISEASE INTERACTIONS
Consult your physician if you have a history of any of the following: high or low blood pressure, alcohol or drug abuse, heart disease, or seizures. Use of venlafaxine may cause complications in patients with liver or kidney disease, since these organs work together to remove the medication from the body.

≡ SIDE EFFECTS ≡

SERIOUS
Headache, changes in or blurred vision, decreased sexual ability or desire, difficulty urinating, itching, skin rash, chest pain, heartbeat irregularities, changes in moods or mental state, extreme drowsiness or fatigue. Call your physician immediately.

COMMON
Fatigue, dizziness or drowsiness, anxiety, dry mouth, changed sense of taste, loss of appetite, nausea, vomiting, chills, diarrhea, constipation, prickly sensation of skin, heartburn, increased sweating, runny nose, stomach gas or pain, insomnia, unusual dreams, weight loss.

LESS COMMON
Frequent yawning, twitching.

VERAPAMIL HYDROCHLORIDE

Available in: Extended-release capsules, tablets, injection
Available OTC? No   **As Generic?** Yes
Drug Class: Calcium channel blocker

▼ USAGE INFORMATION

WHY IT'S PRESCRIBED
To treat high blood pressure (hypertension), angina pectoris (chest pain associated with heart disease), and heartbeat irregularities (cardiac arrhythmias).

HOW IT WORKS
Verapamil interferes with the movement of calcium into heart muscle cells and the smooth muscle cells in the walls of the arteries. This action relaxes blood vessels (causing them to widen), which lowers blood pressure, increases the blood supply to the heart, and decreases the heart's overall workload.

▼ DOSAGE GUIDELINES

RANGE AND FREQUENCY
Adults: 40 to 160 mg, 3 times a day. Your doctor may increase dose as necessary, up to a maximum of 480 mg per day. Extended-release capsules: 200 to 480 mg once a day. Extended-release tablets: 120 mg once a day to 240 mg every 12 hours.

Children: The dose will be determined by a pediatrician.

ONSET OF EFFECT
Oral forms: 1 to 2 hours. Injection: 1 to 5 minutes.

DURATION OF ACTION
Extended-release capsules: 24 hours. Tablets: 8 to 10 hours. Injection: 1 to 6 hours.

DIETARY ADVICE
Take oral forms with food.

STORAGE
Store in a tightly sealed container away from heat and direct light.

MISSED DOSE
Take it as soon as you remember. If it is near the time for the next dose, skip the missed dose and resume your regular dosage schedule. Do not double the next dose.

STOPPING THE DRUG
Do not stop taking this drug suddenly, as this may cause potentially serious health problems. If therapy is to be discontinued, dosage should be reduced gradually, according to doctor's instructions.

PROLONGED USE
Lifetime therapy with verapamil may be necessary; regular medical exams and tests are important in such cases.

▼ PRECAUTIONS

Over 60: Adverse reactions may be more likely and more severe in older patients.

Driving and Hazardous Work: Do not drive or engage in hazardous work until you determine how the medicine affects you.

Alcohol: Avoid alcohol.

Pregnancy: Large doses of verapamil have been shown to cause birth defects in animals; human studies have not been done. Before you take verapamil, tell your doctor if you are pregnant or plan to become pregnant.

Breast Feeding: Verapamil passes into breast milk but has not been reported to cause problems; caution is advised. Consult your doctor for advice.

Infants and Children: Oral doses for children 1 to 15 years old must be determined by your pediatrician.

Special Concerns: In addition to taking verapamil, be sure to follow all special instructions on weight control and diet. Your doctor will advise you about which specific factors are most important for you. Check with your doctor before making changes in your diet. Extended-release forms should not be crushed or chewed.

▼ OVERDOSE

Symptoms: Extremely slow heartbeat and heart palpitations; dizziness or fainting (due to excessively low blood pressure).

What to Do: Call your doctor, emergency medical services (EMS), or the nearest poison control center immediately.

▼ INTERACTIONS

DRUG INTERACTIONS
Consult your physician for specific advice if you are taking acetazolamide, amphotericin B, corticosteroids, dichlorphenamide, diuretics, methazolamide, beta-blockers, carbamazepine, cyclosporine, lithium, procainamide, quinidine, digitalis, disopyramide or the following eye medicines: betaxolol, levobunolol, metipranolol, or timolol.

FOOD INTERACTIONS
Avoid foods high in sodium.

DISEASE INTERACTIONS
Caution is advised when taking verapamil. Consult your doctor if you have any of the following: abnormal heart rhythm or other disorders of the heart and blood vessels, mental depression, or Parkinson's disease. Verapamil may cause complications in patients with liver or kidney disease, since these organs work together to remove the medication from the body.

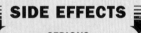

≣ SIDE EFFECTS ≣

SERIOUS
Breathing difficulty, coughing, or wheezing; irregular or pounding heartbeat; chest pain; extreme dizziness; fainting. Call your doctor immediately.

COMMON
Headache, dizziness, constipation, flushing and a feeling of warmth, swelling in the feet, ankles, or calves, heart palpitations.

LESS COMMON
Diarrhea, nausea, unusual fatigue and weakness, skin rash, increased urination, ringing in the ears.

WARFARIN

BRAND NAMES

Coumadin, Panwarfin

Available in: Tablets, injection
Available OTC? No   **As Generic?** Yes
Drug Class: Anticoagulant

▼ USAGE INFORMATION

WHY IT'S PRESCRIBED
To prevent blood clot formation in patients who are suffering from heart, lung, and blood vessel disorders that could likely lead to heart attack, stroke, or other problems.

HOW IT WORKS
Warfarin blocks the action of vitamin K, a compound necessary for blood clotting.

▼ DOSAGE GUIDELINES

RANGE AND FREQUENCY
Adults: To start, 10 to 15 mg daily, taken once a day. Long-term, usually 2 to 10 mg per day, taken once a day. Children: The dose must be determined by a pediatrician. It should be taken at the same time every day.

ONSET OF EFFECT
36 to 48 hours.

DURATION OF ACTION
24 to 96 hours.

DIETARY ADVICE
Warfarin can be taken with liquid or food.

STORAGE
Store in a tightly sealed container away from heat and direct light.

MISSED DOSE
If you miss a dose, take it as soon as you remember, unless it is almost time for the next dose. In that case, skip the missed dose and go back to your regular schedule. Do not double the next dose.

STOPPING THE DRUG
Take it as prescribed for the full treatment period, even if you begin to feel better before the scheduled end of therapy. The decision to stop taking the drug should be made by your doctor.

PROLONGED USE
Regular tests of prothrombin time (a simple test that measures the time it takes for one stage of blood coagulation to occur) are needed when taking this drug. Your doctor may also take stool and urine samples periodically to check for the presence of blood.

▼ PRECAUTIONS

Over 60: Adverse reactions may be more likely and more severe in older patients.

Driving and Hazardous Work: Avoid if you have blurred vision or feel dizzy. Avoid activities that could cause injury.

Alcohol: Use with caution. Alcohol can increase or decrease the effect of warfarin. Usually, consume no more than one drink a day.

Pregnancy: Warfarin may cause birth defects. Do not use during pregnancy.

Breast Feeding: Warfarin passes into breast milk. Do not use while nursing.

Infants and Children: Not recommended for children under 18.

OVERDOSE
Symptoms: Bleeding gums, uncontrolled nosebleeds, blood in the urine or stools.

What to Do: Discontinue the medicine and call your doctor, emergency medical services (EMS), or the nearest poison control right away.

▼ INTERACTIONS

DRUG INTERACTIONS
Consult your doctor for specific advice if you are taking steroid drugs, acetaminophen, allopurinol, aminogluthemide, antibiotics, antiarrhythmic heart drugs, androgens, antacids, antifungal drugs, antihistamines, aspirin, antidiabetic drugs, disulfiram, a nonsteroidal anti-inflammatory drug (NSAID), barbiturates, benzodiazepine tranquilizers, calcium supplements, chloramphenicol, or any cholesterol-lowering drugs.

FOOD INTERACTIONS
Avoid green, leafy vegetables and other foods that are rich in vitamin K (liver, broccoli, cauliflower, kale, spinach, and cabbage). Intake of too much vitamin K can override the anticlotting effect of warfarin and render the drug useless. On the other hand, certain substances can interfere with the absorption of vitamin K so much that normal, healthy clotting (necessary for wounds to heal) is impaired. Megadoses of vitamin E can do this, as can fish oil supplements and foods high in omega-3 fatty acids. These substances can enhance the effect of anticlotting drugs so much that a tendency to hemorrhage may result.

DISEASE INTERACTIONS
Consult your doctor about taking warfarin if you have high blood pressure, diabetes, serious liver or kidney disease, or a severe allergy.

≡ SIDE EFFECTS ≡

SERIOUS
Allergic reaction (marked by wheezing, breathing difficulty, hives, or swelling of lips, tongue, and throat); bleeding into skin and soft tissue; abnormal bleeding from nose, gastrointestinal tract, urinary tract, or uterus; severe infection; excessive or unexpected menstrual bleeding; black vomit; bruises or purple marks on skin. Consult your doctor immediately.

COMMON
No common side effects have been reported.

LESS COMMON
Loss of appetite, unusual weight loss, nausea, vomiting, skin rash, diarrhea, cramping.

ZAFIRLUKAST

Available in: Tablets
Available OTC? No   **As Generic?** No
Drug Class: Leukotriene receptor antagonist

▼ USAGE INFORMATION

WHY IT'S PRESCRIBED
To prevent the symptoms of asthma on a maintenance basis and also to prevent bronchospasm (contraction of the smooth muscle tissue surrounding the airways, which results in narrowing and obstruction of the air passages). Zafirlukast may be used in conjunction with other asthma treatments.

HOW IT WORKS
Zafirlukast blocks receptors for leukotrienes, chemicals that cause inflammation and constriction of the bronchial airways. Unlike bronchodilators, which relieve an acute asthma attack, zafirlukast is taken regularly when no symptoms are present, to reduce the chronic airway inflammation that underlies asthma. This prevents symptomatic asthma attacks.

▼ DOSAGE GUIDELINES

RANGE AND FREQUENCY
Adults and teenagers: 20 mg twice a day. Children ages 7 to 11: 10 mg twice a day. Doses are usually taken in the morning and evening, on an empty stomach (at least 1 hour before or 2 hours after eating).

ONSET OF EFFECT
Within 1 week.

DURATION OF ACTION
Unknown.

DIETARY ADVICE
Zafirlukast should be taken 1 hour before or 2 hours after meals. Taking with a high-fat or high-protein meal reduces its availability in the body by 40%.

STORAGE
Store in a tightly sealed container away from heat and direct light.

MISSED DOSE
Take it as soon as you remember. If it is near the time for the next dose, skip the missed dose and resume your regular dosage schedule. Do not double the next dose.

STOPPING THE DRUG
The decision to stop the drug should be made by a doctor.

PROLONGED USE
No problems are expected. It is important to take zafirlukast every day, even during symptom-free periods.

▼ PRECAUTIONS

Over 60: In clinical trials, mild or moderate infections, primarily of the respiratory tract, occurred more often than expected in older patients. The rate of infection was proportional to the dose of zafirlukast taken. Other adverse reactions were no more likely or more severe in older patients than in younger persons.

Driving and Hazardous Work: Do not drive or engage in hazardous work until you determine how the medication affects you.

Alcohol: No special warnings.

Pregnancy: In some animal studies, zafirlukast caused birth defects and other problems. Human studies have not been done. Before you take zafirlukast, tell your doctor if you are pregnant or plan to become pregnant.

Breast Feeding: Zafirlukast passes into breast milk; do not use it while nursing.

Infants and Children: The safety and effectiveness of zafirlukast in children under the age of 7 have not been established.

Special Concerns: Zafirlukast has no effect on an asthma attack already in progress. In very rare cases, the drug may cause Churg-Strauss syndrome, a tissue disorder that strikes adult asthma patients and, if untreated, can destroy organs. Early symptoms include fever, muscle aches, and weight loss.

OVERDOSE
Symptoms: None.

What to Do: Call your doctor if you suspect an overdose.

▼ INTERACTIONS

DRUG INTERACTIONS
Consult your doctor for specific advice if you are taking aspirin, carbamazepine, cyclosporine, felodipine, isradipine, nicardipine, nifedipine, nimodipine, phenytoin, tolbutamide, erythromycin, terfenadine, theophylline, or warfarin. Patients who are taking warfarin or any other anticoagulant should have their prothrombin time monitored closely, and appropriate changes made in the anticoagulant dosage, when they start taking zafirlukast. Before you take zafirlukast, tell your doctor if you are allergic to any over-the-counter or prescription medicine.

FOOD INTERACTIONS
No known food interactions.

DISEASE INTERACTIONS
Consult your doctor if you have any other medical condition. Use of zafirlukast can cause complications in patients with liver disease, since this organ works to remove the medication from the body.

⧮ SIDE EFFECTS ⧮

SERIOUS
Burning or prickling sensation, skin rash. A rare side effect with high doses is liver dysfunction (symptoms include: abdominal pain, nausea, fatigue, lethargy, itching, yellow discoloration of the eyes or skin, and flu-like symptoms). Call your doctor immediately.

COMMON
Headache.

LESS COMMON
Weakness, abdominal pain, back pain, diarrhea, dizziness, mouth ulcers, nausea, vomiting.

ZALEPLON

Available in: Capsules
Available OTC? No   **As Generic?** No
Drug Class: Sedative/hypnotic

▼ USAGE INFORMATION

WHY IT'S PRESCRIBED
For the short-term treatment of insomnia and other sleep-related problems.

HOW IT WORKS
By depressing activity in the central nervous system (the brain and spinal cord), zaleplon causes drowsiness and mild sedation. Because the drug is metabolized more quickly than similar medications, zaleplon is associated with a lower incidence of such common side effects as daytime drowsiness.

▼ DOSAGE GUIDELINES

RANGE AND FREQUENCY
The appropriate dosage will be determined by your doctor. The recommended dosage for adults: 10 mg. Debilitated patients and people over 60: 5 mg. Zaleplon should only be taken at bedtime or after the patient has gone to bed and has difficulty falling asleep.

ONSET OF EFFECT
Within 1 hour.

DURATION OF ACTION
About 4 hours.

DIETARY ADVICE
Do not take following a heavy, high-fat meal. The absorption of zaleplon may be slowed, thereby reducing the drug's effectiveness.

STORAGE
Store in a tightly sealed container away from moisture, heat, and direct light.

MISSED DOSE
If you forget to take the medication at bedtime and you are unable to fall asleep, you can still take the drug unless it is within 4 hours of when you need to be awake.

STOPPING THE DRUG
The decision to stop taking the drug should be made in consultation with your doctor.

PROLONGED USE
Zaleplon is usually prescribed only for short-term therapy (lasting several days or up to 4 weeks). See your doctor for periodic evaluations if you must take this drug for a longer time. Persistent

insomnia may be a sign of an underlying medical problem.

▼ PRECAUTIONS

Over 60: Adverse reactions may be more likely in older patients. Smaller doses are usually prescribed.

Driving and Hazardous Work: Avoid such activities until you determine how this medication affects you.

Alcohol: Avoid alcohol.

Pregnancy: In large doses zaleplon has been shown to slow the progress of fetal development in animals. Human studies have not been done. Zaleplon is not recommended for use by pregnant women. Before you take zaleplon, be sure to tell your doctor if you are pregnant or plan to become pregnant.

Breast Feeding: Zaleplon passes into breast milk, but its effect on the nursing infant is unknown. Women who are nursing should not take this medication.

Infants and Children: Safety and effectiveness have not been established for patients under age 18.

Special Concerns: When you stop taking zaleplon, you may have trouble falling asleep for the first few nights.

OVERDOSE
Symptoms: Severe drowsiness, breathing difficulty, severe clumsiness or unsteadiness, severe dizziness, severe nausea and vomiting, slow heartbeat, vision problems.

What to Do: Call your doctor, emergency medical services (EMS), or the nearest poison control center immediately.

▼ INTERACTIONS

DRUG INTERACTIONS
Other drugs may interact with zaleplon. Consult your doctor for specific advice if you are taking rifampin, phenytoin, carbamazepine, phenobarbital or other drugs that depress the central nervous system; these include antihistamines, other psychiatric medications, barbiturates, sedatives, cough medicines, decongestants, and painkillers. Be sure your doctor knows about any over-the-counter medication you may take.

FOOD INTERACTIONS
No known food interactions.

DISEASE INTERACTIONS
Caution is advised when taking zaleplon. Consult your doctor if you have a history of drug dependence or alcohol abuse, chronic respiratory disease (including asthma, bronchitis, or emphysema), mental depression, or sleep apnea. Using zaleplon may cause complications in patients with liver disease, since this organ works to remove the medication from the body.

≡ SIDE EFFECTS ≡

SERIOUS
Hallucinations, abnormal thoughts or behavior, confusion or disorientation, unsteadiness, dizziness, lightheadedness, unusual nervousness, agitation, difficulty breathing. Call your doctor immediately.

COMMON
Daytime drowsiness, general pain or discomfort, memory problems, headache.

LESS COMMON
Abdominal pain, weakness, fever.

ZANAMIVIR

Available in: Inhalant
Available OTC? No **As Generic?** No
Drug Class: Antiviral

▼ USAGE INFORMATION

WHY IT'S PRESCRIBED
To treat type A or type B influenza. Zanamivir can reduce the severity of symptoms and shorten the duration of flu episodes.

HOW IT WORKS
Zanamivir is believed to interfere with the synthesis of the viral enzyme neuraminidase, which a virus needs in order to infect cells in the respiratory tract and elsewhere in the body. The drug affects only certain susceptible strains of the influenza type A or type B viruses.

▼ DOSAGE GUIDELINES

RANGE AND FREQUENCY
Adults and teenagers: 2 inhalations (one 5-mg blister per inhalation) every 12 hours for 5 days. On the first day of treatment, 2 doses should be taken if at all possible, provided there is at least 2 hours between doses. On subsequent days, follow the dosage schedule outlined above. Treatment should be initiated within 2 days after the onset of symptoms of the flu.

ONSET OF EFFECT
Unknown.

DURATION OF ACTION
Unknown.

DIETARY ADVICE
No special restrictions.

STORAGE
Store in a tightly sealed container away from heat and direct light.

MISSED DOSE
Take it as soon as you remember that you have missed your dose. If it is near the time for the next dose, skip the missed dose and resume your regular dosage schedule. Do not double the next dose.

STOPPING THE DRUG
It is important to take zanamivir for the full treatment period as prescribed. Do not stop taking the drug before the scheduled end of therapy even if you begin to feel better, as this may lead to a relapse.

PROLONGED USE
If your symptoms do not improve or if they become worse in a few days, you should consult your doctor.

▼ PRECAUTIONS

Over 60: No special problems are expected.

Driving and Hazardous Work: Avoid such activities until you determine how the medicine affects you.

Alcohol: No special warnings.

Pregnancy: Adequate studies have not been completed. Discuss with your doctor the relative risks and benefits of using this drug while pregnant.

Breast Feeding: Zanamivir may pass into breast milk, although it is unknown if this poses any risks to the nursing infant. Consult your doctor for specific advice.

Infants and Children: Zanamivir is not recommended for children under the age of 12.

Special Concerns: Zanamivir should be administered using the Diskhaler device. See your doctor for instructions and a demonstration of the proper use of this device.

OVERDOSE
Symptoms: No specific ones have been reported.

What to Do: If you have any reason to suspect an overdose, call your doctor, emergency medical services (EMS), or the nearest poison control center.

▼ INTERACTIONS

DRUG INTERACTIONS
No known drug interactions.

FOOD INTERACTIONS
No known food interactions.

DISEASE INTERACTIONS
Consult your doctor if you have any respiratory illness, such as chronic obstructive pulmonary disease (COPD) or asthma.

⬇ SIDE EFFECTS ⬇

SERIOUS
There are no serious side effects associated with the use of zanamivir.

COMMON
There are no common side effects associated with the use of zanamivir.

LESS COMMON
Dizziness.

ZIDOVUDINE (AZT)

Available in: Capsules, syrup, injection
Available OTC? No   **As Generic?** No
Drug Class: Antiviral

BRAND NAME

Retrovir

▼ USAGE INFORMATION

WHY IT'S PRESCRIBED
To treat HIV infection in combination with other drugs and to prevent passage of the virus from pregnant women to their babies. Although not a cure for HIV, this drug may suppress the replication of the virus and delay the progression of the disease. Also used to treat HIV-related dementia and HIV-related thrombocytopenia (low platelet count).

HOW IT WORKS
Zidovudine (AZT) interferes with the activity of enzymes needed for the replication of DNA in viral cells, thus preventing the human immunodeficiency virus (HIV) from reproducing.

▼ DOSAGE GUIDELINES

RANGE AND FREQUENCY
For HIV infection—Adults and teenagers: Capsules: 200 mg, 3 times a day, or 300 mg, 2 times a day. Injection (given until oral dose can be taken): Adults and teenagers: 0.9 mg per lb of body weight injected slowly into a vein every 4 hours (6 times a day). To prevent the transmission of HIV to newborns—For pregnant women: Capsules: 100 mg, 5 times a day from 14th week of pregnancy to delivery. Injection: 0.9 mg per lb of body weight for first hour of delivery, followed by 0.45 mg per lb until baby is delivered. For newborns: Syrup: 0.9 mg per lb of body weight starting within 12 hours of birth and continuing for 6 weeks. Higher doses (up to 1,200 mg per day) are sometimes used to treat HIV-related dementia or thrombocytopenia.

ONSET OF EFFECT
Unknown. With most antiretroviral drugs, an early response can be seen within the first few days of therapy, but the maximum effect may take 12 to 16 weeks.

DURATION OF ACTION
Unknown. The effects of zidovudine may be prolonged if the medication is used in combination with other effective drugs and the virus is maximally suppressed.

≡ SIDE EFFECTS ≡

SERIOUS
Anemia (low red blood cell count) causing paleness, fatigue, or shortness of breath; fever. If such symptoms occur, call your doctor right away.

COMMON
Headaches, nausea, muscle aches, insomnia, mood swings, stomach upset, loss of appetite.

LESS COMMON
Bands of discoloration on the fingernails; hepatitis (liver inflammation, which may cause yellowish discoloration of skin and eyes).

DIETARY ADVICE
Take with food to minimize side effects.

STORAGE
Store in a tightly sealed container away from heat and direct light.

MISSED DOSE
Take the drug as soon as you remember. If it is near the time for the next dose, skip the missed dose and resume your regular dosage schedule. Do not double the next dose.

STOPPING THE DRUG
The decision to stop taking the drug should be made in consultation with your doctor.

PROLONGED USE
See your doctor regularly for tests and examinations as long as you take this drug.

▼ PRECAUTIONS

Over 60: No special studies have been done on older patients. A lower dose may be warranted, especially if kidney function is impaired.

Driving and Hazardous Work: Do not drive or engage in hazardous work until you determine how the medicine affects you.

Alcohol: Avoid alcohol if liver function is impaired.

Pregnancy: Zidovudine can decrease the risk of passing the AIDS virus to the unborn child; in animal studies it has not caused birth defects.

Breast Feeding: Women who are infected with HIV should not breast feed to avoid transmitting the virus to an uninfected child.

Infants and Children: The usage and dosage of zidovudine for infants and children must be determined by your doctor.

Special Concerns: Use of zidovudine does not eliminate the risk of passing HIV to other persons. You should take appropriate preventive measures.

OVERDOSE
Symptoms: Sudden nausea and vomiting; headache, dizziness, or drowsiness.

What to Do: Seek medical assistance right away.

▼ INTERACTIONS

DRUG INTERACTIONS
Consult your doctor for specific advice if you are taking amphotericin B (by injection), anticancer agents, thyroid drugs, azathioprine, chloramphenicol, colchicine, cyclophosphamide, flucytosine, ganciclovir, interferon, mercaptopurine, methotrexate, plicamycin, clarithromycin, or probenecid. Also consult your doctor for specific advice if you are taking any other prescription or over-the-counter medication.

FOOD INTERACTIONS
Zidovudine may be better tolerated if taken with food.

DISEASE INTERACTIONS
Caution is advised when taking zidovudine. Consult your doctor if you have anemia or another blood problem or liver disease.

ZOLMITRIPTAN

Available in: Tablets
Available OTC? No   **As Generic?** No
Drug Class: Antimigraine/antiheadache drug

▼ USAGE INFORMATION

WHY IT'S PRESCRIBED
To treat severe, acute migraine headaches. This medication is not intended as a migraine preventive or for use against any other kinds of pain or headache, including basilar and hemiplegic migraines. Your doctor will determine whether zolmitriptan is appropriate in your particular case.

HOW IT WORKS
The exact mechanism of zolmitriptan's action is unknown.

▼ DOSAGE GUIDELINES

RANGE AND FREQUENCY
A single dose ranging from half of a 2.5 mg tablet to one 5 mg tablet is generally effective. If the migraine returns or there is only partial relief, the dose may be repeated once after 2 hours, but no more than 10 mg should be taken in a 24-hour period. Because the individual response to zolmitriptan may vary, your

doctor will determine the appropriate dosage. A general recommendation is to take one 2.5 mg tablet as the initial dose.

ONSET OF EFFECT
Within 2 hours.

DURATION OF ACTION
Up to 24 hours.

DIETARY ADVICE
The medication can be taken with or without food.

STORAGE
Store in a tightly sealed container away from moisture, heat, and direct light.

MISSED DOSE
Not applicable, since the drug is taken only when necessary.

STOPPING THE DRUG
Consult your doctor before discontinuing zolmitriptan.

PROLONGED USE
No special problems are expected. Patients at risk for heart disease should undergo periodic medical tests and evaluation.

▼ PRECAUTIONS

Over 60: Zolmitriptan is not recommended for use in older patients.

Driving and Hazardous Work: Do not drive or engage in dangerous work until you determine how the medication affects you.

Alcohol: No special warnings, although alcohol may trigger or exacerbate migraine headaches.

Pregnancy: Do not use zolmitriptan without first consulting your doctor if you are pregnant or if you suspect you might be pregnant.

Breast Feeding: Zolmitriptan may pass into breast milk; consult your doctor.

Infants and Children: The safety and effectiveness in patients under age 18 have not been established.

Special Concerns: Serious, but rare, heart-related problems may occur after using zolmitriptan. Anyone at risk for unrecognized coronary artery disease—such as postmenopausal women, men over the age of 40, or people with known risk factors for heart disease (hypertension, high blood cholesterol levels, obesity, diabetes, a strong family history of heart disease, or cigarette smoking)—should have the first dose of the medication administered in a doctor's office. Zolmitriptan should not be used by anyone with any symptoms of active heart disease (chest pain or tightness, shortness of breath).

OVERDOSE
Symptoms: Increase in blood pressure resulting in lightheadedness, tension in the neck, fatigue, and loss of coordination.

What to Do: An overdose with zolmitriptan is unlikely. If someone takes a much larger dose than prescribed, call your doctor, emergency medical services (EMS), or the nearest poison control center immediately.

▼ INTERACTIONS

DRUG INTERACTIONS
Do not take zolmitriptan within 24 hours of taking almotriptan, naratriptan, sumatriptan, rizatriptan, ergotamine-containing medication, dihydroergotamine mesylate, or methysergide mesylate. Zolmitriptan and MAO inhibitors such as phenelzine, tranylcypromine, procarbazine, and selegiline should not be used within 14 days of each other. Zolmitriptan should be used with caution in patients taking SSRIs (selective serotonin reuptake inhibitors), which include fluoxetine, fluvoxamine, paroxetine, and sertraline.

FOOD INTERACTIONS
See Dietary Advice.

DISEASE INTERACTIONS
You should not take zolmitriptan if you have a history of angina, heart disease, stroke, uncontrolled hypertension, heartbeat irregularities, or peripheral vascular disease. Zolmitriptan should be used with caution in patients with liver disease or severely impaired kidney function.

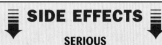

≣ SIDE EFFECTS ≣

SERIOUS
Serious side effects with zolmitriptan are rare. However, zolmitriptan may cause a heart attack, chest pain or tightness, sudden or severe abdominal pain, shortness of breath, wheezing, heartbeat irregularities, swelling of face, eyelids, or lips, skin rash, or hives. Seek emergency medical assistance immediately.

COMMON
Hot flashes or chills, numbness, prickling or tingling sensations, dry mouth, dizziness, drowsiness, weakness.

LESS COMMON
Indigestion, nausea, muscle ache.

ZOLPIDEM TARTRATE

Available in: Tablets
Available OTC? No   **As Generic?** No
Drug Class: Sedative/hypnotic

▼ USAGE INFORMATION

WHY IT'S PRESCRIBED
For the short-term treatment of insomnia.

HOW IT WORKS
Zolpidem depresses activity in the central nervous system (the brain and spinal cord), which causes drowsiness and mild sedation.

▼ DOSAGE GUIDELINES

RANGE AND FREQUENCY
Adults: 10 mg at bedtime. Patients over 60: 5 mg at bedtime.

ONSET OF EFFECT
Within minutes.

DURATION OF ACTION
2 to 4 hours.

DIETARY ADVICE
Zolpidem may be taken without regard to diet, although it generally works faster on an empty stomach.

STORAGE
Store in a tightly sealed container away from heat and direct light.

MISSED DOSE
Take the drug as soon as you remember, unless it is late at night. Do not take the drug unless your schedule permits 7 or 8 hours of sleep.

STOPPING THE DRUG
The decision to stop taking the drug should be made in consultation with your doctor. Discontinuing the drug abruptly may produce withdrawal symptoms (including sleep disruption, nervousness, irritability, diarrhea, abdominal cramps, muscle aches, memory impairment). The dosage should be reduced gradually according to your doctor's instructions.

PROLONGED USE
Zolpidem is usually prescribed only for short-term therapy (lasting several days or up to 2 weeks). See your doctor for periodic evaluations if you must take this medicine for a longer time. Persistent insomnia may be a sign of an underlying medical problem.

▼ PRECAUTIONS

Over 60: Adverse reactions may be more likely and more severe in older patients. Smaller doses usually are prescribed.

Driving and Hazardous Work: Zolpidem may impair mental alertness and physical coordination. Adjust your activities accordingly.

Alcohol: Avoid alcohol.

Pregnancy: In large doses zolpidem has been shown to slow the progress of fetal development in animals. Human studies have not been done. Before you take the drug, be sure to tell your doctor if you are pregnant or plan to become pregnant.

Breast Feeding: Zolpidem passes into breast milk, but its effect on the nursing infant is unknown. Consult your doctor for advice.

Infants and Children: Safety and effectiveness have not been established for patients under age 18.

Special Concerns: When you stop taking zolpidem, you may have trouble falling asleep for the first few nights.

OVERDOSE
Symptoms: Severe drowsiness, breathing difficulty, severe clumsiness or unsteadiness, severe dizziness, severe nausea and vomiting, slow heartbeat, vision problems.

What to Do: Call your doctor, emergency medical services (EMS), or the nearest poison control center immediately.

▼ INTERACTIONS

DRUG INTERACTIONS
Other drugs may interact with zolpidem. Consult your doctor for specific advice if you are taking tricyclic antidepressants (such as amitriptyline, clomipramine, doxepin, or nortriptyline) or other drugs that depress the central nervous system; these include antihistamines, barbiturates, other psychiatric medications, sedatives, cough medicines, decongestants, and painkillers. Be sure your doctor knows about any over-the-counter medication you may take.

FOOD INTERACTIONS
No known food interactions.

DISEASE INTERACTIONS
Caution is advised when taking zolpidem. Consult your doctor if you have a history of alcohol abuse or drug dependence, sleep apnea, chronic respiratory disease (including asthma, bronchitis, or emphysema), or mental depression. Use of zolpidem may cause complications in patients with liver or kidney disease, since these organs work together to remove the medication from the body.

≡ SIDE EFFECTS ≡

SERIOUS
Hallucinations, abnormal thoughts or behavior, confusion or disorientation, unsteadiness, dizziness, lightheadedness, unusual nervousness, agitation, difficulty breathing. Call your doctor immediately.

COMMON
Daytime drowsiness, diarrhea, general pain or discomfort, memory problems, nausea, bizarre or unusually vivid dreams, vomiting.

LESS COMMON
Stomach discomfort, agitation, feelings of panic, convulsions, muscle cramps, nausea, vomiting, unusual fatigue, uncontrolled weeping, worsening of emotional problems, vision problems, dry mouth.

CERTIFIED POISON CONTROL CENTERS

A poison control center can provide valuable instruction in the event of a potential drug overdose or other emergency involving an ingested substance. The places below, listed by state, are all certified by the American Association of Poison Control Centers. Each is staffed 24 hours a day by trained personnel who can answer questions about what to do in the event of a possible drug overdose or poisoning with a toxic substance.

Calling the national toll-free number (800) 222-1222 will connect you directly to a regional poison center for your area. In addition, many hospitals and medical centers provide emergency services within a local area. Keep your area numbers handy in the event of an emergency. In addition, keep a bottle of ipecac syrup on hand, in case you are told to "induce vomiting," as well as a supply of activated charcoal.

Alabama
Alabama Poison Center, Tuscaloosa
(800) 222-1222

Regional Poison Control Center, Birmingham
(800) 222-1222
(205) 939-9720

Arizona
Arizona Poison and Drug Information Center, Tucson
(800) 222-1222
(520) 626-7899

Samaritan Regional Poison Center, Phoenix
(800) 222-1222
(602) 495-6360

California
Central California Regional Poison Control Center, Fresno/Madera
(800) 876-4766 (CA only)
(800) 972-3323 (TTY/TDD)
(559) 622-2300

San Diego Regional Poison Center
(800) 876-4766 (CA only)
(800) 972-3323 (TTY/TDD)
(858) 715-6300

San Francisco Bay Area Regional Poison Control Center
(800) 876-4766 (CA only)
(800) 972-3323 (TTY/TDD)
(415) 502-6000

University of California at Davis Medical Center, Regional Poison Control Center, Sacramento
(800) 876-4766 (CA only)
(800) 972-3323 (TTY/TDD)

(916) 227-1400

Colorado
Rocky Mountain Poison and Drug Center, Denver
(800) 222-1222
(303) 739-1100

Connecticut
Connecticut Regional Poison Center, Farmington
(800) 222-1222
(866) 218-5372 (TTY/TDD)
(860) 679-4540

Delaware
The Poison Control Center, Philadelphia
(800) 222-1222
(215) 590-8789 (TTY/TDD)
(215) 590-2003

District of Columbia
National Capital Poison Center, Washington, D.C.
(800) 222-1222
(202) 362-8563 (TTY/TDD)
(202) 362-3867

Florida
Florida Poison Information Center—Jacksonville
(800) 222-1222
(800) 282-3171 (TTY/TDD)
(904) 244-4465

Florida Poison Information Center, Tampa
(800) 222-1222
(813) 844-7044

Georgia
Georgia Poison Center, Atlanta
(800) 222-1222

(404) 616-9287 (TDD)
(404) 616-9237

Indiana
Indiana Poison Center, Indianapolis
(800) 222-1222
(317) 929-2336 (TTY)
(317) 929-2335

Kentucky
Kentucky Regional Poison Center, Louisville
(800) 222-1222
(502) 629-7264

Louisiana
Louisiana Drug and Poison Information Center, Monroe
(800) 222-1222
(318) 342-3648

Maryland
Maryland Poison Center, Baltimore
(800) 222-1222
(410) 706-1858 (TDD)
(410) 706-7604

Massachusetts
Regional Center for Poison Control and Prevention, Boston
(800) 222-1222
(888) 244-5313 (TTY/TDD)
(617) 355-6609

Michigan
Regional Poison Control Center, Children's Hospital of Michigan, Detroit
(800) 222-1222
(800) 356-3232 (TDD)
(313) 745-5335

Minnesota
Hennepin Regional Poison Center,

Minneapolis
(800) 222-1222
(612) 904-4691 (TTY)
(612) 347-3144

Missouri
Cardinal Glennon Children's Hospital
Regional Poison Center, St. Louis
(800) 222-1222
(314) 772-8300

Montana
Rocky Mountain Poison and Drug
Center, Denver, CO
(800) 222-1222
(303) 739-1100

Nebraska
The Poison Center, Omaha
(800) 222-1222
(402) 955-6976

Nevada
Rocky Mountain Poison and Drug
Center, Denver, CO
(800) 222-1222
(303) 739-1100

New Jersey
New Jersey Poison Information and
Education System, Newark
(800) 222-1222
(973) 926-8008 (TTY/TDD)
(973) 926-7443

New Mexico
New Mexico Poison and Drug
Information Center, Albuquerque
(800) 222-1222
(505) 272-4261

New York
Finger Lakes Regional Poison Center,
Rochester
(800) 222-1222
(716) 273-3854 (TTY)
(716) 273-4155

Hudson Valley Regional Poison Center,
Sleepy Hollow
(800) 222-1222
(914) 366-3031

Long Island Regional Poison Control
Center, Mineola
(800) 222-1222
(516) 747-3323 (TDD Nassau)
(516) 924-8811 (TDD Suffolk)
(516) 663-4574

New York City Poison Control Center
(800) 222-1222
(212) 689-9014 (TDD)
(212) 447-8152
(212) 447-2666

North Carolina
Carolinas Poison Center, Charlotte
(800) 222-1222
(704) 395-3795

Ohio
Central Ohio Poison Center, Columbus
(800) 222-1222
(614) 228-2272 (TTY)
(614) 722-2635

Cincinnati Drug & Poison Information
Center and Regional Poison Control
System
(800) 222-1222
(513) 636-5063

Oregon
Oregon Poison Center, Portland
(800) 222-1222
(503) 494-8600

Pennsylvania
Central Pennsylvania Poison Center,
Hershey
(800) 222-1222
(717) 531-8335 (TTY)
(717) 531-7057

The Poison Control Center, Philadelphia
(800) 222-1222
(215) 590-8789 (TTY/TDD)
(215) 590-2003

Pittsburgh Poison Center
(800) 222-1222
(412) 390-3300

Rhode Island
Regional Center for Poison Control and
Prevention, Boston
(800) 222-1222
(888) 244-5313 (TTY/TDD)
(617) 355-6609

Tennessee
Middle Tennessee Poison Center,
Nashville
(800) 222-1222
(615) 936-2047 (TDD)
(615) 936-0760

Texas
North Texas Poison Center, Dallas
(800) 764-7661 (TX only)
(214) 589-0911

Southeast Texas Poison Center,
Galveston
(800) 764-7661 (TX only)
(409) 765-1420
(800) 764-7661 (TTY/TDD, TX only)
(409) 766-4403

Utah
Utah Poison Control Center, Salt Lake City
(800) 222-1222
(801) 581-7504

Virginia
Blue Ridge Poison Center, Charlottesville
(800) 222-1222
(804) 924-0347

Washington
Washington Poison Center, Seattle
(800) 222-1222
(800) 572-0638 (TDD: WA only)
(206) 517-2394 (TDD)
(206) 517-2350

West Virginia
West Virginia Poison Center, Charleston
(800) 222-1222
(304) 347-1212

Wyoming
The Poison Center, Omaha, NE
(800) 222-1222
(402) 955-6976 (NE & WY only)

HEALTH INFORMATION ORGANIZATIONS

▼

There are hundreds of health information organizations in this country. They offer a range of services, from sending literature on a specific disorder or providing updates on the latest drugs and treatments to making referrals to physicians, hospitals, or local support groups. Some focus on a single disease or area of health; others operate on a national level and offer general advice on a wide range of health issues.

Which type of group or organization is right for you depends on your particular needs. When looking for additional informa-

tion or support, a good place to start is with your doctor, who may be able to recommend specific groups for you to contact. You can also refer to the list of major national health information organizations below. Many have toll-free phone numbers or fax lines. Others can be contacted via the Internet or e-mail. This is a limited listing. There are many more associations that offer valuable patient support. If one organization doesn't have the information you need, a staff member may be able to refer you to another one that does.

Agency for Healthcare Research and Quality (AHRQ)
2101 East Jefferson Street
Rockville, MD 20852-4908
(800) 358-9295
Internet site: http://www.ahrq.gov
An information clearinghouse sponsored by the U.S. Department of Health and Human Services. Offers publications on back pain, HIV infection, living with heart disease, and many other topics.

American Academy of Pediatrics
141 Northwest Point Boulevard
Elk Grove Village, IL 60007-1098
(847) 434-4000
Internet site: http://www.aap.org
Offers child-related publications on antibiotics, safety, first aid, and more.

American Cancer Society (ACS)
1599 Clifton Road, NE
Atlanta, GA 30329-4251
(800) 227-2345
Internet site: http://www.cancer.org
A national organization offering information on the management of all types of cancer. Makes referrals to local self-help organizations.

American Cancer Society
Response Line
(800) 227-2345
Provides publications and information about cancer and its treatment.

American Diabetes Association
1701 North Beauregard Street
Alexandria, VA 22311
(800) DIABETES (342-2383)
Internet site: http://www.diabetes.org
Provides information and public education programs on diabetes.

American Dietetic Association
216 West Jackson Boulevard
Chicago, IL 60606-6995
Nutrition Hotline
(800) 366-1655
Internet site: http://www.eatright.org
Provides recorded nutritional messages from registered dietitians. The organization also answers food and nutrition questions and makes referrals to registered dietitians.

American Heart Association
7272 Greenville Avenue
Dallas, TX 75231
(800) 242-8721
Internet site: http://www.americanheart.org
A national organization with many local branches, offering pamphlets and public education programs on all aspects of cardiovascular health. Check your telephone book for a branch near you.

American Self-Help Clearinghouse
St. Clare's Riverside Medical Center
25 Pocono Road
Denville, NJ 07834
(973) 625-7101
A not-for-profit agency that makes referrals to more than 700 national self-help groups. Also provides information on how to start your own local self-help group.

Arthritis Foundation
P.O. Box 7669
Atlanta, GA 30357-0669
(800) 283-7800
(404) 872-7100
E-mail: help@arthritis.org
Internet site: http://www.arthritis.org
Makes referrals to local chapters and provides information on the causes and treatment of rheumatoid arthritis, osteoarthritis, and other musculoskeletal disorders. Also provides services to improve quality of life for people with arthritis.

Cancer Information Service
Office of Cancer Communications
National Cancer Institute
(800) 4-CANCER (422-6237)
Internet: http://cis.nci.nih.gov/
A hotline of the National Cancer Institute, offering information on cancer, smoking cessation, and other topics.

CDC National AIDS Hotline
(800) 342-AIDS (342-2437)
Sponsored by the Centers for Disease Control and Prevention. Offers publications and referrals to thousands of community-based organizations that deal with AIDS and HIV infection.

CDC National STD Hotline
(800) 227-8922
Sponsored by the Centers for Disease Control and Prevention. Provides anonymous, detailed information on sexually transmitted diseases.

CDC Travel Health Line
(877) FYI-TRIP (394-8747)
Fax-on-command: (888) 232-3299
Internet site: http://www.cdc.gov/travel/
Sponsored by the Centers for Disease Control and Prevention. Detailed health advice tailored to specific international travel destinations.

Centers for Disease Control and Prevention (CDC)
Office of Public Affairs
1600 Clifton Road, NE
Atlanta, GA 30333
(800) 311-3435
(404) 639-3534
Internet site: http://www.cdc.gov
A U.S. government agency dealing with issues of public health, including AIDS and other infectious diseases, environmental concerns, and occupational safety.

Consumer Health Information Research Institute (CHIRI)
300 East Pinkhill Road
Independence, MO 64057
(816) 228-4595
A nonprofit organization that answers consumer questions on health-related fraud and quackery.

Food and Drug Administration (FDA)
5600 Fishers Lane
Rockville, MD 20857
(888) INFO-FDA (463-6332)
Internet site: http://www.fda.gov
The U.S. government agency that aims to protect consumers against impure and unsafe foods, drugs, and cosmetics. Answers questions, listens to complaints, and makes referrals to other appropriate agencies. Offers FDA publications on drug labeling, safe use of medications, food and nutrition, and other topics.

National Cancer Institute
National Institutes of Health
9000 Rockville Pike
Bethesda, MD 20892
(301) 435-3848
CancerFax: (301) 402-5874
Internet site: http://www.nci.nih.gov
A branch of the National Institutes of Health that provides information on dozens of types of cancers.

National Eye Institute
2020 Vision Place
Bethesda, MD 20892-3655
(301) 496-5248
E-mail: 2020@nei.nih.gov
Internet site: http://www.nei.nih.gov
A branch of the National Institutes of Health that provides information on various eye ailments.

National Heart, Lung, and Blood Institute
Office of Prevention, Education, and Control
31 Center Drive, MSC 2480
Bethesda, MD 20892-2480
(301) 496-0554
Internet site: http://www.nhlbi.nih.gov
A branch of the National Institutes of Health that provides written material on cardiovascular and respiratory health.

National Institute of Allergy and Infectious Diseases (NIAID)
NIAID Office of Communications and Public Liaison
31 Center Drive MSC 2520
Bethesda, MD 20892-2520
(301) 496-5717
Internet site: http://www.niaid.nih.gov
Provides information on pollen allergies, dust allergies, sexually transmitted diseases, and other topics.

National Institute of Arthritis and Musculoskeletal and Skin Diseases (NIAMS)
Information Clearinghouse
1 AMS Circle
Bethesda, MD 20892-3675
(301) 495-4484
(877) 22-NIAMS (226-4267)
Internet site: http:/www.nih.gov/niams/
A branch of the National Institutes of Health, offering information on arthritis, osteoporosis, various skin diseases, and other topics.

National Institute of Child Health and Human Development
(800) 370-2943
Internet site: http://www.nichd.nih.gov/
A branch of the National Institutes of Health that provides information on issues of child health and development.

National Institute of Diabetes and Digestive and Kidney Disorders (NIDDK)
(301) 496-3583
Internet site: http://www.niddk.nih.gov/
A branch of the National Institutes of Health that offers information on diabetes, digestive disorders, endocrine and metabolic disorders, kidney disease, nutrition and obesity, and urologic disease.

National Institute on Aging
31 Center Drive, MSC 2292
Bethesda, MD 20892
(800) 222-2225
301-496-1752
Internet site: http://www.nih.gov/nia/
A branch of the National Institutes of Health that provides information and publications on arthritis, accident prevention, incontinence, cancer, menopause, osteoporosis, nutrition, heart disease, and other topics of interest to older adults.

National Institutes of Health
9000 Rockville Pike
Bethesda, MD 20892
(301) 496-4461
Fax: (301) 496-0017
Internet site: http://www.nih.gov
The principal medical research arm of the U.S. government. Makes referrals to appropriate federal agencies.

National Institute of Mental Health (NIMH)
NIMH Public Inquiries
6001 Executive Boulevard, Rm. 8184, MSC 9663
Bethesda, MD 20892-9663
(301) 443-4513
Internet site: http:/www.nimh.nih.gov/
Makes referrals to local mental health associations and offers publications on depression, bipolar disorder, anxiety, phobias, panic disorder, Alzheimer's disease, and other conditions.

National Library of Medicine
Public Health Service
National Institutes of Health
8600 Rockville Pike
Bethesda, MD 20894
(888) FIND-NLM (346-3656)
(301) 594-5983
Internet site: http://www.nlm.nih.gov/
One of the world's largest health science libraries. Open to the public. Offers reference services to general consumers.

National Self-Help Clearinghouse (NSHC)
365 Fifth Avenue
Suite 3300
New York, NY 10016
(212) 817-1822
Internet site: http://www.selfhelpweb.org/
Provides referral services to local self-help groups and organizations.

The Office on Women's Health
Room 730B
Humphrey Building
200 Independence Avenue, SW
Washington, DC 20201
(202) 690-7650
http://www.4woman.gov/owh/
A branch of the Department of Health and Human Services. Provides general fact sheets on various issues in women's health.

GLOSSARY OF DRUG TERMS

▼

ACE inhibitor: An abbreviation for angiotensin-converting enzyme inhibitor, a type of *antihypertensive* drug. ACE inhibitors prevent the formation of angiotensin II, a naturally occurring substance that constricts blood vessels, thus causing blood pressure to rise.

active ingredient: The chemical component of a drug preparation that exerts the desired therapeutic effects. The active ingredient is commonly what we think of as the "drug." Drugs contain *inactive ingredients* as well, such as the binders and colorings added to a pill to hold it together and give it its characteristic color.

addiction: A term used to describe physical dependence on a drug; psychological factors may also play a role in addiction.

adverse reaction: A harmful and unintended response to a drug.

agonist: A drug or other compound that stimulates activity in specific cells, setting into motion particular chemical reactions and bodily processes.

allergic drug reaction: An exaggerated immune response to a drug, which can result in hives, itching, or, in serious cases, shock and breathing difficulty. People who are allergic to one drug, such as penicillin, may also be allergic to chemically related drugs in the same drug class.

aminoglycoside: One of a group of chemically related *antibiotics* that is used to treat a variety of infections.

amphetamine: One of a group of drugs, related to the generic parent drug amphetamine, that stimulates the central nervous system.

analgesic: An agent that relieves pain. Some examples of analgesics include *narcotics, NSAIDs* (which have other properties in addition to pain relief), and a varied group of miscellaneous pain-relievers, such as acetaminophen.

anaphylaxis: An acute allergic reaction to a drug or venom, as from a bee sting, that may be marked by swollen airways and severe difficulty in breathing.

androgen: A male sex hormone, such as testosterone, that is administered for cancer, certain endocrine disorders, and a few other conditions.

anesthetic: A drug that eliminates the sensation of pain.

angiotensin-converting enzyme inhibitor: See *ACE inhibitor.*

anorectic: A drug that suppresses appetite. Some drugs suppress appetite as a *side effect.*

antacid: A drug that counteracts stomach acids. Antacids are used to relieve indigestion, heartburn, peptic ulcers, and a few other gastrointestinal disorders.

antagonist: A drug or other compound that inhibits chemical activity in specific cells, suppressing particular physiological reactions and bodily processes.

antianginal: A drug, such as a *nitrate*, that relieves the chest pain caused by insufficient flow of heart blood, a characteristic of angina.

antianxiety agent: A psychiatric drug, also called an anxiolytic, that relieves anxiety. These drugs also help to relax muscles and to treat insomnia.

antiarrhythmic: A drug used to correct heart rhythm abnormalities.

antiasthmatic: A drug used in the treatment of asthma.

antibacterial: A drug used specifically to combat bacterial infections, as opposed to infections caused by other microorganisms, such as fungi and viruses. Also commonly referred to as an *antibiotic.*

antibiotic: A drug that kills or inhibits the growth of infectious bacteria or other germs. Some antibiotics are naturally produced by bacteria, fungi, and other microorganisms; others are synthetic (man-made).

antibody: A protein produced by the immune system that normally acts to neutralize or eliminate foreign substances in the body. A *drug allergy* is associated with an overactive response of an antibody to a particular drug.

anticancer agent: A drug used to combat cancer.

anticlotting agent: A general term describing a drug that inhibits the clotting of blood. These drugs are sometimes referred to as *anticoagulants.*

anticoagulant: A drug that blocks the activity of certain blood clotting factors that promote the formation of fibrin, a protein essential in the formation of blood clots. Anticoagulant drugs can either impede the formation of a clot or prevent an already formed clot from breaking away, traveling to a narrow blood vessel, and stopping circulation in a critical organ.

anticonvulsant: A drug used to control seizures or convulsions, typically those brought on by epilepsy.

antidementia drug: A drug that slows the progression of Alzheimer's disease and other related forms of mental deterioration.

antidepressant: A drug that elevates mood and relieves depression. Types of antidepressants include *tricyclic antidepressants, monoamine oxidase (MAO) inhibitors*, and *selective serotonin reuptake inhibitors*.

antidiabetic agent: A drug used to treat diabetes.

antidiarrheal agent: A drug that relieves diarrhea.

antidote: A compound that counteracts *poisoning*.

antiemetic: A drug used to stop or prevent vomiting.

antifungal: A drug that combats fungal infections, such as athlete's foot or nail fungus. *Topical* antifungals are applied externally to the skin, hair, or nails. *Systemic* antifungals are taken orally or by injection; typically they help to fight fungal infections affecting the bloodstream or other internal organs or tissues.

antiglaucoma agent: A drug used to treat glaucoma, the buildup of excessive pressure in the eye. This condition is a common cause of blindness in older people.

antigout agent: A type of drug that serves to relieve gout (a painful arthritic condition of the joints) by limiting the buildup of uric acid, a metabolic waste product.

antihistamine: A drug that blocks the actions of *histamine*. Such drugs relieve allergies, hay fever, hives, rashes, itching, cold symptoms, and motion sickness.

antihypertensive: A drug that lowers blood pressure in people with high blood pressure (hypertension), a condition that increases the risk for stroke, heart disease, and many other ailments. Different types of antihypertensives are prescribed for people with mildly elevated blood pressure and for those with extremely high blood pressure.

antihypotensive: A drug that elevates blood pressure in people who have dangerously low blood pressure (hypotension).

anti-infective: A drug used to treat infections, including those caused by bacteria (*antibacterials*), fungi (*antifungals*), viruses (*antivirals*), parasites (*antiparasitics*), and other disease-causing microorganisms.

anti-inflammatory: A drug used to reduce the swelling, redness, or pain caused by inflammation, an immune reaction to injury that can occur either inside the body (for example, arthritic joints) or on a localized external area (for example, skin rash). Some anti-inflammatory drugs are *steroids*; others are nonsteroidal (see *NSAIDs*).

antimalarial: An *antiparasitic* drug used specifically to treat or prevent malaria, a mosquito-borne illness caused by the plasmodia parasite.

antimanic drug: A medication that relieves the mental and physical hyperactivity and incapacitating mania and mood elevation that are characteristic of manic-depressive illness (bipolar disorder).

antimicrobial agent: A general term for a drug used to treat infections due to microorganisms, such as bacteria, fungi, and viruses. This group of drugs includes *anti-infectives, antibiotics, antifungals*, and *antivirals*.

antimigraine drug: A drug that relieves or prevents migraine headaches.

antinauseant: A medication that relieves or prevents the queasy sensations of nausea.

antineoplastic agent: A drug used to counter the growth and spread of tumors and malignant cells.

antiobesity agent: A drug that works to promote weight loss through any of various mechanisms. Some of the antiobesity drugs are *serotonergics*.

antiparasitic: A drug used to treat infestations of parasites, including worms and amoebas.

antiparkinsonism agent: A drug used to relieve the trembling and rigidity of Parkinson's disease and other related disorders. These drugs are also called antiparkinsonian agents.

antiplatelet agent: A drug that reduces the tendency of blood cells called platelets to clump together and form clots where the normal flow of blood is disrupted. For example, blood flow may be impaired by fatty deposits in the coronary arteries of someone who has heart disease, predisposing that person to a heart attack. Aspirin, in low doses, is the most widely prescribed antiplatelet drug.

antiproliferative: A drug that suppresses the excess proliferation of skin cells that occurs in certain skin disorders, such as psoriasis.

antipruritic: A drug that is used to relieve itching.

antipsoriatic: A drug used to treat psoriasis, a chronic skin and joint condition marked by scaly red patches. In some cases, this medication is also used for arthritis.

antipsychotic: A drug used to treat severe psychiatric disorders, such as schizophrenia and others that cause hallucinations or delusions.

antipyretic: A drug used to reduce fever (elevated body temperature).

antireflux agent: A drug that alleviates gastroesophageal reflux (commonly known as heartburn).

antirheumatic: A drug used to treat rheumatoid arthritis, a serious, recurring form of arthritis marked by pain and inflammation of the joints.

antiseptic: A drug or other substance that arrests the growth and action of bacteria and other microorganisms. Also called a germicide.

antispasmodic: A drug used to reduce involuntary muscle spasms, such as those that can occur in the gastrointestinal tract or bladder.

antitubercular agent: A type of drug used in the treatment and prevention of tuberculosis.

antitussive: A cough suppressant.

antiurolithic: A drug used in the treatment of kidney stones, a relatively common disorder that is marked by

the formation of small, hard pellets in the urinary tract.

antiviral: A drug used to combat infections caused by viruses, such as AIDS.

anxiolytic: See *antianxiety agent.*

aplastic anemia: A rare but potentially fatal side effect of certain drugs characterized by suppression of the bone marrow, resulting in the inability to produce adequate amounts of essential blood components.

autonomic nervous system: The part of the nervous system that controls smooth muscle (the type that surrounds blood vessels and other structures), heart muscle, and many of the body's so-called involuntary actions, such as glandular secretions, the motion of the gastrointestinal tract, and the contraction or dilation of blood vessels. Many drugs, such as some used for hypertension, act through the autonomic nervous system. Because this system has such wide-ranging effects, drugs that affect it typically produce a wide variety of side effects in addition to their desired therapeutic actions.

azalide: A type of *antibiotic* used to fight infections.

barbiturate: One of a class of related drugs that are used as *hypnotics*, *sedatives*, and *antispasmodics* to induce sleep, relieve anxiety, and relax the muscles.

behavior modifier: A drug that can facilitate a behavior change, such as stopping excessive drinking or quitting smoking.

benzodiazepine: One of a class of related *antianxiety* drugs used as tranquilizers. Examples include diazepam (brand name Valium) and

alprazolam (brand name Xanax); many end with the suffix "-epam" or "-olam."

beta-blocker: A drug that inhibits chemical activity in specialized nervous system structures called beta receptors, which are found in the heart, the airways, and other areas. Beta-blockers are commonly used as *antihypertensive* drugs; they lower blood pressure by slowing the heart rate and reducing the force of the heartbeat. They are also sometimes used to treat angina, abnormal heart rhythm, anxiety, glaucoma, and other disorders.

bioavailability: A scientific term for the degree and rate at which a substance, such as a drug, is absorbed into the body and becomes available to exert therapeutic effects.

bioequivalent: A scientific term for drugs that have equivalent chemical properties, so that equal amounts of each drug are delivered to the body in a similar time frame. Generic drugs, for example, are bioequivalent to brand name drugs.

bone resorption inhibitor: A drug that suppresses the normal breakdown of bone. These drugs are useful for treating high blood calcium levels (hypercalcemia) or bone disorders such as Paget's disease.

brand name: The name chosen by a drug manufacturer to market a drug. Prozac, for example, is the brand name for the antidepressant drug with the *generic name* fluoxetine.

brand name drug: A drug that is sold under a registered *brand name.*

broad-spectrum antibiotic: An antibiotic drug that is active against a wide range of infectious bacteria.

bronchodilator: A drug that prompts the bronchial air passages to expand, making it easier to breathe. Bronchodilators are primarily used to treat asthma and related conditions.

calcium channel blocker: A type of *antihypertensive* drug that induces the muscle surrounding blood vessels to relax. It does this by decreasing the movement of calcium ions through muscle cell membranes, thus causing blood vessels to dilate and blood pressure to fall.

caplets: Oblong, capsule-shaped tablets that are generally easier to swallow than round pills.

cardiac glycoside: See *digitalis drug*.

catecholamine: One of a group of chemical messengers that have wide-spread effects on the body, such as speeding up the heart, raising blood pressure, and increasing respiration. Man-made catecholamines have been prepared as drugs, primarily for use in emergency situations.

centrally acting: A drug or other agent that works through the *central nervous system* to produce its desired therapeutic effects.

central nervous system (CNS): The part of the nervous system consisting of the brain and spinal cord.

cephalosporin: One of a group of chemically related *antibiotics,* originally derived from a fungus and since enhanced with the production of man-made versions, that are widely used to treat a variety of infections.

chelating agent: A drug that binds with metals, reducing their concentration in body tissues. Toxic levels of metals can build up in cases of lead poisoning or in such conditions as Wilson's disease, a hereditary disorder marked by the buildup of copper in the body.

chemotherapy: The use of drugs to combat cancer or other conditions.

clearance: The rate at which a drug is passed through the kidneys and into the urine. The term *renal clearance* is sometimes used instead. ("Renal" stands for something related to, involving, or affecting the kidneys.)

contraceptive: A drug or device used to prevent pregnancy.

contraindication: A disease or condition that either completely precludes the use of a certain drug or means that the drug should be used with special caution.

corticosteroid: A type of anti-inflammatory drug that mimics the actions of powerful naturally occurring substances called *steroids*, which are released by the adrenal glands and have numerous and widespread effects on the body. Corticosteroids are available in many forms, including *inhalant, ophthalmic, otic, topical,* and *systemic* preparations. They are used to treat asthma, allergies, skin inflammations, inflammatory bowel disease, some forms of cancer, and other disorders.

cytotoxic drug: A drug that works by killing rapidly dividing cells, typically those associated with cancer.

decongestant: A drug that relieves nasal or sinus congestion resulting from colds or allergies.

dependence: Addiction to a drug, or the need to continue to use a drug, because of psychological or physical factors. *Narcotics,* for example, commonly lead to dependence.

desensitization: A medical treatment for a drug allergy that aims to lessen sensitivity and improve *tolerance* to the drug by administering, over time, a series of gradually increased doses.

digitalis drug: A type of drug that slows the heartbeat and increases the force with which the heart beats, thereby improving the pumping action of the heart and relieving the symptoms of congestive heart failure. Also known as a cardiac glycoside.

diuretic: A drug that alters kidney function by drawing water from the body and increasing the total output of urine.

divided doses: Doses of a drug given at intervals that are spaced throughout the day, rather than as a single dose.

drug allergy: An allergic reaction to a specific drug, such as *penicillin,* or to a drug component. Responses can range from mild (for example, a skin rash) to severe (shock, difficulty breathing, and other complications associated with *anaphylaxis*). Those with a drug allergy should avoid use of the drug as well as substances that are chemically related to the drug. Such individuals should also inform their doctors, dentist, and others of the drug allergy (regardless of severity).

drug class: A group of drugs that have similar chemical structures and actions on or within the body. There are many different classes of drugs. Although members of a drug class have similar properties, there are variations among them that may make one particular drug preferable for a specific disorder or patient over other drugs in the same class.

drug fever: An adverse drug reaction marked by elevated body temperature, resulting from an allergic reaction or other causes.

drug interaction: Reciprocal activity or influence between two or more drugs that may alter the effects of one or all of the drugs involved. Drug interactions vary widely. They may increase–or decrease–the amount of active drug, the effectiveness of a drug, and the likelihood of adverse side effects. Responses to a drug interaction can range from clinically inapparent or mild to life-threatening.

drug rash: A skin rash resulting from an allergic reaction to a particular medication, usually appearing during the first few days after taking it. Drug rashes can occur with either *topical* or *systemic* preparations.

electrolyte: A chemical, such as calcium, potassium, or sodium, dissolved in blood or cellular fluids, that acts as a vital messenger for many bodily processes. Electrolytes are essential, for example, in maintaining heart rhythm and kidney function. Certain drugs can disrupt electrolyte levels.

elixir: A form of liquid medication that consists of a drug mixed in a flavored alcohol solution.

emollient: A drug preparation or other substance that is applied to the skin to soothe and soften the area. Many emollients can also be applied to the lips and *mucous membranes.*

estrogen: A female sex hormone, produced by the ovaries, that has multiple effects, including stimulating the reproductive cycle and the development of female secondary sex characteristics. Various forms of estrogen are used as drugs for treating menopause symptoms, breast cancer, and other conditions.

estrogen replacement therapy: The use of supplemental *estrogen*, one of the female sex hormones produced by the ovaries, to relieve the adverse effects of menopause.

expectorant: A type of drug used in cough preparations that promotes the discharge and expulsion of mucus or phlegm from the throat and airways.

Food and Drug Administration (FDA): The U.S. governmental agency that regulates and monitors food and drug safety. Its functions include ruling on the safety of new drugs before they become available to the public, reclassifying drugs from prescription to *OTC* status, regulating food and drug labeling, and establishing safe limits for additives.

food interactions: An action between a specific food and a drug, which may influence the amount of drug available in the body for therapeutic effects. Because of food interactions, some drugs should not be taken with meals in general, or with specific foods in particular.

g or gm: An abbreviation for *gram.*

generic drug: A copycat version of a *brand name drug.* Generic drugs are chemically equivalent to brand name drugs but cost loss. Generics, which cannot be marketed until the exclusive patent for the brand name drug has expired (usually after about 20 years), are normally sold simply under the drug's *generic name.*

generic name: The scientific name for a drug. Generic names, as opposed to *brand names*, are nonproprietary and are recognized worldwide.

gram (g): A metric measure of weight, sometimes used in drug dosages. There are about 454 grams in a pound.

growth hormone: A naturally occurring chemical secreted by the pituitary gland that promotes growth by acting through a number of intermediaries on various body tissues. Synthetic versions of the hormone are available as drugs and are usually administered by injection to children. Also called somatotropic hormone or somatotropin.

habituation: A term used to describe psychological dependence on a drug.

histamine: A compound produced by cells in the stomach, skin, respiratory tract, and elsewhere. Histamine aids digestion by triggering stomach acid secretion. It also plays a central role in allergic reactions, causing inflammation, hives, itching, and constriction of the airways.

histamine (H1) blocker: A type of *antihistamine* used to treat hay fever and other allergies.

histamine (H2) blocker: A drug that binds to a specialized receptor in the stomach wall termed an H2 receptor, thereby preventing the release of *histamine*. In the digestive tract, histamine triggers stomach acid secretion. The drugs in this group are commonly used to treat heartburn, ulcers, and other digestive disorders.

hormone: Chemicals, secreted by various organs, that are typically carried by the bloodstream and exert their effects on cells and tissues throughout the body. Some hormones have been synthesized and are used as drugs to regulate the menstrual cycle, promote growth, combat cancer, and treat other conditions.

hypersensitivity: An exaggerated response to a drug, or a drug-related allergic reaction.

hypnotic: A drug that is used primarily to induce sleep (for example, a *benzodiazepine*).

hypoglycemic agent: A drug that lowers blood sugar levels, commonly used in the treatment of diabetes.

immunization: Stimulation of the immune system to produce antibodies against a specific disease, thereby conferring protection against it, through the oral or injectable administration of a *vaccine*, a *toxoid*, or cells or blood serum from infected persons. The term is sometimes used interchangeably with *vaccination*.

immunosuppressant: A drug that suppresses the immune system. Such an effect may be desirable to prevent the immune system from rejecting a new organ following a transplant, and sometimes in the treatment of certain cancers, the autoimmune disease rheumatoid arthritis, or other serious medical conditions.

implant: A capsule that is implanted under the skin and that slowly releases a drug into the body for an extended period.

inactive ingredient: A substance, such as a coloring, flavoring, binder, gelatin capsule coating, or preservative, that does not have any therapeutic effects but that is combined with an active drug compound during the manufacturing process to make a medication. Most manufacturers list the inactive ingredients alphabetically on the label's ingredients list.

indication: The disorder, condition, disease, or symptom for which a drug is prescribed or approved for use by the Food and Drug Administration.

inhalant: A drug preparation that is inhaled through the mouth or nose.

interferon: A naturally occurring substance that activates the body's immune response. Interferons have been synthesized for use as anti-cancer agents and also as drugs for various other purposes.

intramuscular: Into the muscle. Some medications and vaccines are formulated as solutions that are injected into a muscle. The body then absorbs the drug from the muscle.

intravenous: Into the vein. Many drugs are formulated as solutions for injection or slow drip into a vein, where they gain immediate access to the bloodstream. The drug is then carried by the blood to other parts of the body.

jaundice: A liver disorder, marked by yellow discoloration of the skin and eyes, that may be the result of liver disease, an allergic reaction to a drug, or even an adverse reaction to a drug that affects the liver. Jaundice is often reversible, but its cause should always be investigated because of the liver's crucial function in the body.

keratolytic: A medication used to treat certain skin conditions, such as acne, that causes the layer of dead skin on its uppermost surface to peel.

kg: An abbreviation for *kilogram*.

kilogram (kg): A metric unit of weight equal to about 2.2 pounds. Some drug doses are prescribed per kg of body weight.

laxative: One of a group of drugs that relieves constipation by adding bulk to stools (bulk-forming laxative), softening stools (stool softener), lubricating the gastrointestinal tract (lubricant), or increasing intestinal tract motility (stimulant).

lipid-lowering drug: A medication that lowers harmful blood cholesterol levels and helps to reduce the risk of heart disease. Also called a cholesterol-lowering drug.

local: An effect that is felt within a restricted portion or area of the body. Drugs that tend to act locally—including most *topical* agents applied to the skin, *inhalants* that act on the airways, and *ophthalmic* preparations applied to the eyes—generally produce less serious *side effects* than *systemic* drugs, which act on multiple sites throughout the body.

loop diuretic: One of a class of *diuretic* drugs commonly prescribed for the treatment of high blood pressure. Loop diuretics act on the part of the kidneys known as the loop of Henle to block the reabsorption of sodium and water into the bloodstream. This action leads to an increased amount of fluid (urine) leaving the body.

macrolide: One of a group of *antibiotics* that are active against various infectious microorganisms and that share a characteristic chemical ring structure.

MAO inhibitor: See *monoamine oxidase inhibitor.*

mast-cell stabilizer: A drug that prevents the release of *histamine* from specialized cells (mast cells) in the respiratory passages, thus reducing inflammation of the airways. Mast-cell stabilizers are commonly used in the treatment of asthma.

mcg: An abbreviation for *microgram.*

mEq: An abbreviation for *milliequiv-alent.*

metered-dose inhaler: A device, commonly used by patients with asthma, that converts liquid medicine into an aerosol spray. The spray can then be breathed in through the mouth, delivering a standard dose of medication to the airways.

mg: An abbreviation for *milligram.*

microgram (mcg): A metric measure of weight, equal to one-millionth of a *gram*, that is sometimes used in drug dosages.

milliequivalent (mEq): A chemical unit of measure that is sometimes used to indicate dosages of vitamins and some drugs.

milligram (mg): A metric measure of weight, equal to one-thousandth of a *gram*, that is commonly used in drug dosages.

milliliter (mL): A metric measure of volume, equal to one-thousandth of a liter, that is sometimes used in dosing recommendations for liquid medications. There are about 5 mL in a teaspoon, 15 mL in a tablespoon, 30 mL in one fluid ounce, and 240 mL in one cup (8 fluid ounces).

mineral: An inorganic substance, found in the earth's crust, that plays a crucial role in the human body for enzyme synthesis, regulation of heart rhythm, bone formation, digestion, and other metabolic processes. Humans constantly replenish their mineral supply with food and water.

miotic: A drug that causes constriction of the pupils (miosis).

mL: An abbreviation for *milliliter.*

monoamine oxidase (MAO) inhibitor: An *antidepressant* drug that elevates mood by blocking the actions of the nervous system enzyme, monoamine oxidase, thereby increasing levels of specialized substances called mono-amines in the brain.

mucolytic: A type of medication that is used in the treatment of coughs to thin and break up excessive mucus secretions.

mucous membrane: The pink and shiny skin-like layers that line the lips, mouth, vagina, eyelids, stomach, gastrointestinal and urinary tracts, and other cavities and passages in the body. The mucous membranes secrete the thick and slippery fluid called mucus, which lubricates and protects these tissues. Some drugs are formulated as *topical* prepara-tions for application specifically to the mucous membranes.

narcotic: A drug that acts on the *central nervous system* and that is used primarily to diminish pain but which has numerous effects on the body, including drowsiness and mental clouding (without loss of con-sciousness), slowed breathing, and decreased motility of the gastrointes-tinal tract. Also sometimes called an opiate or opioid.

nebulizer: A device that uses com-pressed air to convert liquid medica-tions into extremely fine aerosolized mists that can deeply penetrate the lungs when inhaled through the mouth or nose. A nebulizer is particu-larly effective for dilating constricted bronchial tubes, making it easier to breathe. Nebulizers are frequently used in the form of *metered-dose inhalers,* hand-held devices designed

to deliver a standardized dose of the medication.

nephrotoxic: Poisonous, or toxic, to the kidneys. Because a number of medications are considered potentially nephrotoxic, the function and health of the kidneys should be closely mon-itored while taking such drugs.

neuropathy: An adverse side effect of certain drugs that is caused by dam-age to nerves and marked by burning, tingling, pain, or numbness in the fingers, toes, limbs, or other areas.

neurotoxicity: A scientific term for the nerve damage that can occur as a side effect of certain drugs or *toxins.*

nitrates: A group of *antianginal* drugs that dilate the heart's blood vessels, making it easier for blood to flow through them.

nonsteroidal anti-inflammatory drug: See *NSAID.*

NSAID: An abbreviation for a non-steroidal anti-inflammatory drug. NSAIDs reduce pain and inflammation in damaged tissues in such conditions as arthritis and headache by blocking the production of specialized *hor-mone*-like fatty acids known as *prostaglandins.*

off-label use: A common—and legiti-mate—practice in which a doctor prescribes one or more drugs for a disease, symptom, or condition that has not been specifically approved by the *FDA*. Once a drug has been approved for one *indication*, doctors are then free to prescribe the drug for other purposes.

ointment: A semisolid drug prepara-tion, usually having a greasy or fatty base, typically applied to the skin.

ophthalmic: A drug that has been formulated for administration onto or around the eye.

opiate or opioid: A morphine-like pain-relieving drug chemically related to opium. See *narcotic*.

oral agent: A drug in solid (such as a pill or capsule) or liquid form that is meant to be ingested by swallowing.

orthostatic hypotension: A dramatic drop in blood pressure upon sitting or standing up, especially if coming to an upright position quickly. Symptoms include faintness, dizziness, and loss of balance. Various *antihypertensive* agents and other drugs can cause this type of very low blood pressure.

OTC: A common abbreviation for *over-the-counter* drugs.

otic: A drug that has been formulated for administration into or onto the surface of the ear.

ototoxicity: A scientific term for the damage to structures in the ear and loss of hearing that can occur as an adverse reaction to certain drugs (for example, *aminoglycoside antibiotics*) and *toxins*.

over-the-counter (OTC): A drug that is allowed to be sold without a prescription—for example, at a pharmacy, supermarket, or convenience store. An increasing number of drugs that were formerly available only by *prescription* can now be purchased OTC, although the dose is typically lower than that of the prescription version.

overdose: Excessive accumulation of a drug in the body, resulting in toxic levels that can be extremely dangerous. An accidental overdose is of particular concern in children, older adults, and those who have kidney, liver, or other diseases that may impair their ability to process and excrete a drug. An intentional overdose is a concern in depressed patients attempting suicide.

parenteral: A medication that is designed to be administered by a route other than orally (through the gastrointestinal tract), such as by injection into the muscles (*intramuscular*) or veins (*intravenous*) or through the skin (*subcutaneous*).

parkinsonism: A nervous disorder that can result as a side effect of certain drugs. Symptoms resemble those of Parkinson's disease and include generalized weakness; a rigid, mask-like facial expression; trembling or tremors in the hands, arms, or legs; and a rigid posture and shuffling gait.

penicillin: One of a group of *antibiotics* (first mass-produced for clinical use in the 1940s) that are widely used against a range of infections. Many derivatives of penicillin, such as amoxicillin, have since been synthesized; their names end with the suffix "-illin."

peripherally acting: A drug or other agent that works on or near the surface or periphery of the body, often via the *peripheral nervous system*.

peripheral nervous system: The part of the nervous system outside of the brain and spinal cord, such as the nerves leading to the muscles, skin, and internal organs.

pharmacist: A professional who is licensed to dispense *prescription* medicines.

photosensitivity: An adverse *side effect* of certain medications marked by a decreased tolerance to the sun's ultraviolet rays, resulting in a tendency for exposed skin to sunburn easily.

pioneer drug: The first version of a new, *brand name* drug.

poisoning: Illness, injury, or death due to exposure to a drug or toxin. Depending on the toxic qualities of the substance and its potency, small or large amounts can cause poisoning.

potassium-sparing diuretic: A mild *diuretic* drug commonly prescribed for the treatment of high blood pressure. Such drugs act on the kidneys to block the reabsorption of sodium and water by the bloodstream, leading to an increase in the volume of urine. Potassium-sparing diuretics help to prevent excessive loss of the electrolyte potassium, a common problem with other types of diuretics.

prescription: An instruction by a physician that directs a pharmacist to dispense a particular drug in a specific formulation and dose. Prescription medications, unlike *over-the-counter* drugs, require the physician's approval, usually in written form.

priapism: A medical term for a condition characterized by prolonged and painful erection of the penis, resulting from an obstructed outflow of blood in this organ. In some cases, priapism occurs as a side effect or reaction to a medication and is only relieved once the medication is stopped.

progestin: A general term for progesterone, a female sex *hormone* produced by the ovaries that helps to regulate menstruation. Synthetic versions of progestin have been prepared as drugs for use as *contraceptives* and in the treatment of menopause, certain cancers, abnormal uterine bleeding, and other conditions.

prostaglandin: One of a group of chemicals, occurring naturally in the body, that produce a wide range of effects, such as inducing pain and inflammation, stimulating contractions of the uterus during labor, and protecting the stomach's lining. Some drugs, such as misoprostol, are man-made prostaglandins. Other drugs, such as *NSAIDs*, counteract the effects of certain prostaglandins.

protease inhibitor drug: A drug that blocks production of a key enzyme, protease, which the virus that causes AIDS (the HIV virus) needs in order to replicate. These drugs have helped to keep AIDS from developing in countless HIV-infected individuals.

renal clearance: The rate at which a drug is passed through the kidneys and into the urine. "Renal" stands for something related to, involving, or affecting the kidneys. Some sources refer to renal clearance as *clearance*.

retinoid: A man-made derivative of vitamin A used to treat acne, skin wrinkling, and other skin conditions. Tretinoin is a classic example of a retinoid drug.

Reye or Reye's syndrome: A rare but swift and potentially fatal condition in children and teenagers marked by liver degeneration and swelling of the brain. The illness is thought to be related to the administration of aspirin to children under age 16 who have signs and symptoms of the chicken pox, the flu, or a flu-like viral illness.

sedative: A drug that has a calming or tranquilizing effect, used primarily to reduce anxiety or nervousness.

selective serotonin reuptake inhibitor (SSRI): One of a newer class of *antidepressant* drugs that elevates mood by indirectly increasing the levels of a specialized chemical in the brain (a neurotransmitter) called serotonin. Various SSRI medications are currently being sold (by prescription only) and are used by large numbers of individuals. Among the commonly recognized SSRI medications are fluoxetine (Prozac) and sertraline (Zoloft).

serotonergic: A drug that increases the supply of a nervous system chemical in the brain called serotonin. Some serotonergics are used as *antiobesity agents* because they help make the patient feel satiated (full).

serotonin-blocker: A drug that blocks activity of the nervous system chemical serotonin in the brain. This effect may help to stimulate appetite or relieve certain types of headache.

side effect: A secondary, and often adverse, effect of a drug. Side effects are known and predictable responses to a specific drug, though usually only a small number of individuals taking the drug will experience them.

soft tissue: A general term for internal body parts other than bones and joints, such as muscles and the tissue under the skin. Soft tissue can become infected by microorganisms such as bacteria; *anti-infectives* are used to treat such infections.

solution: A mixture of one or more drugs that are dissolved in a liquid.

spacer: A device commonly used in conjunction with a *metered-dose inhaler* that attaches to the inhaler's mouthpiece and acts as a reservoir to hold the airborne medicine. The use of a spacer helps to ensure that a standard dose of the medication is delivered to airways.

SPF: An abbreviation for Sun Protection Factor, which indicates the relative ability of a sunscreen to block out the sun's damaging ultraviolet rays. Experts recommend using an SPF of at least 15, which will allow a person to remain in the sun without sustaining ultraviolet burn damage for 15 times longer, on average, than if no sunscreen were applied.

SSRI: See *selective serotonin reuptake inhibitor*.

stability: The chemical properties of a drug that assure it will not decompose readily during storage, so that it will remain potent and effective through the expiration date.

statin: One of a group of drugs that lowers harmful serum cholesterol levels by inhibiting a critical enzyme needed for the manufacture of cholesterol in the liver. Statins are also known as HMG-CoA reductase inhibitors.

steroid: A naturally occurring compound or drug that has far-ranging effects on numerous body processes. Some steroids are *hormones*—either sex hormones (for example, testosterone) or adrenal gland hormones (for example, prednisone). The terms steroid and *corticosteroid* are often used interchangeably.

stool softener: A type of *laxative* that bulks up and softens the consistency of fecal matter, thus easing the passage of stool and relieving constipation, hemorrhoid pain, and related discomforts.

subcutaneous: Under the skin. A number of medications are designed to be injected or surgically inserted just under the skin. Examples include various fertility drugs, anti-HIV medicines, and drugs used to treat chronic headache. When a choice in *parenteral* administration is available, subcutaneous injection is often chosen over *intramuscular injection*, which can be quite painful and less well absorbed.

sulfa drug: One of a class of bacteria-inhibiting drugs (specifically, *antibiotics*) that is created synthetically in the laboratory and is chemically very closely related to the compound known as sulfanilamide.

sulfonylurea: One of a class of chemically related and commonly used oral medications designed to treat diabetes by means of reducing and controlling the level of sugar in the blood. (Poor blood sugar control is a serious aspect of diabetes that can cause numerous complications.)

superinfection: A dangerous *side effect* of certain *antibiotics* that is marked by the emergence of a secondary infection during the course of antibiotic therapy. It can occur when antibiotics alter the normal balance of microbes in the respiratory, gastrointestinal, or urinary tracts, allowing certain potentially hazardous microorganisms to predominate and flourish.

suspension: A form of liquid medication, often cloudy in appearance, that consists of a solid (typically, a powder) that is dispersed into water (or another liquid medium) but in which the solid remains undissolved.

sympatholytic: An *antihypertensive* drug that acts on the *peripheral nervous system* to block nerve signals that trigger the constriction of blood vessels, thus causing the blood vessels to dilate and blood pressure to decline. Drugs that are sympatholytic include the *beta-blockers* and other medications used for treating high blood pressure.

sympathomimetic: A drug that acts on the nervous system and stimulates the involuntary activities of the organs, glands, muscles, and other structures in the body. A sympathomimetic drug such as albuterol dilates the respiratory passages and help to relieve asthma.

syrup: A form of liquid medication consisting of a drug dissolved in a concentrated sugar solution.

systemic: Affecting the body in general, as opposed to a limited *local* area. Drugs taken orally or injected *intravenously*, for example, are sometimes referred to as systemic medications, since they are widely distributed throughout the body by the bloodstream. In contrast, most medications applied *topically* to the skin, or dropped into the ears or eyes, would generally be considered non-systemic, or local, preparations.

tardive dyskinesia: A medical term for an irreversible nervous condition, marked by unusual involuntary movements of the mouth, tongue, neck, lips, and sometimes fingers, that can occur after prolonged treatment with potent *antipsychotic* drugs.

tetracycline: A type of *antibiotic* medication synthesized or derived from a certain Streptomyces microorganism. Because tetracycline is effective against a wide range of infections, it is considered a "broad-spectrum" antibiotic.

thiazide: A type of *diuretic* drug commonly prescribed for the treatment of high blood pressure. These drugs act on the kidneys to block the reabsorption of sodium and water by the bloodstream, leading to an increase in the volume and output of urine.

thrombolytic agent: A drug that dissolves blood clots, also known as thrombi. These medications are typically administered in a hospital by *intravenous* injection—for example, to dissolve a blood clot that is blocking a coronary artery and causing a heart attack.

tolerance: The body's adaptation to a drug, so that the drug's effects are lessened with continued use. Tolerance may work beneficially; for example, a *side effect* may become much less pronounced with continued use of a drug. On the other hand, drugs such as painkillers may become less effective as a person's tolerance develops, and higher and higher doses may be required.

topical: Designed to be applied to and act locally on a restricted area of the body, such as the application of a cream medication to the skin, an *ointment* to the eyelid, or an *anesthetic* injection to the gums. Topical drug preparations generally have fewer *side effects* than s*ystemic* drugs, which are distributed widely throughout the body.

toxin: A poisonous substance that has adverse effects on the body. Some toxins are produced by disease-causing bacteria or by certain plants (for example, mushrooms) or animals (such as snakes). Affected persons are sometimes inoculated with antitoxins, which neutralize the effects of toxins.

toxoid: A substance, derived from bacteria and used for *vaccination* against certain diseases, that is capable of combating or neutralizing the toxic effects of certain infectious microorganisms.

tranquilizer: An *antianxiety* drug that is used to induce sedation and relieve mental disturbance (such as anxiety and tension) in people as well as in animals.

transdermal patch: A drug-containing adhesive bandage that is worn on the skin and slowly releases medication over an extended period of time. Examples of drugs widely used in this form include nicotine, which is used to encourage smoking cessation, and nitroglycerin, which controls angina (chest pain).

tricyclic antidepressant: A common type of *antidepressant* medication characterized by a three-ring chemical structure that increases the activity of specialized substances called catecholamines in the brain. Amitriptyline hydrochloride (brand name Elavil) is one of several well-known tricyclic antidepressants.

tyramines: Substances found in certain foods and drinks, including aged cheeses, salami, dark chocolate, over- ripe fruits (especially bananas), and some red wines, that can cause a dangerous elevation of blood pressure in people who take take medications known as *MAO inhibitors*.

uricosuric drug: A drug that prevents recurrent gout attacks by promoting the excretion of uric acid in the urine.

vaccination: The oral or injectable administration of killed or inactivated microorganisms (*vaccines*) for the purpose of conferring immunity against a particular disease. The term is sometimes used interchangeably with *immunization*.

vaccine: A preparation of dead or inactivated bacteria, viruses, or *toxins* that stimulate the immune system to produce long-term *antibodies* against a particular infectious microorganism. By triggering the formation of these antibodies, the vaccine serves to prevent the disease from causing illness in the future. Commonly administered vaccines include the polio vaccine (to prevent polio) and the measles- mumps-rubella vaccine (to prevent these three illnesses).

vasodilator: A drug that causes the blood vessels to widen (dilate), increasing the amount of blood that can flow through them.

vitamin: An organic substance that plays an essential role in regulating cell functions. Most vitamins must be ingested because the body cannot manufacture them.

xanthine: A type of drug that opens bronchial air passages and makes breathing easier in patients with asthma and related conditions. A commonly used xanthine is theophylline, which is sold under numerous brand names.

ACKNOWLEDGMENTS

▼

MEDICAL CONSULTANTS

Chief of Medical
Advisory Board
Simeon Margolis, M.D., Ph.D.
*Professor of Medicine and
Biological Chemistry
Johns Hopkins
School of Medicine*

Franklin Adkinson, M.D.
Asthma and Allergy Medicine

Frank Anania, M.D.
*Gastroenterology and
Hepatology*

Lawrence Appel, M.D.
Internal Medicine

Paul Auwaerter, M.D.
*Internal Medicine and
Infectious Disease*

William Bell, M.D.
Hematology

Ivan Borrello, M.D.
Oncology

Steven Brant, M.D.
Gastroenterology

Richard Chaisson, M.D.
Infectious Disease

Lawrence Cheskin, M.D.
Gastroenterology and Nutrition

Bernard Cohen, M.D.
Dermatology

David Cromwell, M.D.
Gastroenterology

E. Claire Dees, M.D.
Oncology

Phillip Dennis, M.D.
Oncology

Adrian Dobs, M.D.
Endocrinology

Christopher Earley, M.D.
Neurology

David Essayan, M.D.
Allergy and Immunology

John Flynn, M.D.
*Internal Medicine and
Rheumatology*

Joel Gallant, M.D.
Infectious Disease (HIV/AIDS)

Mary Lawrence Harris, M.D.
Gastroenterology

Bradley Hinz, M.D.
Ophthalmology

Thomas Inglesby, M.D.
*Internal Medicine and
Infectious Disease*

Suzanne Jan de Beur, M.D.
Endocrinology

Christopher Karp, M.D.
Parasitology

Beth Kirkpatrick, M.D.
Infectious Disease

Susan Koch, M.D.
Dermatology

Alan Krasner, M.D.
Endocrinology

Julie Krop, M.D.
Endocrinology and Metabolism

Ralph Kuncl, M.D.
Neurology

John Lawrence, M.D.
Cardiovascular Medicine

Linda Lee, M.D.
Gastroenterology

Ronald Lesser, M.D.
Neurology

John Lipsey, M.D.
Psychiatry

Dan Martin, M.D.
*Internal Medicine and
Rheumatology*

William Moss, M.D.
Immunology

Patrick Murphy, M.D.
Infectious Disease

Philip Norman, M.D.
Allergy and Immunology

Steve O'Connell, M.D.
Ophthalmology

Paul O'Donnell, M.D.
Oncology

Peter Pak, M.D.
Cardiology

Marco Pappagallo, M.D.
*Neurology (Chronic Pain
Management)*

Wendy Post, M.D.
Cardiovascular Medicine

Charles Pound, M.D.
Urology

Thomas Preziosi, M.D.
Neurology

Peter Rabins, M.D.
Neuropsychiatry

Stuart Ray, M.D.
*Internal Medicine and
Infectious Disease*

Jon Resar, M.D.
Cardiovascular Medicine

Beryl Rosenstein, M.D.
Pulmonary Medicine

Walter Royal, M.D.
Neurology and Virology

Christopher Saudek, M.D.
Endocrinology and Metabolism

Eduardo Sotomayor, M.D.
Oncology

Jerry Spivak, M.D.
Hematology

Timothy Sterling, M.D.
Infectious Disease

Francisco Tausk, M.D.
Dermatology

Peter Terry, M.D.
Asthma and Allergy Medicine

Chloe Thio, M.D.
Infectious Disease

Jason Thompson, M.D.
Nephrology

Thomas Traill, M.D.
Cardiovascular Medicine

Glenn Treisman, M.D.
Psychiatry

John Ulatowski, M.D.
Neurology

Edward Wallach, M.D.
Obstetrics and Gynecology

Gary Wand, M.D.
Endocrinology

James Weiss, M.D.
Cardiovascular Medicine

James Weisz, M.D.
Ophthalmology

Elizabeth Whitmore, M.D.
Dermatology

INDEX

▼

GENERIC drug names appear in capital letters.

GENERIC drug names appear in capital letters.

GENERIC drug names appear in capital letters.

GENERIC drug names appear in capital letters.